A Surgeon's Gu
to Anaesthesia and
Peri-operative Care

A Surgeon's Guide to Anaesthesia and Peri-operative Care

Edited by

Jane Sturgess
Consultant Neuroanaesthetist, Addenbrooke's Hospital,
Cambridge University Hospitals NHS Foundation Trust,
Cambridge, UK

Justin Davies
Consultant Colorectal Surgeon, Addenbrooke's Hospital,
Cambridge University Hospitals NHS Foundation Trust,
Cambridge, UK

Kamen Valchanov
Consultant Anaesthetist, Papworth Hospital,
Cambridge, UK

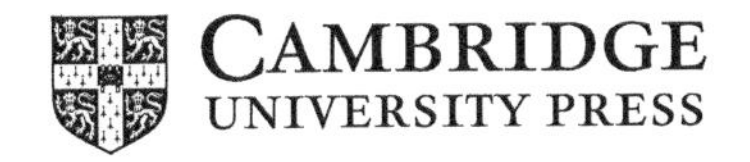

CAMBRIDGE
UNIVERSITY PRESS

University Printing House, Cambridge CB2 8BS, United Kingdom

Cambridge University Press is part of the University of Cambridge.

It furthers the University's mission by disseminating knowledge in the pursuit of education, learning and research at the highest international levels of excellence.

www.cambridge.org
Information on this title: www.cambridge.org/9781107698079

First published 2014

Printed in the United Kingdom by Clays, St Ives plc

A catalogue record for this publication is available from the British Library

Library of Congress Cataloguing in Publication data
A surgeon's guide to anaesthesia and peri-operative care / edited by Jane Sturgess, Justin Davies, Kamen Valchanov.
p. ; cm.
Includes bibliographical references and index.
ISBN 978-1-107-69807-9 (Paperback)
I. Sturgess, Jane, editor of compilation. II. Davies, Justin, editor of compilation. III. Valchanov, Kamen, editor of compilation.
[DNLM: 1. Anaesthesia–methods. 2. General Surgery–methods. 3. Peri-operative Care–methods. WO 200]
RD81
617.9′6–dc23 2013046224

ISBN 978-1-107-69807-9 Paperback

Contents

List of contributors vii
Foreword: Professor Michael Parker ix

Section I – Basic sciences

1. **General physiology** 1
Kamen Valchanov

2. **System-specific physiology** 13
Jane Sturgess

3. **Pain and analgesia** 35
David Sapsford

4. **Local anaesthetics** 48
David Tew

5. **Sedation** 59
Justin Davies and Jane Sturgess

6. **Physics and measurement** 63
Ari Ercole

Section II – Anaesthesia and peri-operative care for surgical specialties

7. **Cardiothoracic cases** 77
Kamen Valchanov and Pedro Catarino

8. **Colorectal cases** 91
Jane Sturgess and Justin Davies

9. **Upper gastrointestinal cases** 102
Mark Abrahams and Richard Hardwick

10. **Hepatobiliary and pancreatic cases** 116
Hemantha Alawattegama and Paul Gibbs

11. **Endocrine cases** 125
Pete Hambly and Radu Mihai

12. **Vascular cases** 137
Fay Gilder and Paul Hayes

13. **Organ transplant cases** 147
Nicola Jones and Christopher J.E. Watson

14. **Otorhinology, head and neck cases** 161
Helen Smith and Neil Donnelly

15. **Paediatric cases** 168
Simon Whyte and Sonia Butterworth

16. **Plastic, reconstructive and cosmetic cases** 181
Andrew Bailey and Charles Malata

17. **Neurosurgery cases** 197
Jane Sturgess and Ramez Kirollos

18. **Trauma cases** 208
Rhys Thomas and Wayne Sapsford

19. **Orthopaedic cases** 223
David Tew and Alan Norrish

20. **Urology cases** 236
Hemantha Alawattegama and Manit Arya

21. **Bariatric cases** 246
Michael Margarson and Christopher Pring

Section III – At a glance

22. **Scoring systems** 259
Jane Sturgess and Justin Davies

23. **Modes of mechanical ventilation** 269
Kamen Valchanov

24. **Fluids** 273
Jane Sturgess

25. **Coagulation** 277
Jane Sturgess

26. **Pre-operative echocardiography** 281
Kamen Valchanov

27. **Common drugs and doses** 285
Jane Sturgess

28. **Physiology and risk in special circumstances** 288
Jane Sturgess

29. **Medicolegal aspects of consent** 294
Kamen Valchanov

30. **Nerve injury** 298
Jane Sturgess

31. **Pre-operative investigations** 302
Joseph E. Arrowsmith

32. **Enhanced recovery** 310
Jane Sturgess

33. **Post-operative cognitive dysfunction** 312
Ram Adapa

List of abbreviations 317
Index 320

Contributors

Mark Abrahams
Consultant Anaesthetist, Addenbrooke's Hospital, Cambridge University Hospitals NHS Foundation Trust, Cambridge, UK

Ram Adapa
Consultant Anaesthetist and Honorary Visiting Senior Research Fellow, Addenbrooke's Hospital, Cambridge University Hospitals NHS Foundation Trust, Cambridge, UK

Hemantha Alawattegama
Consultant Anaesthetist, Addenbrooke's Hospital, Cambridge University Hospitals NHS Foundation Trust, Cambridge, UK

Joseph E. Arrowsmith
Consultant Anaesthetist, Papworth Hospital, Cambridge, UK

Manit Arya
Senior Lecturer and Consultant Urological Surgeon, Division of Surgery and Interventional Science, University College London, London, UK

Andrew Bailey
Consultant Anaesthetist, Addenbrooke's Hospital, Cambridge University Hospitals NHS Foundation Trust, Cambridge, UK

Sonia Butterworth
Consultant Paediatric Surgeon, and Clinical Assistant Professor of Surgery, BC Children's Hospital, Vancouver, BC, Canada

Pedro Catarino
Consultant Cardiothoracic Surgeon, Papworth Hospital, Cambridge, UK

Justin Davies
Consultant Colorectal Surgeon, Addenbrooke's Hospital, Cambridge University Hospitals NHS Foundation Trust, Cambridge, UK

Neil Donnelly
Consultant ENT Surgeon, Addenbrooke's Hospital, Cambridge University Hospitals NHS Foundation Trust, Cambridge, UK

Ari Ercole
Consultant in Anaesthesia and Intensive Care, Addenbrooke's Hospital, Cambridge University Hospitals NHS Trust, Cambridge, UK

Paul Gibbs
Consultant HPB and Transplant Surgeon, Addenbrooke's Hospital, Cambridge University Hospitals NHS Foundation Trust, Cambridge, UK

Fay Gilder
Consultant Anaesthetist, Addenbrooke's Hospital, Cambridge University Hospitals NHS Foundation Trust, Cambridge, UK

Pete Hambly
Consultant Anaesthetist, John Radcliffe Hospital, Oxford, UK

Richard Hardwick
Consultant Surgeon, Addenbrooke's Hospital, Cambridge University Hospitals NHS Foundation Trust, Cambridge, UK

Paul Hayes
Consultant Vascular Surgeon, Addenbrooke's Hospital, Cambridge University Hospitals NHS Foundation Trust, Cambridge, UK

Nicola Jones
Consultant in Anaesthesia and Critical Care, Papworth Hospital, Cambridge, UK

Ramez Kirollos
Consultant Neurosurgeon, Addenbrooke's Hospital, Cambridge University Hospitals NHS Foundation Trust, Cambridge, UK

Charles Malata
Consultant in Plastic and Reconstructive Surgery, Addenbrooke's Hospital, Cambridge University Hospitals NHS Foundation Trust, Cambridge, UK

Michael Margarson
Consultant Anaesthetist and Director of Critical Care, St Richard's Hospital, Chichester, UK

Radu Mihai
Consultant in Endocrine Surgery, Honorary Senior Clinical Lecturer, John Radcliffe Hospital, Oxford, UK

Alan Norrish
Consultant Orthopaedic Surgeon, Addenbrooke's Hospital, Cambridge University Hospitals NHS Foundation Trust, Cambridge, UK

Christopher Pring
Consultant Surgeon, Department of Bariatric Surgery, St Richard's Hospital, Chichester, UK

David Sapsford
Consultant Anaesthetist, Addenbrooke's Hospital, Cambridge University Hospitals NHS Foundation Trust, Cambridge, UK

Wayne Sapsford
Consultant Vascular and Trauma Surgeon, Barts Health NHS Trust and Homerton University Hospital NHS Foundation Trust, and RAF Consultant Adviser in Surgery, The Royal London Hospital, London, UK

Helen Smith
Consultant Anaesthetist, Addenbrooke's Hospital, Cambridge University Hospitals NHS Foundation Trust, Cambridge, UK

Jane Sturgess
Consultant Neuroanaesthetist, Addenbrooke's Hospital, Cambridge University Hospitals NHS Foundation Trust, Cambridge, UK

David Tew
Consultant Anaesthetist, Addenbrooke's Hospital, Cambridge University Hospitals NHS Foundation Trust, Cambridge, UK

Rhys Thomas
Consultant Trauma Anaesthetist and Pre-Hospital Care, 16th Air Assault Medical Regiment; Honorary Consultant Anaesthetist, Swansea Morriston NHS Trust (AMBU Health Board), Swansea, UK

Kamen Valchanov
Consultant Anaesthetist, Papworth Hospital, Cambridge, UK

Christopher J.E. Watson
Professor of Transplantation, University of Cambridge and Honorary Consultant Surgeon, Addenbrooke's Hospital, Cambridge, UK

Simon Whyte
Associate Head and Clinical Assistant Professor of Paediatric Anaesthesia, BC Children's Hospital, Vancouver, BC, Canada

Foreword

Successful outcome from surgery does not come about because of a surgeon's encyclopaedic knowledge of surgical conditions, nor from his or her masterly ability as a technical operator, although both of these components surely contribute. Good outcome is the result of multiple factors within a team framework, all contributing to the end result of surgery. Implicit within these constituents is the close relationship between the surgeon and the anaesthetist and the understanding each has of the complexities and difficulties with which the other might have to contend throughout the period of an operation, which includes the pre- and post-operative phases.

This book serves to inform surgeons of the intricacies and minutiae of anaesthesia in all aspects, ranging from day care local anaesthesia to cardiac bypass techniques. It is comprehensive and yet eminently readable and informative. The early chapters on basic physiology, combined with later chapters on fluids and commonly used drugs and dosages are fundamental to any trainee or practising surgeon and are beautifully composed. To miss these gems would be akin to ignoring the basic science lectures that are so important in the understanding of all medicine and surgery.

Subsequent chapters relate to specialty specific surgical fields and are particularly interesting and suitably detailed. In addition, there are chapters on associated subjects such as enhanced recovery, post-operative cognitive dysfunction and medico-legal aspects of consent. The editors have gone to considerable trouble to find authors with the specific knowledge and interests to produce a concise and yet wide-ranging book, which leaves the surgical reader admirably informed about his or her colleague's armamentarium of anaesthetic approaches, potential pitfalls and rescue strategies.

At this stage in my career I can only state that I wish this book had been written 40 years ago!

Michael Parker
Professor of Laparoscopic and Colorectal Surgery,
Council member, Royal College of Surgeons of England

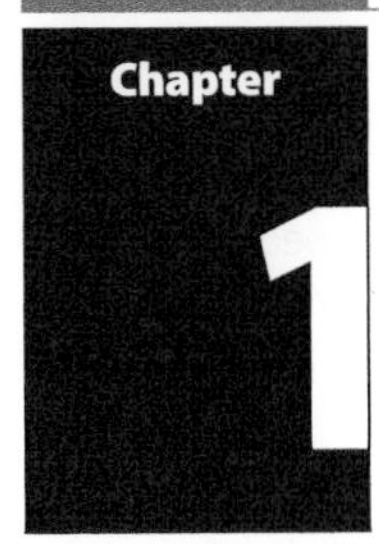

General physiology

Kamen Valchanov

Physiology along with anatomy and pharmacology are the foundations of modern medicine. These sciences have evolved dramatically over the last century and it is no longer possible for the ordinary medic to be an expert in the three of these basic sciences and be an expert in their own field too. However, a sound understanding of the basic principles of physiology, anatomy and pharmacology is necessary for safe practice. In the modern world of ultrafast information exchange, data not known by the medical practitioners can easily be acquired by the touch of a button on a smart phone. The smart phone, however, is unlikely to treat a patient, and it is the medic who can make an educated decision on the next course of action. In this chapter we will discuss some of the basic physiology concepts underpinning modern surgical practice. Many of those are referred to in the second section of the book dealing with individual surgical specialties.

Homeostasis

Homeostasis is a property of a system that regulates its internal environment and maintains stable constant conditions. In biological terms, homeostasis refers to maintaining optimal conditions for cell function, i.e. temperature, pH, water and ion content.

A stable pH is important for optimal function of intracellular enzyme systems and all processes to maintain a cell's integrity. Acid–base stability in all cells is achieved with the provision of oxygen, nutrients, and removal of waste products, including CO_2, at an optimal temperature. Maintaining homeostasis is a property of most physiological systems. It can be considered at a cellular level where it is necessary to maintain individual cellular function and cell wall integrity, or it can be considered on a larger scale, concerning the whole organism/body. In the latter, the cardiovascular system regulates blood flow to all tissues, from maintenance of organism blood pressure to local tissue vessel diameter. Respiratory homeostasis maintains gas delivery and waste gas clearance from tissues. And renal and neuroendocrine systems maintain the milieu in which the body functions, namely appropriate energy supply, pH environment, temperature and hydration status.

Osmosis

Osmosis is the spontaneous movement of solvent through a partially permeable membrane into a region of higher solute concentration, in the direction that tends to equalise the solute concentrations on both sides. Osmosis is a concept fundamental to the oncotic

A Surgeon's Guide to Anaesthesia and Peri-operative Care, ed. Jane Sturgess, Justin Davies and Kamen Valchanov. Published by Cambridge University Press.

Table 1.1 Mechanism by which substances move across cell membranes

Process	Summary of action	Common sites of action
Osmosis	Movement of water from an area of low solute concentration to high solute concentration across a semipermeable membrane	All vessels, causes tissue oedema if low intravascular albumin (low solute) concentration
Diffusion	Movement of ions from high concentration to low concentration. It is a slow process and inefficient as it must occur over great distances	All vessels, very important for K^+ which is predominantly intracellular. If plasma K^+ is low, intracellular compartments will mobilise to the plasma compartment – therefore low plasma concentration = VERY low whole body potassium
Filtration	Requires a pressure gradient across the membrane to be traversed. Molecules move from high pressure to low pressure	The kidney, all substances part of the 'ultrafiltrate' in Bowman's capsule. Important amino acids, elements for electrolyte, fluid and acid–base balance etc. are reabsorbed later in the nephron
Active transport	Molecules are transported across membranes regardless of the transmembrane concentration gradient. It is an energy-dependent process	The brain for glucose, amino acids in the kidney (reabsorption), gastric acid in the stomach
Exocytosis	Formation of membrane-enclosed vesicles that move to the cell membrane and discharge their contents. It is energy-dependent	Hormones from the posterior pituitary, pancreatic enzymes, acetylcholine at the neuromuscular junction

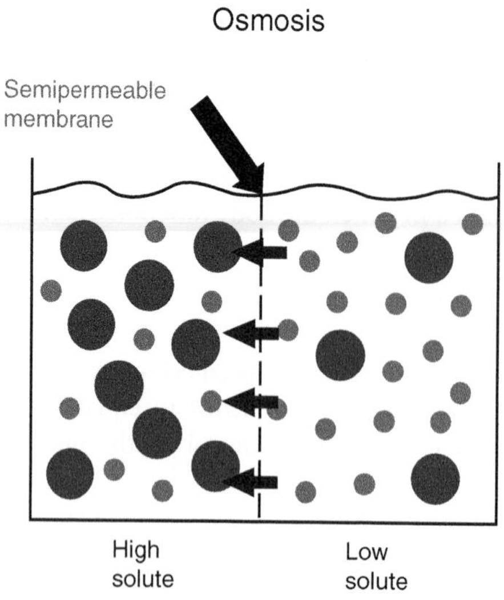

Osmosis

Semipermeable membrane

High solute

Low solute

Figure 1.1 Osmosis is the spontaneous movement of solvent through a partially permeable membrane into a region of higher solute concentration.

pressure across the capillary wall (Figure 1.1). The capillary wall acts as a membrane that is impermeable to colloids (plasma proteins, albumin) yet permeable to water. The colloid osmotic pressure owing to the plasma colloids is called oncotic pressure. Water can also be moved across the capillary wall through the mechanism of filtration, i.e. under a pressure difference. In cases where the intravascular colloid (albumin) content is reduced or colloids from the intravascular bed have leaked into the interstitium (e.g. sepsis) the oncotic balance is disrupted, thus drawing water from the vasculature into the extracelluar compartment, producing oedema. It is therefore important that the homeostasis of oncotic pressure is maintained constant in order to avoid oedema.

Thermoregulation

Thermoregulation involves a group of processes that maintain constant optimal temperature for cell function. Humans are homeothermic animals. Tight control of the balance between heat production and loss is essential to maintain normal body functions.

In humans the normal body temperature is considered to be 37 °C, and undergoes circadian fluctuation from 0.5 to 0.7 °C. Temperature regulation is less precise in children. Pregnancy leads to increased basal temperature. This precise balance is regulated by a specialised thermoregulation centre located in the hypothalamus. Disease processes or exercise can lead to impaired thermoregulation and the bodily processes function in different but not normal conditions.

Heat is produced by muscular exercise, assimilation of food and all vital processes of the basal metabolic rate. Many chemical reactions (synthesis and breakdown) lead to a final product/s and heat release. These can be augmented in times of need, by release of hormones (e.g. thyroid, anabolic, catecholamines). Fat is a source of heat that can release heat energy quickly. In particular, brown fat in children can be very efficient.

Heat is lost from the body by radiation, conduction and vaporisation (and evaporation) of water from the respiratory tract and skin. These are discussed in more detail in Chapter 6 Physics and measurement. Radiation and conduction remove 70% of the heat, vaporisation and sweating 27%, respiration 2%, and urination and defaecation 1%.

Fever is of particular interest in medicine. Along with pain it is the commonest and oldest marker of disease. For fever to occur, thermoregulation has to fail, and inflammatory cytokines (pyrogens) produce heat-releasing reactions. An interesting and fortunately rare condition in peri-operative medicine is malignant hyperthermia. It is a result of a mutation in the ryanodine receptor leading to excess release of calcium from muscle. This is triggered by volatile anaesthetic agents or succinylcholine, and if untreated, can be fatal. Prompt recognition and treatment can save lives, and almost always involves cancellation of surgery and post-operative intensive care.

Hypothermia is common in hospitals. It is a result of patients' disease conditions, and their inability to compensate for the increased exposure to low ambient temperature. The multitude of patient exposures for surgery, including patient transfer, air conditioning, application of cold fluids internally and externally and exposed body cavities during surgery may all contribute to hypothermia. Along with reduced metabolic demand, the reduced body temperature results in impaired bodily functions, including cognition, coagulation, immunity and cardio-respiratory function. At temperatures of 32 °C and below, the heart develops arrhythmias and asystole may ensue. The National Institute for Health and Clinical Excellence (NICE) produced guideline 65 in 2008 to prevent inadvertent peri-operative hypothermia in adults. Many warming blankets and other devices are now available to help prevent inadvertent peri-operative hypothermia.

Metabolic pathways

Precise balance between energy production and consumption in the body is essential. Hormones regulate the metabolic processes producing energy and heat (thermal energy). They also regulate the energy-consuming processes. The first law of thermodynamics states that energy is neither created nor destroyed; it merely changes its form. As such there must be a balance between caloric intake and energy output. The imbalance leads to obesity or starvation.

The energy metabolism consists of basal metabolic rate plus the metabolism for additional functions. The basal metabolic rate is the energy required for support of all basic functions and maintenance of cell wall integrity, which cannot be switched off. This is traditionally the metabolic rate during sleep in a room at comfortable temperature. Any additional activity, such as exercise, stress, surgery or intensive intellectual processes, requires additional energy.

At a cellular level the energy storage is in the form of high-energy phosphate compounds, mostly adenosine triphosphate (ATP) in the mitochondria. Upon aerobic hydrolysis to adenosine diphosphate (ADP) there is a release of energy required for muscle contraction, active transport and synthesis. Further hydrolysis to adenosine monophosphate (AMP) releases more energy. Another energy-rich phosphate is the muscle creatine phosphate.

During exercise, the energy demand increases over the basal metabolic rate and additional ATP energy release is required. A similar condition occurs in patients undergoing surgery. Because of the stress induced by surgery, an array of metabotropic hormones are released, all metabolic processes are augmented, inflammatory mediators released, heat is lost, the heart rate increases and glycogen is released from the liver. Additional utilisation of oxygen is required, and additional CO_2 is produced. This explains why patients with critically impaired cardio-respiratory function can live comfortably at home with few symptoms, whereas they can rapidly deteriorate or die as a result of even minor surgical stress (Figure 1.2).

Carbohydrate metabolism

Carbohydrates are an important dietary source of energy. The commonly ingested carbohydrates are hexoses (glucose, galactose, fructose). These are quickly converted to glucose in the circulation after ingestion. The glucose is then distributed and absorbed by most tissues by the action of molecules called glucose transporters. These facilitate diffusion by concentration gradients. Only gut and kidneys take up glucose by energy-dependent active transport. Once the glucose enters the cells it undergoes transformation to glucose-6-phosphate. The glucose-6-phosphate is either converted into glycogen in the liver (glycogenesis), or broken down (glycolysis) to produce energy. The liver glycogen serves as an energy store (of carbohydrate). On the other hand the glycolysis, through several enzymatic breakdowns, produces pyruvate, which is used in the citric acid cycle in the mitochondria, thereby generating ATP (Figure 1.3). Some of the pyruvate is converted to lactate (catalysed by NADH) in the absence of oxygen. When the oxygen supply is restored the accumulated lactate is converted back to pyruvate.

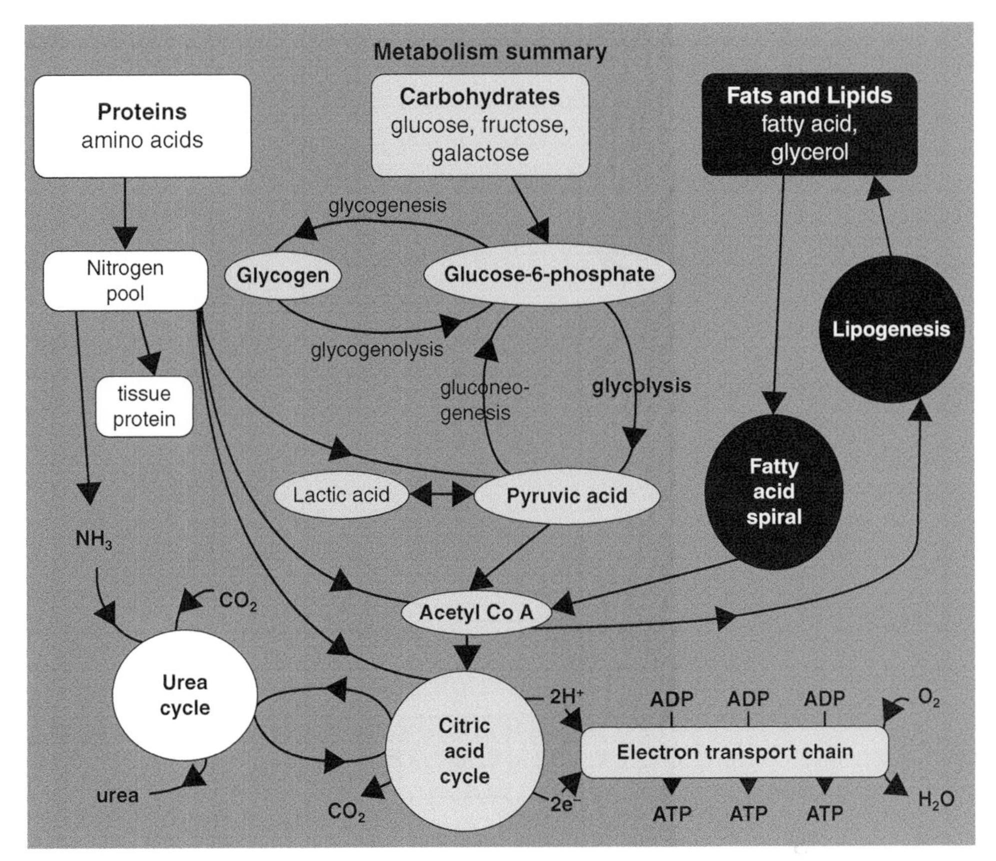

Figure 1.2 Metabolism summary. The main energy source in the body is carbohydrate aerobic breakdown. In addition to this, the fatty acid breakdown can also produce acetyl Co A for the citric cycle, feeding electrons for ATP production, but this pathway is less generous in its supply and only used as a secondary pathway. Finally, the protein breakdown can also be used for energy production but is least efficient.

These processes are hormonally regulated. The main player is insulin. Insulin enhances tissue take up of glucose from the circulation and increases glycogen storage. It also regulates the aerobic glucose breakdown to the citric acid cycle. The deficiency of insulin conversely causes glycogen breakdown and glucose release in the circulation. Glucagon has the opposite effects, forcing glycogenolysis. Similar actions are produced by cortisol and adrenaline. In a clinical situation like septic shock, or after the stress of major surgery, augmented release of adrenaline and cortisol and relative deficiency of insulin impair glucose metabolism. The patient presents with hyperglycaemia and lactic acidosis (as a result of hypoperfusion of tissues and anaerobic carbohydrate metabolism and liver dysfunction with reduced lactic metabolism).

The highly efficient energy release of triphosphate resynthesis is an oxygen-demanding process (aerobic). However, under special circumstances, when there is an oxygen debt, anaerobic (oxygen independent) pathways release energy through carbohydrate breakdown to lactic acid (e.g. during excessive exercise, or tissue hypoxia from pathological causes). During exercise the anaerobic pathways are self-limiting because of build up of lactic acid and decline of pH. On the other hand the body cannot easily compensate for iatrogenic

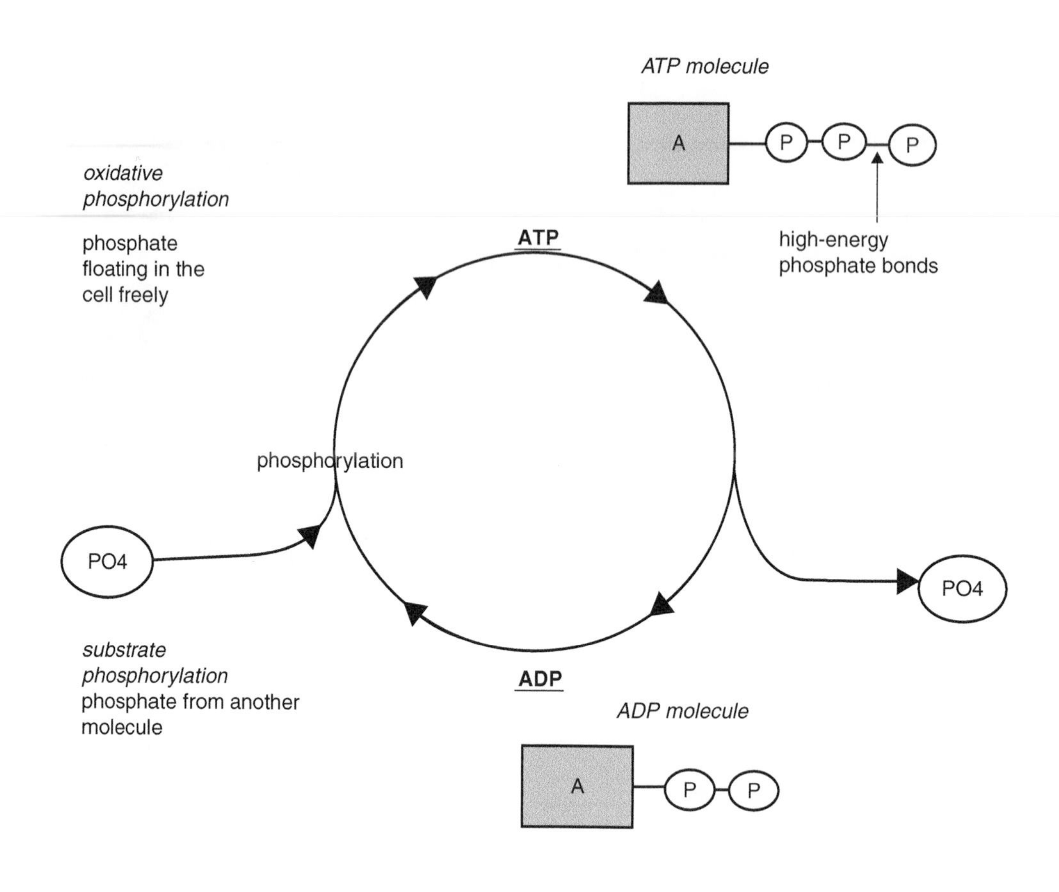

Figure 1.3 ATP synthesis and breakdown is achieved through phosphorylation and dephosphorylation of the adenosine molecule.

anaerobic conditions. For example after application of limb tourniquets or aortic cross clamp there is a substantial lactic acid build up in the distal tissues, which is released into the circulation once the tourniquets or clamp are released, resulting in acidosis and increased respiratory rate. The second insult to the cardiovascular system is the return of cold blood with an elevated potassium concentration. This ischaemic time needs to be limited for two reasons: to avoid tissue necrosis, and to preclude overwhelming acidosis on reperfusion. Similar effects are seen when reperfusing donated organs with prolonged cold ischaemic times, and cardiac arrest has occurred in the recipient. This is often quickly resolved with simple measures and CPR, but can result in death.

Arterial blood gas analysis

Arterial blood gas analysis is one of the most useful monitoring tools in modern medicine. It provides information about pH, oxygen and CO_2 tension, and allows a number of calculated values, including HCO_3^- and base excess. The importance of these will be discussed below.

The pH is a crucial number defining acid–base balance. It represents the balance between all bases and acids and hence the metabolic milieu of the cellular metabolism. The pH is defined as a negative logarithm to the base of 10 of the hydrogen ion concentration, and its normal value is 7.4 (equivalent to 40 pmol/l H^+). The value is a scalar; it has no measurement unit, it is a mere number. Interestingly, H^+ concentrations are expressed in $\times.10^{-8}$ – $\times.10^{-7}$ mmol/l, which are challenging to calculate. In 1909, the Danish chemist Sorensen introduced the pH as a tool for simplifying these long numbers in his PhD, and it is still used by the rest of the world now.

A pH more than 7.44 is called alkalosis, and less than 7.36 acidosis. The acid–base balance is governed by respiratory and metabolic function. The respiratory function can affect it by maintaining the blood CO_2 tension. Therefore, hypercarbia (pCO_2 greater than 6 kPa) causes respiratory acidosis. The respiratory acidosis is compensated if pH remains normal (7.36 –7.44), and this can be achieved by metabolic compensation, i.e. increasing HCO_3 concentration. Conversely, hypocarbia (pCO_2 lower than 4.5 kPa) causes respiratory alkalosis. The respiratory alkalosis can be compensated if the pH remains normal, and this can be achieved by metabolic compensation, i.e. reducing HCO_3 concentrations. The metabolic pathways of regulating acid–base status involve blood buffering and renal excretion of solutes, but revolve around the HCO_3 concentration in the blood. Metabolic acidosis is caused by low HCO_3 concentrations (less than 21 mmol/l) and can be compensated if the pH is normal and there is a respiratory compensation by hypocarbia. Conversely, metabolic alkalosis is represented by high HCO_3 concentrations (greater than 26 mmol/l), and can be respiratory compensated by hypercarbia. The best way of making sense of this is by analysis using a Davenport diagram (Figure 1.4).

The easiest way of analysing arterial blood gases is by using only three variables (pH, pCO_2 and HCO_3). If the pH is less than 7.4 then the primary problem is likely to be acidosis, compensated or uncompensated. A typical example of compensated metabolic acidosis is: pH 7.38, pCO_2 4.4 kPa, and HCO_3 19 mmol/l. If the pH is more than 7.4 then the primary problem is likely to be alkalosis. A typical example of decompensated metabolic alkalosis is pH 7.5 pCO_2 6.5 kPa, and HCO_3 31 mmol/l.

Normal arterial blood gas values are:

	Low	High
pH	7.36	7.44
pCO_2	4.6 kPa	6 kPa
pO_2	10 kPa	13 kPA
HCO_3	21 mmol/l	26 mmol/l
Sats	95%	100%
BE	-2.5 mmol/l	+2.5 mmol/l

Another calculated value in the arterial blood gas analysis is base excess. Base excess is a fictitious value as it does not exist in real life, and yet it governs so much decision-making in UK intensive care units. It is defined as the amount of acid which needs to be added to a solution to reduce the pH to 7.4. Conversely, the base deficit is the amount of base that needs to be added to a solution to increase the pH to 7.4. During cardiopulmonary bypass

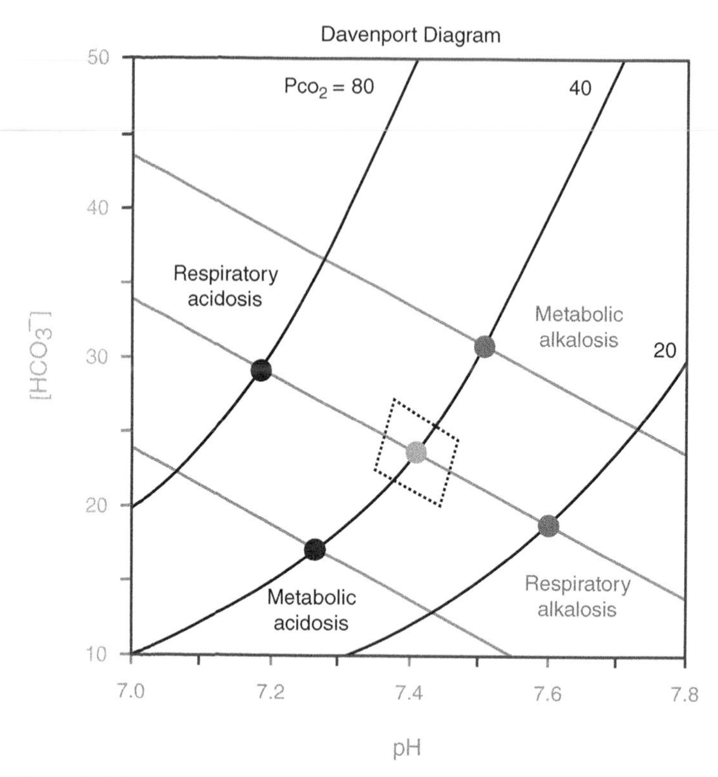

Figure 1.4 Davenport diagram.

when the base excess is less than -5, i.e. there is base deficit, the perfusionists would normally add HCO_3 to treat the number. On the other hand the same number in most UK intensive care units will be left untreated, and in fact adding $NaHCO_3$ is frowned upon. It is not known if treating base deficit by the addition of $NaHCO_3$ worsens prognosis, but it does not address the primary question, i.e. the reason for acidosis.

Sepsis and septic shock

Sepsis is a clinical syndrome characterised by a multisystem response to a microbial pathogenic insult consisting of a mosaic of interconnected biochemical, cellular, and organ–organ interactions. The Surviving Sepsis campaign defines it also as:

> 'Presence of inflammation together with systemic manifestations of infection.'

Severe sepsis is defined as:

> 'Sepsis plus sepsis-induced organ dysfunction or tissue hypoperfusion.'

Septic shock is defined as:

> 'Sepsis-induced tissue hypoperfusion persisting despite adequate fluid resuscitation.'

Table 1.2 Diagnostic criteria for sepsis: infection, documented or suspected, and some of the following:

General variables	Fever (> 38.3 °C) Hypothermia (core temperature < 36 °C) Heart rate > 90/min – one or more than two SD above the normal value for age Tachypnoea Altered mental status Significant oedema or positive fluid balance (> 20 mL/kg over 24 hrs) Hyperglycaemia (plasma glucose > 140 mg/dL or 7.7 mmol/l) in the absence of diabetes
Inflammatory variables	Leukocytosis (WBC count > 12,000 μl^{-1}) Leukopenia (WBC count < 4000 μl^{-1}) Normal WBC count with greater than 10% immature forms Plasma C-reactive protein more than two SD above the normal value Plasma procalcitonin more than two SD above the normal value
Haemodynamic variables	Arterial hypotension (SBP < 90 mm Hg, MAP < 70 mm Hg, or a SBP decrease > 40 mm Hg in adults or less than two SD below normal for age)
Organ dysfunction variables	Arterial hypoxaemia (Pao_2/Fio_2 < 300) Acute oliguria (urine output < 0.5 mL/kg/hr for at least 2 hrs despite adequate fluid resuscitation) Creatinine increase > 0.5 mg/dL or 44.2 µmol/l Coagulation abnormalities (INR > 1.5 or aPTT > 60 s) Ileus (absent bowel sounds) Thrombocytopenia (platelet count < 100,000 μl^{-1}) Hyperbilirubinaemia (plasma total bilirubin > 4 mg/dl or 70 µmol/l)
Tissue perfusion variables	Hyperlactataemia (> 1 mmol/l) Decreased capillary refill or mottling

Another term used in sepsis literature is SIRS (systemic inflammatory response syndrome): the diagnosis requires four derangements –

1. Temperature < 36 °C or >38 °C
2. Heart rate > 90 bpm
3. Respiratory rate > 20 bpm (or PCO_2 < 4.3 kPa)
4. White blood cells < 4.10^9/l or > 10.10^9/l

Systemic inflammatory response syndrome is a syndrome which reflects the generalised body reaction to an insult. While it is a reliable feature of the septic process there are conditions resembling sepsis by definition and fulfilling the SIRS criteria. A typical condition is pancreatitis where, owing to autolysis and release of digestive hormones in the circulation, a sterile inflammatory cascade produces a generalised septic response.

The general diagnostic criteria for sepsis are summarised in Table 1.2. This is a condition that requires prompt treatment. The simplified recommendations for the treatment include:

A. Initial resuscitation: with volume against a haemodynamic target;
B. Diagnosis: septic screen and imaging for potential source of infection;

C. Antimicrobial therapy;
D. Source control: where source is found, targeted treatment including surgery to be considered early.

Fluid balance and replacement

The human body relies on a well-balanced intravascular volume to maintain optimal circulation for different circumstances. This in turn ensures sufficient oxygen tissue supply and CO_2 clearance. The circulating blood volume is tightly regulated by neural, hormonal and renal systems. Additionally, blood is regulated in its haemoglobin content, osmolality and solute concentrations.

Cardiac output is governed by cardiac pump function, peripheral vascular resistance and circulating blood volume. These factors also interact with lung function. Cardiac output itself depends on pre-load, heart rate, myocardial contractility and afterload.

Pre-load is largely represented by the total circulating blood volume. Afterload is represented by the peripheral vascular resistance and, to a lesser extent, circulating blood volume. These parameters are frequently altered in the peri-operative period. The circulating blood volume can be diminished (owing to blood loss) or redistributed (owing to reduction of peripheral vascular resistance or plasma volume sequestration in abdominal organs). Maintaining a physiological state of the body fluid compartments as far as possible would mean a careful and adequate substitution of actual fluid losses. There are two types: fluid losses through urine, digestive tract and insensible losses; surgery-related fluid losses, i.e. pre-operative dehydration, bleeding and fluid redistribution.

When choosing fluid replacement regimes in the peri-operative setting two facts need to be born in mind:

1. The extracellular deficit after usual fasting is low;
2. The basal fluid loss via insensible perspiration is approximately 0.5 ml/kg/h, extending to 1 ml/kg/h during major abdominal surgery.

Therefore volume loading in pre-operatively euvolaemic patients is not necessary. In fact overhydration can lead to oedema, slow recovery, and potentially lead to peri-operative complications and higher mortality. Fluid use should be targeted at replacing lost volume only.

Colloids and crystalloids

Volume replacement in the peri-operative period could be achieved by either crystalloid or colloid solutions. Colloids are solutions containing substances that are evenly dispersed throughout. Crystalloids are solutions containing substances that can pass through a semipermeable membrane. All have advantages and disadvantages, as discussed below. Over the last half century, scientists have been trying to develop blood substitutes with oxygen-carrying capacity in addition to volume expansion properties. Fluorocarbons and synthetic haemoglobins have been studied, but none are currently in clinical use. Please see Chapter 24 'Fluids' for further information.

Crystalloid solutions

Normal saline (0.9% NaCl): Contains 154 mmol/l Na^+ and 154 mmol/l Cl^-, pH 5.0. It stays in the circulation for a short time (30–60 minutes), and can produce oedema when it exits the vascular bed. It can also cause hyperchloraemic metabolic acidosis.

Hartmann's (Ringer's lactate) solution (Na^+ 131 mmol/l, K^+ 5 mmol/l, Ca^{2+} 2 mmol/l, Cl^- 111 mmol/l, lactate 29 mmol/l, pH 6.5): It is cheap, produces no immune sensitivity or coagulopathy, is a balanced solution, and hence does not produce acidosis. Unfortunately it contains lactate.

Dextrose saline (4% dextrose/0.18% saline): It contains Na^+ 30 mmol/l, Cl^- 30 mmol/l, dextrose 40 g. It is an excellent maintenance solution designed to meet hydration and metabolic requirements for post-operative paediatric patients.

5% dextrose: It contains dextrose 50 g, pH 4. It is an excellent energy-providing maintenance fluid. Shortly after infusing intravenously the dextrose leaves the circulation, and the remainder is hypotonic water; hence excessive use leads to oedema.

Colloid solutions

Blood: While using packed red cells is the most natural method of volume expansion, there are numerous problems associated with safety of blood transfusion, and the possible immunological sequelae thereafter.

Albumin 4.5%: It contains Na^+ 160 mmol/l, K^+ 2 mmol/l, Cl^- 136 mmol/l, albumin 45 g, pH 7.4. It is expensive. Because of its negative charge it binds to endothelial surfaces, drugs and inflammatory mediators. Its role was questioned in the 1990s because of a controversial meta-analysis.

Gelatins (Gelofusine, Haemacel): These are plasma expanders with a shorter half-life than starches. They can be allergogenic, impair haemostasis and renal function. Gelofusine contains Na^+ 154 mmol/l, Cl^- 125 mmol/l, gelatin 40 g, pH 7.4.

Starches (HES 6%, Voluven, Volulyte, Tetraspan): Hydroxy ethyl starch is an efficient and long-lasting volume expander. Voluven has been withdrawn from the market owing to safety concerns. These products can cause renal failure and impair coagulation.

Evidence and modern science: some researchers have published dozens of studies 'proving' the benefit and safety of colloid solutions. However, subsequent investigations suggested that some such studies involved forged signatures of co-authors, trials conducted without approval, failure to obtain consent and even fabricating entire studies. A substantial number of meta-analyses studies and systematic reviews of colloids were subsequently withdrawn by journals.

Massive blood loss

Massive blood loss is an infrequent occurrence in medical practice but its management can test any doctor to the edge of their abilities. It is defined as loss of one circulating volume in 24 hours. A normal circulating volume is estimated at 7% of ideal body weight in adults and 8–9% in children. Such bleeding has numerous implications: there is low circulating volume (low pre-load, and reduced perfusion to non-vital organs); anaemia (low oxygen-carrying capacity); loss of clotting factors (perpetuating further bleeding); loss of plasma protein (low oncotic pressure and oedema); stress response (surge of adrenaline, cortisol and other hormones); cooling through volume replacement; and a multitude of other factors. It has to be remembered that the treatment of this condition is life-saving and hence urgent. The priority is to restore circulatory volume and halt bleeding. The best volume replacement in such cases is packed red cells. Further, transfusion of platelets and fresh frozen plasma restores most of the clotting abnormalities, but fibrinogen, cryoprecipitate and other clotting factors (like Factor VII and XIII) may be required. Then warming up and preserving organ function is the next priority. After the first set of blood products administered, clotting tests and full blood count need to be checked and the laboratory involved in guiding the type of products required. All of these transfusions, while life-saving, produce a complex immunological response in most patients, which could impact in later life.

Further reading

Chappell D, Jacob M, Hofmann-Keifer, *et al.* A rational approach to peri-operative fluid management. *Anesthesiology* 2008; **109**: 723–40.

Finfer SR, Vincent J-L. Severe sepsis and septic shock. *NEJM* 2013; **369**: 840–51.

Ganong WG. *Review of Medical Physiology.* Lange: McGraw-Hill, 2001.

Namas R, Zamora R, Namas R, *et al.* Sepsis: Something old, something new, and systems view. *I Crit Care* 2012; **27**: 314e1.

NICE Clinical Guideline 65. The management of inadvertent peri-operative hypothermia in adults. London: NICE, 2008.

Stainsby D, LacLennan S, Hamilton PJ. Management of massive blood loss: a template guideline. *Br J Anaesth* 2000; **85**: 487–91.

Surviving Sepsis Campaign: International guidelines for management of severe sepsis and septic shock: 2012. http://www.sccm.org/Documents/SSC-Guidelines.pdf.

West, JB. *Respiratory Physiology: The Essentials.* 6th edn. USA: Lippincott, Williams & Wilkins, 2000.

Basic sciences

System-specific physiology

Jane Sturgess

This chapter will aim to give an overview of system-specific physiology. It includes sections on respiratory, cardiovascular, renal and central nervous system physiology.

Respiratory physiology

Control of ventilation

Ventilation is controlled by a number of centres and receptors, that act upon each other in a controlled fashion via positive and negative feedback. Central control arises from the respiratory centre in the medulla oblongata, the dorsal neurons are predominantly concerned with inspiration, and the ventral neurons with expiration. Other areas of the brain that have input to the respiratory centre include the pneumotaxic centre in the pons, the cerebral cortex and the hypothalamus.

Chemoreceptors are located in the brain and in the peripheral circulation. When activated they feedback to the respiratory centre (Fig 2.1).

Hypoventilation results in an increase in blood pCO_2 and causes a respiratory acidosis. The pCO_2 and hydrogen ion concentration [H+] are intimately related, as can be seen from the equation:

$$CO_2 + H_2O \Leftrightarrow H_2CO_3 \Leftrightarrow HCO_3^- + H^+$$

A rise in blood pCO_2 causes a subsequent rise in $[H^+]$ in the blood and cerebrospinal fluid (CSF). Central chemoreceptors in the medulla respond to changes in cerebrospinal fluid hydrogen ion concentration. An increase in $[H^+]$ stimulates the receptor, and drives ventilation. This central response to increased pCO_2 (via the increased $[H^+]$ in the CSF) is greater than that generated by activation of peripheral chemoreceptors. Patients with chronic lung disease and persistently elevated $PaCO_2$ should have acidic CSF and a constant increase in respiratory drive, yet this is not the case. Homeostasis is the mechanism by which the body acts to maintain a stable internal environment. The CSF pH is returned to normal by diffusion of bicarbonate ions into CSF. In the longer term repeated stimulation of the central chemoreceptors leads to a loss of sensitivity to $PaCO_2$ in this group of patients.

A Surgeon's Guide to Anaesthesia and Peri-operative Care, ed. Jane Sturgess, Justin Davies and Kamen Valchanov. Published by Cambridge University Press.

Table 2.1 Cause and effect site for increased ventilation

Effect site	Stimulus
Cerebral cortex	Anticipated exercise
Hypothalamus	Fear, pain, anxiety
Medulla	CSF H^+ concentration
Aortic and carotid body chemoreceptors	Low pO_2 tension Low blood flow
Carotid body chemoreceptors	Increased pCO_2 tension
Carotid and aortic body baroreceptors	Low blood pressure

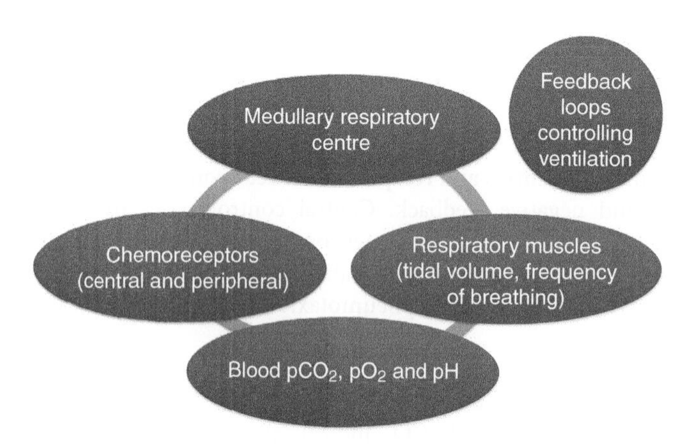

Figure 2.1 Diagram to show the feedback loops controlling ventilation.

Peripheral chemoreceptors are located in the carotid and aortic bodies and have a rapid response rate. They receive a high blood flow and respond primarily to a decrease in PaO_2 (oxygen tension – not concentration). This is important because low oxygen concentration (e.g. anaemia) does *not* stimulate ventilation via the peripheral chemoreceptors but low oxygen tension does. A fall in blood flow to the chemoreceptors, and blood pressure to the baroreceptors also stimulates ventilation – e.g. acute haemorrhage.

Increased $PaCO_2$ tension and $[H^+]$ concentration stimulate ventilation via central mechanisms and by action on the peripherally located carotid bodies.

Anaesthetic drugs (inhaled anaesthetics, barbiturates and opioids) depress the normal ventilatory response to hypoxia, hypercapnia and acidosis.

Lung functions

The lung has many functions in addition to ventilation and these are summarised as:

a. Gas exchange
b. Acid–base balance
c. Filter – blood clots, micro gas bubbles
d. Serves as a blood reservoir

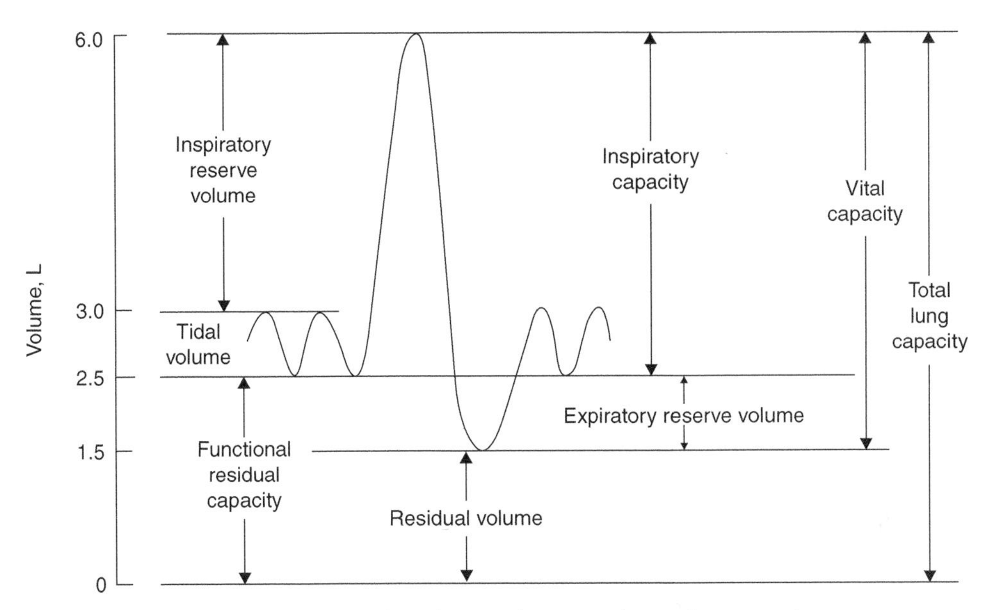

Figure 2.2 Spirometry: diagram showing the volumes and capacities that can be measured.

e. Converts angiotensin I to angiotensin II by angiotensin-converting enzyme
f. Produces immunoglobulin A to protect against respiratory infection
g. Drug metabolism

Spirometry

The lung has the ability to distend and relax. This is why we can measure the various volumes and capacities during lung function testing, and make an assessment of respiratory function. Lung function tests include spirometry (see Figure 2.2 and Table 2.2), flow volume loops and peak expiratory flow rates.

Flow volume loops

The flow volume loop presents information of lung performance (see Figure 2.3) and produces characteristic shapes according to the pathology that exists. It can also be used to record the response to treatment – e.g. does an obstructive pattern return towards normal after the use of bronchodilator? It can also help to identify if there is a fixed or variable large airway obstruction or if it is intra- or extra-thoracic (see Figure 11.3).

Respiratory failure

Definition of respiratory failure

Respiratory failure occurs when gas exchange is sufficiently impaired to cause hypoxaemia.

Type I. Hypoxaemia with normal or low carbon dioxide levels.

- Caused by damage to/problems with lung tissue, e.g. atelectasis, sputum plug, aspiration. The remaining normal lung participates in gas exchange. Carbon

Table 2.2 Examples of lung volumes: based on a 70 kg man

Term	Abbreviation	Volume	Importance
Inspiratory reserve volume	IRV	3000 ml	Extra lung volume that can be achieved with a deep inspiration
Tidal volume	TV	500 ml	Resting
Residual volume	RV	1500 ml	Lung volume at end expiration – oxygen reserve
Expiratory reserve volume	ERV	1000 ml	Extra lung volume available for a full forced expiration
Functional residual capacity	FRC	2500 ml	Potential oxygen reserve (ERV+RV)
Inspiratory capacity	IC	3500 ml	Potential inspiration (IRC+TV)
Vital capacity	VC	4500 ml	Lung that changes volume, or that can collapse (IRV+TV+ERV)
Total lung capacity	TLC	6000 ml	(IRV+TV+ERV+RV)

N.B. A lung capacity is the product of two or more lung volumes, shown in brackets.

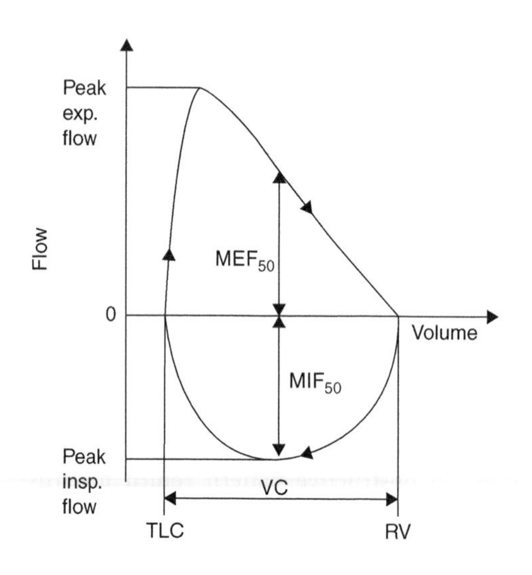

Figure 2.3 Figure showing a normal flow volume loop with lung volumes indicated. TLC = total lung capacity, VC = vital capacity, RV = residual volume, MEF_{50} = maximal expiratory flow rate at 50% of vital capacity. MIF_{50} = maximal inspiratory flow rate at 50% vital capacity. In normal lungs MEF_{50} should equal MIF_{50}.

dioxide excretion requires less functioning tissue than is needed for adequate oxygenation of the blood.

Type II. Hypoxaemia with hypercapnia. These patients will have a respiratory acidosis.

- Otherwise known as ventilatory failure, when alveolar ventilation is insufficient to permit adequate gas exchange. It can be caused by reduced ventilatory effort, e.g. opiate

Table 2.3 Causes of post-operative respiratory failure

Iatrogenic		Pathological	
Drugs	Residual paralysis Opiate suppression of rate/ cough/depth High regional anaesthesia Fluid overload	Pre-existing respiratory disease	Obstructive sleep apnoea COPD/O_2 toxicity/ Exacerbation of asthma Poor cough, reduced lung capacity Sputum plug/secretions
Atelectasis	Diaphragmatic splinting – laparosopic surgery Poor analgesia	Pre-existing cardiac disease	Cardiac failure and pulmonary oedema Myocardial infarction
Procedural	Pneumothorax after CVP insertion Bronchial placement of nasogastric tube and feed	Atelectasis Increased work of breathing Aspiration	Obesity Increased intra-abdominal pressure Sepsis

Table 2.4 The cause of post-operative respiratory failure, an explanation and the likely ABG results

Cause	Explanation	Likely ABG abnormality
Opiate overdose	Depression of central respiratory centres and peripheral chemoreceptor feedback mechanisms	Low PaO_2, high $PaCO_2$, low pH
Atelectasis	Loss of lung volume. Ventilation–perfusion mismatch	Low PaO_2, low $PaCO_2$, normal pH
Secretion retention/ sputum plug	Obstructed lung. No ventilation but good perfusion. Ventilation–perfusion mismatch	Low PaO_2, low $PaCO_2$, normal pH
Pulmonary embolus	Ventilated lung. Obstructed circulation. Increasing inspired oxygen of minimal benefit in massive PE.	Low PaO_2, low $PaCO_2$, possibly elevated $PaCO_2$
Post-operative pneumonia	Loss of lung volume. No ventilation. Depending on severity, perfusion maintained. In severe cases, hypoxic pulmonary vasoconstriction will occur in affected areas.	Low PaO_2, low $PaCO_2$ (but will become high $PaCO_2$ as the patient fatigues). The pH may be elevated early on and then lowered as patient fatigues or when compounded by sepsis

overdose, pain, high epidural block *or* owing to inability to overcome increased resistance to ventilation, e.g. abdominal distension.

Arterial blood gases: please see Chapter 1 'General Physiology' for further explanation of arterial blood gas analysis.

ARDS (acute respiratory distress syndrome)

Definition

Acute respiratory failure with non-cardiogenic pulmonary oedema occurring secondary to severe insults to the lungs or other organs.

Causes of ARDS

1. Sepsis syndrome
2. Severe multiple trauma
3. Aspiration

Criteria for diagnosis of ARDS

1. Bilateral lung infiltrates
2. No evidence of elevated left atrial pressure
3. $PaO_2/FiO_2 < 200$ mm Hg/or 300 according to Berlin criteria

Pathophysiology of ARDS

- Increased capillary permeability
- Protein-rich fluid accumulates inside the alveoli and diffuse alveolar damage occurs
- Inflammation of lung tissue and microcirculation caused by neutrophil activation (and other pro-inflammatory mediators)
- Decreased lung compliance (caused by decreased lung volume rather than lung stiffness) and pulmonary hypertension occur
- A proliferation phase (usually within 72 hours) and then a resolution phase follow
- Some patients fail to enter resolution phase and progress to lung fibrosis with worsening lung compliance and increasing hypoxia, ventilator dependence and mortality

Management of ARDS

ITU management and 'open lung ventilation'.

- Low tidal volume ventilation (6 ml/kg) – accepting hypercapnia and respiratory acidosis
- PEEP – higher levels may improve lung function and oxygenation, but have not shown any mortality improvement
- Prone positioning – used as a rescue measure for resistant hypoxaemia, no survival benefit demonstrated
- High frequency ventilation – ultra-low tidal volumes. Inconclusive results to date and awaiting a large RCT

Supportive treatment

- Fluids – conservative fluid management improves oxygenation but not mortality or non-pulmonary organ failure
- Transfusion – massive transfusion may have been the initial cause and may worsen the situation by detrimental immunomodulatory effects
- Sedation – required for mechanical ventilation
- Paralysis – may decrease the oxygen demand from striated muscles, and improve ventilator mechanics, but requires sedation, and may make weaning from mechanical ventilation more difficult. Useful in severe hypoxaemia

- Nutrition – started early can decrease length of ITU stay and 28-day mortality
- Inhaled pulmonary vasodilators – inhaled nitric oxide is expensive, difficult to use, and has no effect on mortality. Inhaled prostacyclin improves oxygenation but does not reduce duration of mechanical ventilation or mortality
- Other agents considered but without impact on mortality are vasoconstrictors, anti-inflammatories (including corticosteroids) and beta agonists
- ECMO – improves oxygenation in refractory hypoxaemia. Allows better gas exchange with ventilator protective strategies. Benefits on outcome awaited in RCTs

Ventilation modes (IPPV, CPAP, PEEP) and effects on oxygenation and CVS: see Chapter 23 Modes of mechanical ventilation.

Cardiovascular physiology

Autoregulation

Autoregulation can be local or neuronal and serves to maintain adequate

(i) oxygen and nutrient delivery
(ii) removal of metabolic waste products in times of need.

It acts to redistribute blood flow away from tissues with low need, and towards tissues with high metabolic demands.

Local mechanisms for autoregulation are

(i) myogenic
(ii) in response to the tissue milieu, e.g. O_2 deficiency, increased metabolites (for example K^+ and lactic acid)
(iii) in response to vasoactive substances (for example prostacyclin, adenosine)

The trigger acts directly on the blood vessels supplying and draining the tissue to cause either vasodilatation or constriction, thus maintaining adequate tissue blood flow.

Neuronal control of autoregulation can be central or via reflexes and use sympathetic or parasympathetic fibres, and acts to ensure appropriate distribution of blood flow throughout the body, e.g. during exercise or haemorrhage.

Cardiac pressure cycle

Control of cardiac output

Cardiac output (CO) is the volume of blood ejected from the heart per minute, and as such can be calculated by multiplying the heart rate (HR) (bpm – beats per minute) by the stroke volume (SV). The stroke volume is the measured difference between the end diastolic volume (EDV) and the end systolic volume (ESV), and is affected by the filling of the ventricle (pre-load), the contractility of the ventricle, and the ease with which the ventricle can eject the blood (afterload) (Fig 2.4 and 2.6).

$$CO = HR \times SV$$
$$SV = EDV - ESV$$

When considering stroke volume it is also important to understand contractility. According to the Frank Starling law (in the healthy heart), the greater the stretch of the cardiac muscle

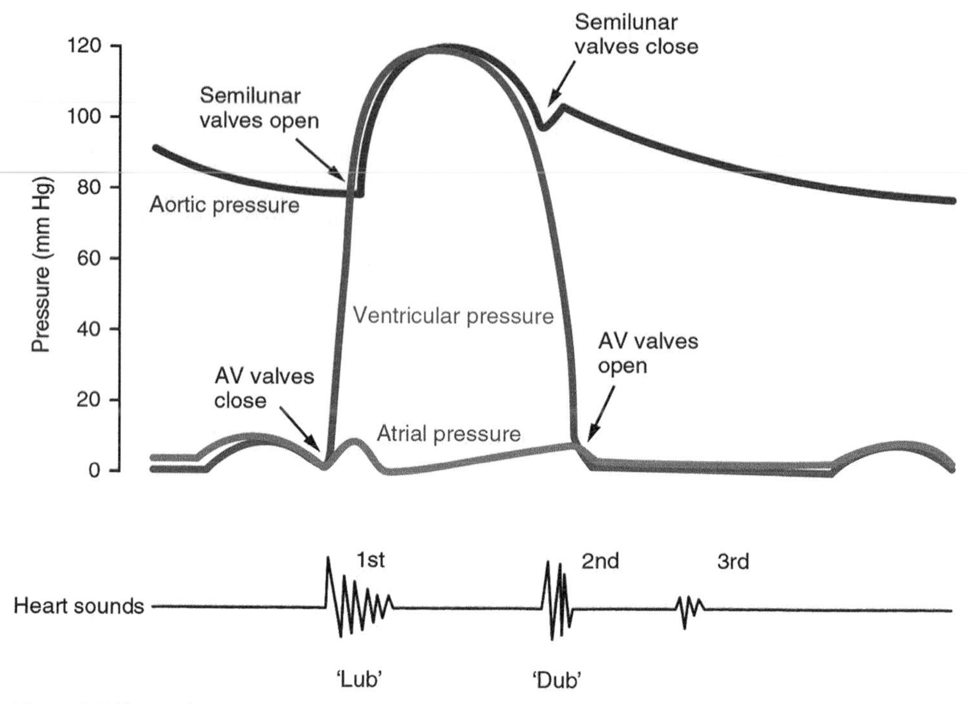

Figure 2.4 The cardiac pressure cycle.

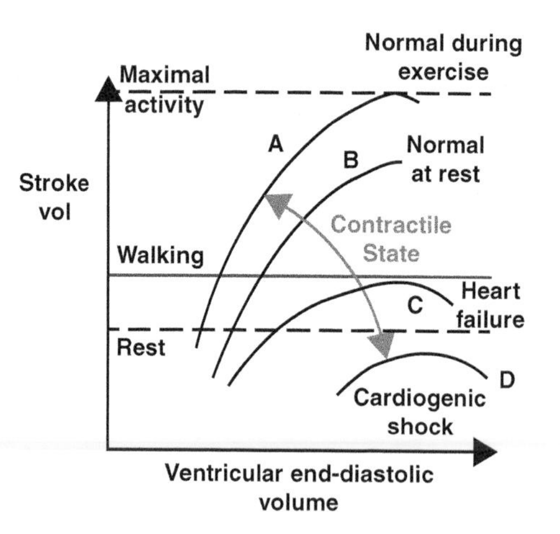

Figure 2.5 Figure to show the Frank Starling curves in normal resting state, during exercise and in heart failure.

fibre, the greater the force of contraction. In other words, a well-filled ventricle contracts more forcefully than an underfilled ventricle. There is an upper limit to the benefits realised, after which the muscle fibre is overstretched and unable to generate a contractive force. This leads to a fall in contractility, stroke volume and cardiac output.

In the failing heart cautious volume resuscitation can improve stroke volume and cardiac output but to a lesser degree. To move the failing heart curve (C) on the graph to the normal heart curve (B) would require fluid and positive inotropic drugs (see Figure 2.5).

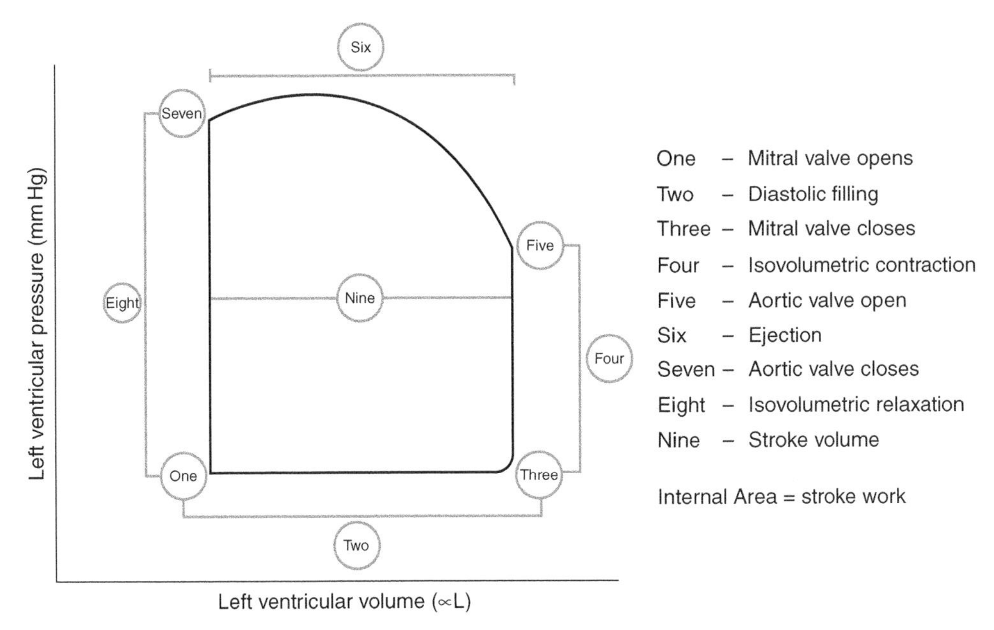

Figure 2.6 Figure to show the changes in volume and pressure during normal ventricular contraction.

Blood pressure (BP) is a product of the cardiac output and the systemic vascular resistance (SVR).

$$BP = CO \times SVR$$

Blood pressure and its physiological control mechanisms

Blood pressure is controlled from a central centre within three areas in the medulla; the centre responds to input from peripheral chemo- and baroreceptors via a feedback mechanism. The renin–angiotensin system is triggered by changes in blood flow to the juxtaglomerular apparatus. The changes in blood pressure caused by activation of the renin–angiotensin pathway feedback to peripheral and central receptors.

Other substances in the body that can affect blood pressure control are:

- Epinephrine and norepinephrine from the adrenal medulla (inotropic, chronotropic and vasoconstriction)
- Anti-diuretic hormone (increases blood volume)
- Atrial natriuretic peptide (diuretic, loss of volume)
- Nitric oxide (vasodilatation)

Blood pressure can also be altered by changes to cardiac output or systemic vascular resistance.

Changes to blood pressure by pathological processes affecting stroke volume:

- Hypovolaemic patients have decreased pre-load and reduced stroke volume. A compensatory tachycardia is mounted to maintain blood pressure
- Pump failure (e.g. myocardial infarction, cardiac failure) reduces stroke volume. Profound hypotension can occur if unable to increase the heart rate

Table 2.5 Summary of mechanisms of blood pressure control

Sensor	Sensor location	Action	Method of action
Cardiac centre	Medulla oblongata	Increased heart rate and contractility to increase cardiac output	Sympathetic nerves, anterior roots of T1–T4
Cardiac centre	Medulla oblongata	Decreased heart rate to decrease cardiac output	Parasympathetic vagus nerve, inhibitory post-ganglionic fibres terminating in the atria
Vasomotor centre	Medulla oblongata	Regulates blood vessel diameter	Sympathetic vasomotor nerves
Baroreceptors	Carotid sinus, aortic arch, right atrium	Feedback to cardiac and vasomotor centres. Local action	Detect intravascular pressure
Chemoreceptors	Carotid bodies, aortic bodies	Respond to hypoxia and hypercapnia as a surrogate measure of perfusion	
Kidneys	Juxtaglomerular apparatus	Adjusts blood volume by water and sodium reabsorption or secretion, and regulation of blood vessel diameter	Activation of the renin–angiotensin–aldosterone system

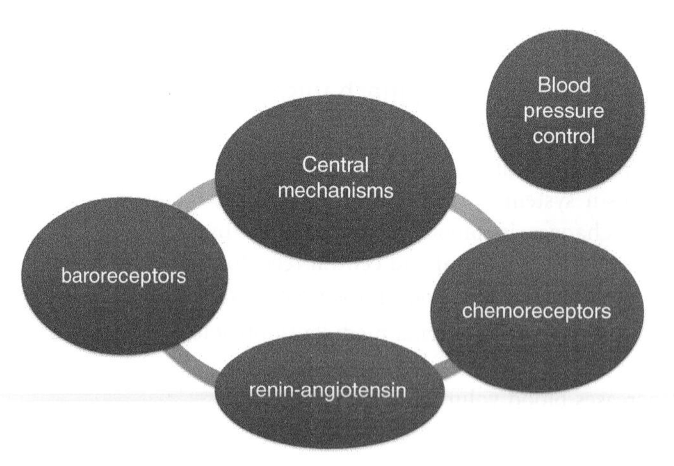

Figure 2.7 Figure to demonstrate the main mechanisms that influence the feedback loop for blood pressure control.

- Increased afterload (e.g. unnecessary vasopressors) can decrease stroke volume. In this scenario blood pressure may well be maintained but organ perfusion will be reduced, and the patient is still in shock

Decreased systemic vascular resistance (e.g. sepsis, anaphylaxis, high epidural blockade, neurogenic shock) causes a fall in blood pressure.

Table 2.6 Examples of pathologies that change stroke volume or heart rate and the effect on blood pressure

Initial problem	Reason	Effect
• Decreased pre-load, e.g. hypovolaemia • Decreased contractility, e.g. MI • Increased afterload with an empty circulation or failing pump (may maintain BP for a period before hypotension as the pump fails) • OR decreased afterload, e.g. sepsis or high epidural block	Decreased cardiac output caused by decreased stroke volume	HYPOTENSION
• Bradycardia caused by drugs (opiate overdose) or heart block • Tachycardia caused by pain or rhythm disturbance AF/SVT	Decreased cardiac output owing to heart rate	

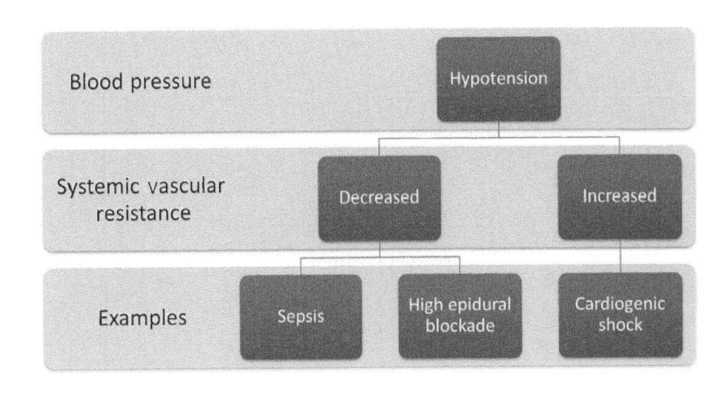

Figure 2.8 Diagram to demonstrate hypotension caused by changes in systemic vascular resistance.

Renal physiology

The kidney regulates fluid and electrolyte balance in the body. It receives 20% of cardiac output and produces 180 l ultrafiltrate per day, which is concentrated into urine (about 1.5 l per day). The minimum amount of urine in 24 hours required to clear waste products is 430 ml. The functional unit of the kidney is the nephron, which is one cell thick and has cortical and medullary components.

Other kidney functions are:

a. Excretion of metabolic waste products (urea, creatinine, uric acid, bilirubin)
b. Excretion of chemicals – e.g. drugs like penicillin
c. Acid–base balance
d. Hormone production – renin, erythropoietin, 1,25 di-hydroxyvitamin D3
e. Action on the renin–angiotensin–aldosterone system
f. Gluconeogenesis

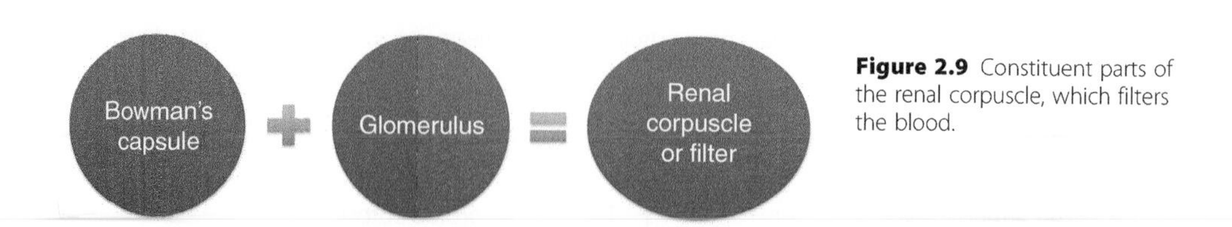

Figure 2.9 Constituent parts of the renal corpuscle, which filters the blood.

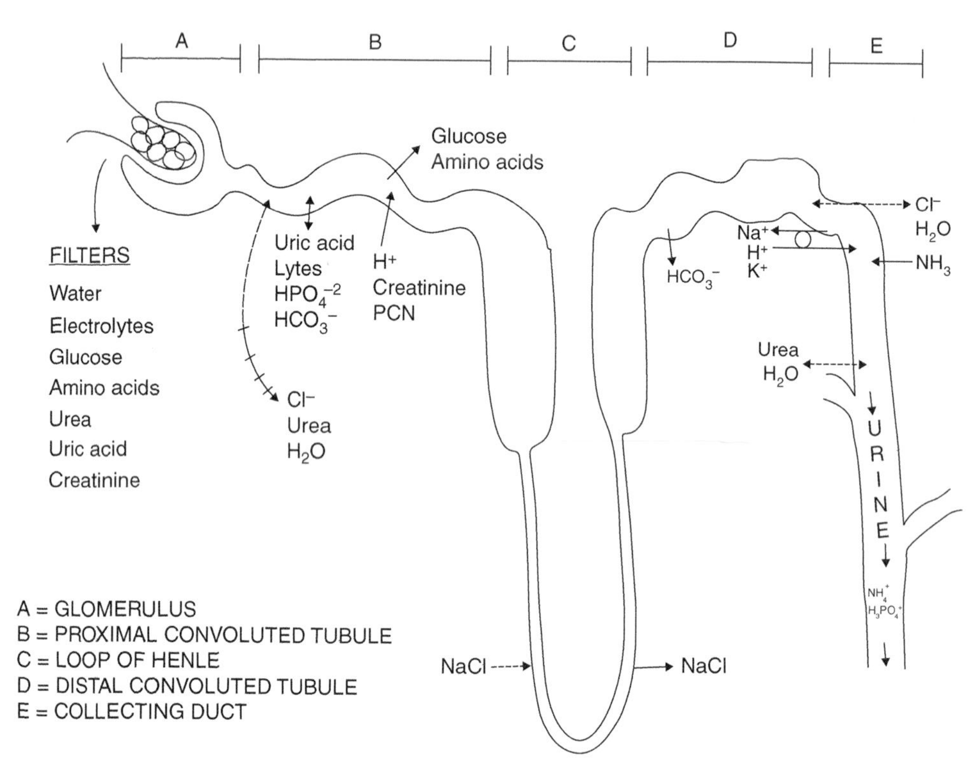

Figure 2.10 Line diagram of the nephron.

Acid–base balance

The kidney contributes, alongside the lungs, in controlling the acid–base balance of the body, either by removing hydrogen ions or by reabsorbing bicarbonate. The failing kidney can be responsible for a metabolic acidosis, and patients with chronic renal failure will often demonstrate low plasma bicarbonate in combination with elevated hydrogen ion concentration. The lungs are able to respond to acidosis rapidly with an increased respiratory rate. The response from the kidneys requires an intra-cellular reaction to occur and is somewhat slower.

Counter-current multiplier (loop of Henle)

The loop of Henle starts in the cortex of the kidney and dips deep into the medulla (Figure 2.12). The thick ascending limb is impermeable to water so the filtrate delivered

Table 2.7 Functional parts of the nephron, and their action on electrolytes, acid–base balance and glucose

	H_2O	Na^+	K^+	H^+	$HCO3^-$	G
Renal corpuscle	U	U	U	U	U	U
Proximal convoluted tubule	R (65%)	R (65%)	R (55%)	S	R	R
Descending loop of Henle	R (10%)	R (25%)	R (30%)	-	-	-
Ascending loop of Henle	x	R	-	-	-	-
Distal convoluted tubule	R(Ald)	R (Ald)	S/R	S	R	-
Collecting duct	R (ADH)	-	S/R	-	-	-

G = Glucose, R=Reabsorption, S=Secretion, U=Ultra filtrated, ADH = Anti-diuretic hormone, Ald = Aldosterone.

Table 2.8 Anatomical sections of the kidney and their function

Anatomical section	Function
Renal corpuscle	Acts to produce a plasma ultrafiltrate, low in protein
Proximal convoluted tubule	Reabsorbs up to 65% of the ultrafiltrate. Conserves fluid. Secretes calcitriol for calcium balance
Descending loop of Henle Ascending loop of Henle	Acts to develop an increasing osmotic gradient in the depth of the medulla. It does this by reabsorbing sodium, with variable permeability/impermeability to water. This will allow concentration of urine in the collecting ducts
Distal convoluted tubule	Maintenance of body electrolytes by balancing secretion and reabsorption
Collecting duct	Permits water reabsorption under the influence of ADH, and production of concentrated urine as the duct passes through the medulla

Table 2.9 Hormonal functions of the kidney

Hormones acting on the kidney		Hormones secreted by the kidney	
Angiotensin II	Converted from angiotensin I in pulmonary capillaries	Renin	From the granular cells of the juxtaglomerular apparatus
Aldosterone	Adrenal cortex, stimulated by angiotensin II, hyperkalaemia and ACTH	Erythropoietin	Produced in response to a drop in PO_2 by cells in the juxtaglomerular apparatus. 10–15% made in the liver
Anti-diuretic hormone	Synthesised in hypothalamus and secreted from posterior pituitary	1,25 dihydroxyvitamin D3	Produced in the proximal convoluted tubule in response to hypocalcaemia
Atrial natriuretic peptide	Released from distended stretched cardiac atrial cells		

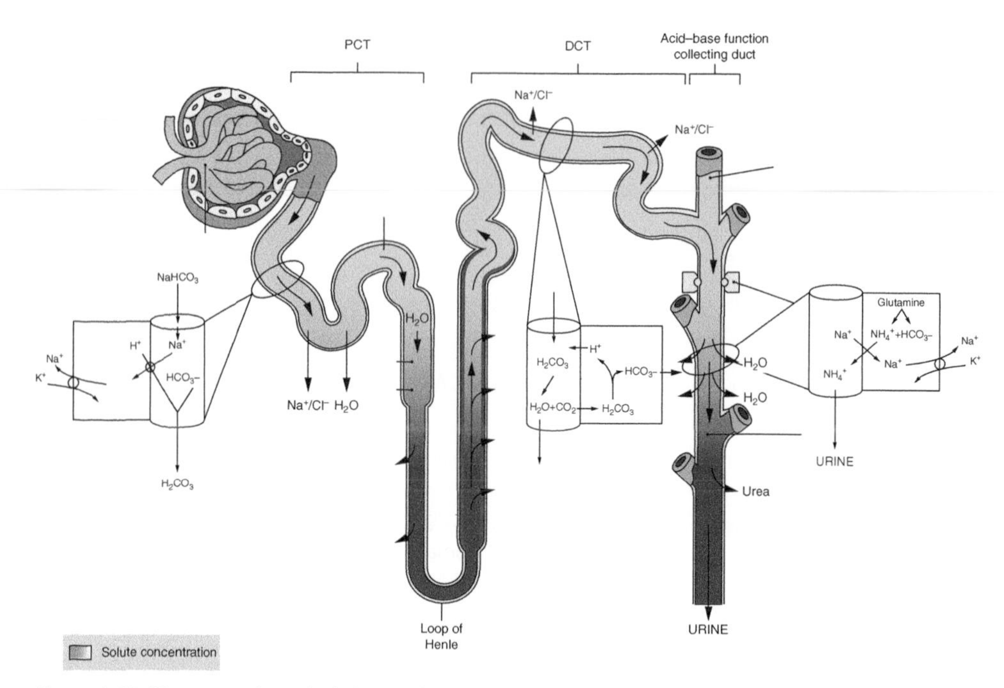

Figure 2.11 Diagram to show the kidney's role in acid–base balance. PCT = proximal convoluted tubule, DCT = distal convoluted tubule, CD = collecting duct. The glomerular filtrate passes through the cylinder from the left-hand side of the image. Intracellular chemical reactions occur in the tubular cells, sodium and bicarbonate pass into the blood/plasma, and NH_4^+ into the urine.

to the DCT and CD is dilute. On the other hand, sodium is actively secreted from the thick ascending limb into the medulla of the kidney. This has two consequences; the first is an even more dilute filtrate within the DCT and CD. The second is a very hyper-osmolar environment within the renal medulla. The collecting duct passes through this hypertonic area on route to the renal pelvis and is the last stage in the formation of urine. Water passes across the collecting duct cell walls into the very concentrated medulla. This passage is enhanced by ADH, and concentrated urine is produced.

Renal autoregulation

As with other organ systems, autoregulation is under a number of control mechanisms. These are myogenic – responding to pressure or metabolic changes – in response to local metabolites, or from central control. In the case of the kidney the local mechanism is via tubuloglomerular feedback, which can activate the renin–angiotensin–aldosterone system. This system links in to feedback mechanisms for central blood pressure control, and therefore maintenance of renal blood flow.

Renin–angiotensin system (Figure 2.13 and 2.14)

Angiotensinogen is a large protein made in the liver. Renin is produced by the juxtaglomerular cells in response to perceived hypovolaemia. It is inhibited by angiotensin II as part of a negative feedback loop. Renin is a proteolytic enzyme that splits the angiotensinogen to

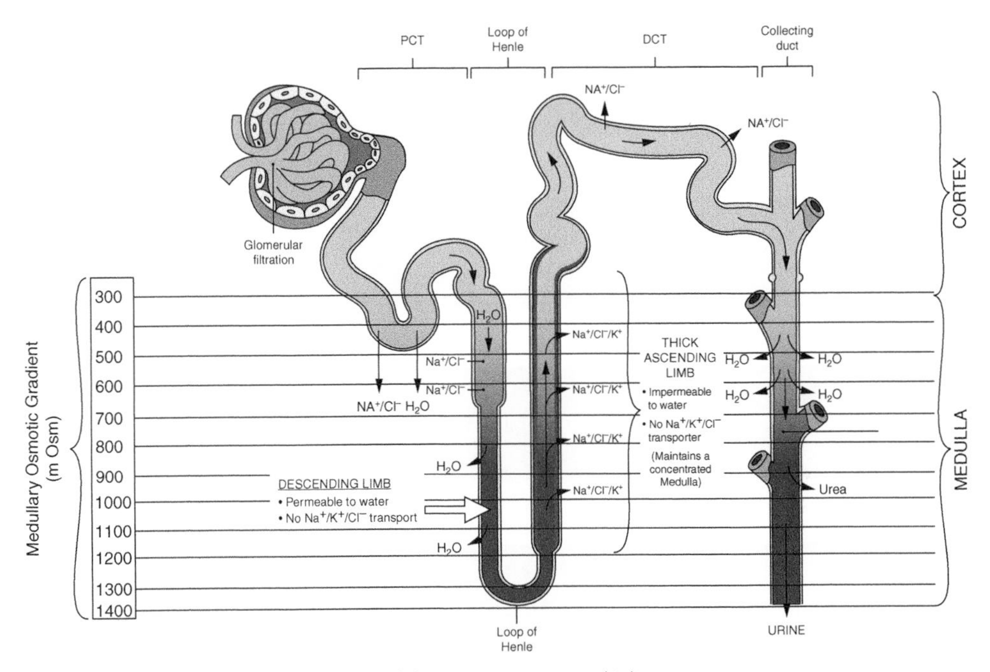

Figure 2.12 Diagram to show the nature of the counter-current multiplier.

form angiotensin I. Endothelial peptidases break it down further until it becomes a group of inactive peptides.

Angiotensin II is the active compound that acts directly and indirectly on the kidney.

Angiotensin II acts to preserve circulating volume by:

(i) Stimulating sodium reabsorption
(ii) Increasing sympathetic activity and therefore increasing SVR, CO and BP
(iii) Affecting renal blood flow and decreases glomerular filtration rate
(iv) Increasing thirst and water intake
(v) Stimulating aldosterone release. Aldosterone promotes sodium and potassium reabsorption

Causes of poor urine output and acute kidney injury/failure

When assessing patients for low urine output the first step is to assess fluid balance and look for signs of an obstructed outflow tract.

Pre-renal

A fall in renal blood flow provides less substrate for ultrafiltration, and in acute cases can lead to low urine output.

All shock states with a fall in cardiac output lead to a fall in renal blood flow.

This is the most common cause of poor urine output for surgical patients.

- **Hypovolaemic shock** – fluid loss (diarrhoea and vomiting, bowel obstruction, high output stomas, diabetes insipidus, burns), concealed haemorrhage (GI haemorrhage,

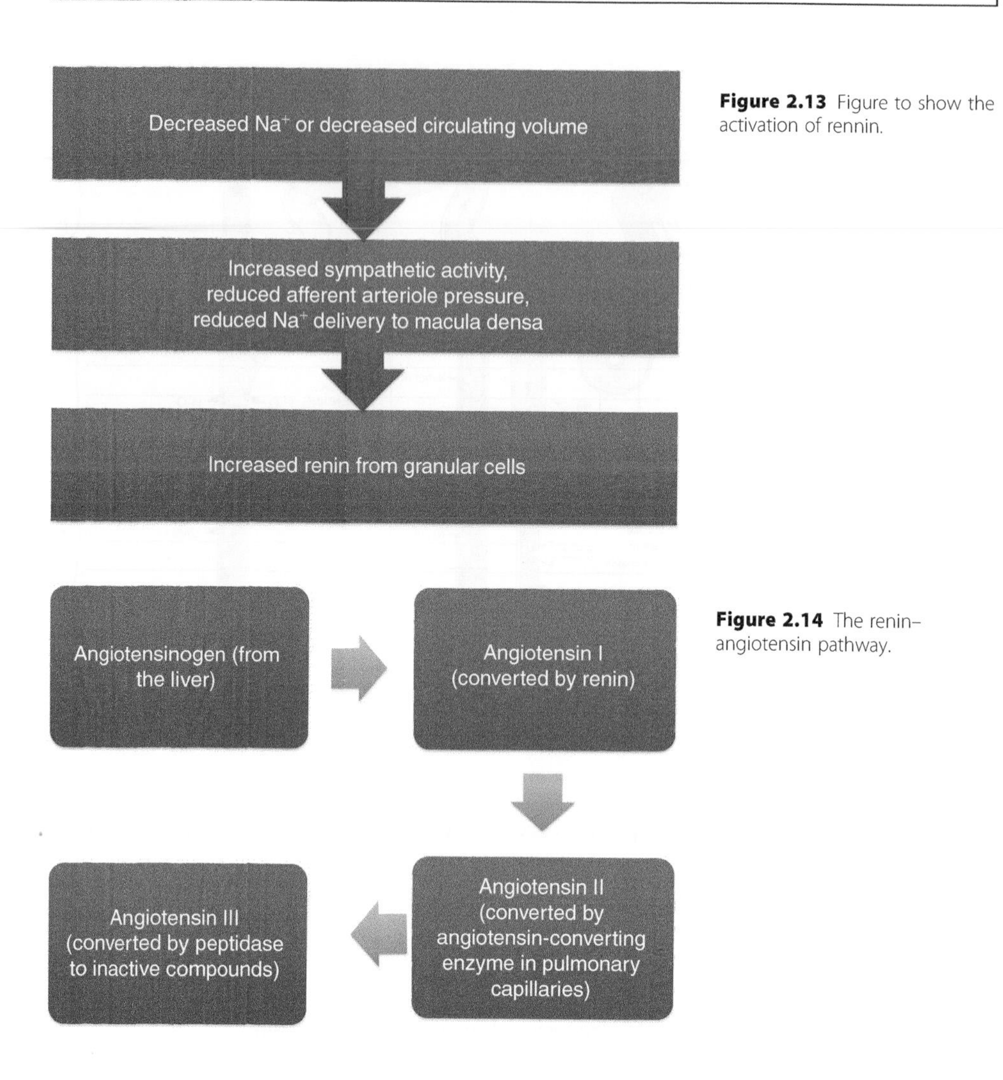

Figure 2.13 Figure to show the activation of rennin.

Figure 2.14 The renin–angiotensin pathway.

retroperitoneal, intra-thoracic), overt haemorrhage (traumatic injury, vascular injury), inadequate fluid replacement (intra-op, post-op)

- **Cardiogenic shock** – myocardial infarction, arrhythmia, pulmonary embolus
- **Septic shock** – pancreatitis, faecal contamination of the intra-abdominal compartment, post-operative pneumonia

Other causes of pre-renal acute renal failure are renal artery occlusion (aortic dissection, thrombus) and hepatorenal syndrome.

If a pre-renal cause for reduced urine output is identified and acted upon early enough, with restoration of circulating volume, progression to acute tubular necrosis and established acute renal failure can be avoided.

Renal

The least common cause of poor urine output in the acutely unwell surgical patient, but it should prompt a review of the drug chart. Medication-induced injury most frequently causes an acute interstitial nephritis, the commonest culprits are NSAIDs, antibiotics (penicillins, aminoglycosides, cephalosporins). Other drugs that can cause renal failure are diuretics (thiazides and furosemide), antihypertensives (ACE inhibitors).

Trauma patients with rhabdomyolysis and myoglobinuria may develop acute renal failure caused by deposition of myoglobin within the nephron.

Post-renal

The second most common cause of poor urine output. Obstruction to the outflow of the kidney causes an acute drop in urine output.

If a patient is catheterised the catheter should be flushed and a bladder washout performed. A bladder scan is also useful to check the residual volume.

- **Kidney** – stones in the calyx, pelvi-ureteric junction (PUJ) or vesico-ureteric junction (VUJ), obstruction (stenosis), external compression of the ureter by retroperitoneal mass or fibrosis
- **Bladder** – clot, debris from infection, stone
- **Urethra** – prostate, stricture, stone
- **Catheter** – clot, debris, lubricating gel used on insertion, clamp, failure of irrigation

Types of renal failure

Acute kidney injury/AKI (previously described as acute renal failure)

Rapid loss of renal function and uraemia over hours or days, often with oliguria/anuria. Signs such as hypertension and anaemia are absent. Acute electrolyte imbalance with hyperkalaemia is common. AKI is reversible if treated appropriately. Kidneys are normal size on imaging.

Treatment is often in the HDU and includes:

1. Treating the cause – stop drug, treat sepsis, remove obstruction
2. Volume resuscitation
3. Blood pressure support to maintain renal blood flow
4. Consider diuretics – furosemide
5. Renal replacement therapy (dialysis or haemofiltration) may be necessary

The phases of acute kidney injury are:

1. Onset phase
2. Oliguric phase
3. Diuretic phase
4. Recovery phase

Chronic renal failure

Slowly progressive and irreversible uraemia, with secondary signs such as hypertension, anaemia, compensated metabolic acidosis and secondary hyperparathyroidism. Urine may still be produced but of poor quality. Patients may be dialysis dependent.

Imaging and biopsy displays abnormal (often shrunken) kidneys.

Acute kidney injury can occur to those with stable chronic renal failure, and lead to a further deterioration in function.

Central nervous system physiology

Normal intracranial pressure (ICP) is between 5–15 mmHg when lying down.

Physiology of space occupying lesions

The cranium forms a rigid box containing brain (1400 g/1400 ml/80%), CSF (150 ml/10%), and blood (150 ml/10%). Any change in the volume of one constituent will affect the volume of the others. If no change in volume is possible the intracranial pressure will be affected (Monro–Kellie Doctrine). It can be seen that a similar change in intracranial volume (A vs. B) caused by blood/oedema/tumour can cause a very different change in pressure P1 vs. P2 (Figure 2.15).

As intracranial pressure rises, there is a need to increase mean arterial pressure to maintain cerebral perfusion pressure.

$$CPP = MAP - ICP$$

If intracranial pressure is presumed to be high, say 25 mmHg, it can be seen that a mean arterial pressure (MAP) of 60 would only produce a cerebral perfusion pressure (CPP) of 35 mmHg. This is the reason for guidelines that recommend maintaining a MAP of 90 mmHg in the brain-injured patient, thereby providing a CPP of 65 mmHg.

The Cushing's reflex is an exaggerated physiological response to maintain CPP when the ICP rises dramatically. It causes severe hypertension and bradycardia and is a late sign signalling impending brain stem herniation.

There are surgical and medical methods to decrease intracranial pressure from space occupying lesions and the method adopted depends on the cause of the space occupying lesion.

Surgical methods include removal of the lesion (where possible) – haematoma, tumour, abscess. If the lesion cannot be removed (i.e. the lesion is brain swelling secondary to head injury, vasopasm, hyperperfusion, peri-lesional oedema) then CSF can be removed with an external ventricular drain (or eventually a CSF diversion procedure, e.g. shunt).

Medical methods may be pharmacological (see Table 2.10) or manipulation of physiology (see autoregulation of cerebral blood flow).

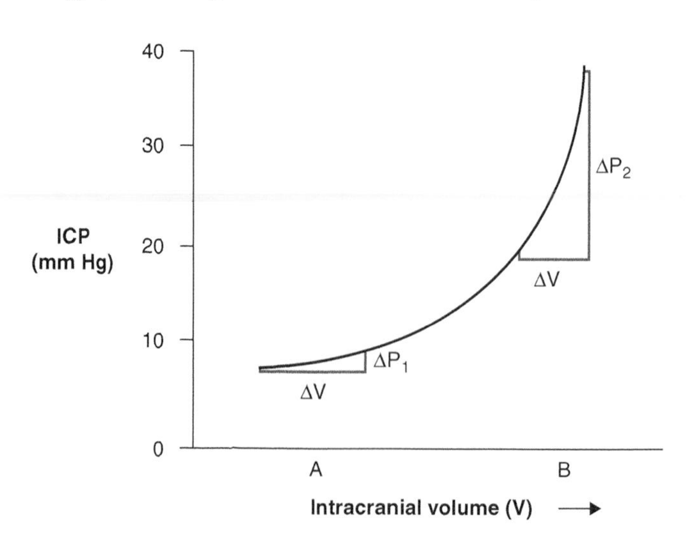

Figure 2.15 Graph to show the change in ICP according to the volume of intracranial contents.

Table 2.10 Medical methods to decrease ICP

Drug	Mechanism
Steroid – dexamethasone	Decreases oedema, very useful for reducing the oedema surrounding a tumour
Osmotic agent – mannitol, hypertonic saline, furosemide	Decrease brain water content. Some concern that if the blood–brain barrier is injured then mannitol will enter brain tissue and result in rebound intracranial hypertension
Anti-epileptics	Decrease brain energy requirements
Anaesthetics	Can decrease brain energy requirements to basal levels
Analgesics	Prevent pain and physiological response to pain
Paralysing agents	Decrease body energy requirements

Table 2.11 Causes of iatrogenic post-operative confusion

Iatrogenic causes of post-operative confusion	
Drugs	Anaesthetic Opiate Parasympathetico-mimetics (e.g. atropine) Benzodiazepines Withdrawal Residual paralysis
Urinary retention	
Cerebral oedema	Prolonged head down position

Table 2.12 Causes of pathological post-operative confusion

Pathological causes of post-operative confusion	
Intracranial SOL	Oedema Pneumocephalus Haematoma Tumour CSF
Seizures	Convulsant/tonic–clonic Non-convulsant
Vascular	Vasospasm Aneurysm rupture Hyperperfusion Cerebrovascular accident
Respiratory	Hypoxia Hypercarbia
Cardiovascular	Hypotension Arrhythmia

Auto-regulation and maintenance of cerebral blood flow

It is arguable that the brain circulation has the tightest control of all organs. This is to permit a steady supply of oxygen and glucose to the brain, an organ that depends upon oxidative metabolism and is without energy reserves.

Auto-regulation is controlled locally and globally in the healthy brain. Active brain areas will have higher oxygen demand and carbon dioxide production, leading to increased regional blood flow. This is described as flow metabolism coupling, in other words the flow to tissues is coupled to their metabolic requirements. Most of the volatile anaesthetic agents disrupt this coupling in a dose-dependent fashion, with sevoflurane causing the least effect. Intravenous anaesthetic agents (propofol, thiopentone) do not un-couple flow-metabolism in the cerebral circulation.

Mean arterial blood pressure

Global auto-regulation is represented in Figure 2.16. A number of points become apparent:

1. Cerebral blood flow (CBF) is steady at 50 ml/100g/min between mean arterial blood pressures of 50 and 150 mmHg in the healthy individual
2. As the mean arterial pressure increases, the intra-luminal diameter of supplying vessels decreases (see top line of Figure 2.16), cerebrovascular resistance (CVR) increases, and cerebral blood volume (CBV) decreases
3. As the mean arterial pressure decreases, the supplying vessels dilate, CVR decreases and CBV increases

The auto-regulation curve is shifted to the right in patients with chronic hypertension, to maintain uniform blood supply across a higher range of mean arterial pressure. This is of particular importance when deciding on blood pressure target during hypotensive anaesthesia for certain surgical procedures, e.g. middle ear surgery, shoulder surgery. A slightly higher blood pressure may be required to maintain cerebral perfusion.

These changes can be employed in times of raised intra-cranial pressure to manipulate the ICP. Elevating the mean arterial pressure will not only maintain CPP (discussed earlier), but will also decrease CBV and reduce ICP.

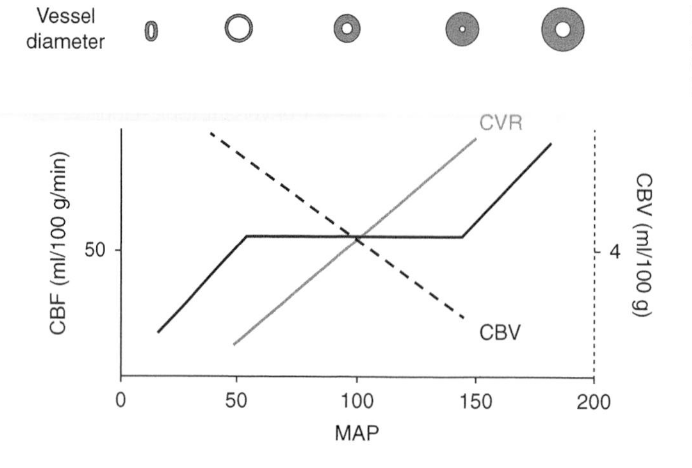

Figure 2.16 Figure to show global cerebral autoregulation of cerebral blood flow in the healthy brain.

Table 2.13 How to manipulate physiology to reduce intracranial pressure in acute head injury

Physical measures to ensure free drainage of cerebral blood (and reduce CBV)	Head up, neck neutral, endotracheal tube secured with tape rather than ties, low intra-thoracic pressure (treat chest pathology)
Maintain CPP by augmenting MAP	Fluid resuscitation, then consider vasopressor support. Aim for MAP 90 mmHg
Reduce CBV by control of $PaCO_2$	Intubation and ventilation to control $PaCO_2$, aim for $PaCO_2$ 4.5–5.0 kPa. Hyperventilation can be used in emergencies for short periods to 4.0 kPa
Maintain CBF at normal levels by control of PaO_2	Intubation and ventilation to prevent hypoxia. Maintain PaO_2 at 11 kPa
Maintain normoglycaemia	The brain is dependent on glucose as its energy source. Hyperglycaemia has also been shown to cause central neuronal injury
Consider moderate hypothermia	Evidence is still lacking, but many centres use moderate hypothermia in malignant raised ICP
Monitoring	Invasive BP, central venous pressure, ICP

How is auto-regulation different in patients with acute head injury?

Auto-regulation depends, in part, upon the endothelium being intact, and able to respond to a physiological trigger. This is not always the case in patients with acute head injury. It appears from studies that the optimum CPP is 70–90 mmHg, but may still vary between (and in) individuals. Above 90 mmHg CPP auto-regulation may be impaired with no further vasoconstriction, meaning a further increase in MAP causes a direct increase in CBF and CBV, and therefore an increase in ICP.

This may also be the case in patients with tumour, subarachnoid haemorrhage and stroke.

Cerebral blood flow, cerebral blood volume and $PaCO_2$

The $PaCO_2$ has a direct effect on the cerebral vasculature. An increase in $PaCO_2$ leads to cerebral vasodilatation whereas a decrease in $PaCO_2$ leads to cerebral vasoconstriction. In the normotensive patient a $PaCO_2$ of 10.5 kPa doubles cerebral blood flow, a $PaCO_2$ of 2.5 kPa halves cerebral blood flow (normal $PaCO_2$ is 5 kPa). The vasoreactivity occurs rapidly in a linear fashion and can be used to control intracranial pressure in emergencies, for example the acutely head injured patient with a unilateral dilated pupil can be hyperventilated to reduce cerebral blood volume, thereby decreasing ICP. It can be seen from the figure that the reduction in CBV is coupled to a reduction in CBF, which may cause harm by an increase in the volume of ischaemic tissue.

Hyperventilation should only be used as a temporary measure to effect rapid control of life-threatening elevations in ICP, while other measures are being started. Clearly hypoventilation must be avoided at all costs.

It should be remembered that the responsiveness of the vessel wall depends upon the presence of normo- or hypertension – the response is obtunded with mild hypotension and obliterated with severe hypotension.

Cerebral blood flow, cerebral blood volume and PaO_2

Arteriolar tone is also affected, but to a lesser degree in clinical situations, by PaO_2. Cerebral blood flow is maintained at 50 ml/100 g/min until the patient becomes hypoxic. There is no increase in cerebral blood flow with increases in PaO_2, but when the PaO_2 falls below 6.7 kPa there is a sudden and steep increase in cerebral blood flow in response to vasodilatation.

Section I

Basic sciences

Chapter 3

Pain and analgesia

David Sapsford

'Pain insists upon being attended to. God whispers to us in our pleasures, speaks in our consciences, but shouts in our pains. It is his megaphone to rouse a deaf world.'
- C. S. Lewis.

Introduction

Pain is an unpleasant sensation to a noxious stimulus, a stressor that can threaten the individual's homeostatic state. The physiological and behavioural adaptive responses to this stress have evolved to preserve life. However, the persistence of this stress response with its concomitant over-stimulation of the sympathetic nervous system, energy depletion and the anomalous hormonal imbalance may be life-threatening.

Effective pain control is an essential component of high-quality care of the surgical patient. Despite advances in the knowledge of pathophysiology, pharmacology, and techniques of post-operative pain control, numerous surgical procedures take place every year where patients continue to experience unnecessary discomfort.

Pain! The fifth vital sign

As the fifth vital sign pain should be measured as frequently as other vital signs visible at the end of the bed. It should be recorded on the standard observation chart, and algorithms should be in place to set thresholds for intervention. Pain that becomes uncontrolled can alert the physician to a change in the pathology or progression of the underlying condition.

This chapter will cover: the transference of the pain signal (transduction, transmission, perception and modulation); the analgesic response (stress release of pro-opiomelanocortin cleaved into ACTH (adreno-corticotrophic hormone), and encephalins); the reflex escape response (the sympathetic nervous system and neuroendocrine system); and the effects of physiological changes.

A Surgeon's Guide to Anaesthesia and Peri-operative Care, ed. Jane Sturgess, Justin Davies and Kamen Valchanov. Published by Cambridge University Press.

Role of the anaesthetist and surgeon

Enhanced recovery has benefits for both the patient and the health organisation; it can only be achieved by effective peri-operative medicine in assessing, preparing and optimising the patient for surgery. This will include adjusting pain therapy and may involve pre-emptive analgesia. It will not be realised without precise information, timely intervention, accurate measurement and control; all these rely on effective communication.

Effective communication between the surgeon and anaesthetist creates a working pain team

In these times of day of surgery admission it is essential that surgeons are aware of the complexities of pain control; the patient groups that can cause problems; the drug interactions; and the possibility of pre-operative optimisation and pre-emptive manoeuvres that will produce high-quality post-operative recovery. It is notable that few patients arrive at surgery without analgesic medication as a significant part of their past medical history.

Pain control requires communication between the patient and the pain team, necessitating precise pre-operative assessment

Central principles

Definition

Pain is defined by the International Association for the Study of Pain as

> **'An unpleasant sensory and emotional experience associated with actual or potential tissue damage, or described in terms of such damage.'**

Pain is personal; there is no outward objective signal that can be used as a monitor of change or efficacy of therapy. This is an active area of research and somatosensory evoked potentials could be useful in the future.

Pain is what the patient says it is! (McCaffery, 1968)

Pain is often divided into acute and chronic. Acute pain is that which is experienced immediately after tissue damage and it has a causal relationship which indicates an organic disease; it resolves with treatment of the cause, and opioids are typically indicated. Chronic or persistent pain may serve no useful function, with an unclear cause; it is resistant to many forms of therapy, opioids are less effective (except for their dissociative and sedative effect, producing tolerance of symptoms), and there may be a secondary, possibly unknown, purpose to the symptom.

Acute pain is different from chronic pain

- Acute pain (physiological) has a purpose
- Chronic pain (pathological) will not kill your patient!

However it is becoming apparent that this is a spurious distinction and the two conditions appear to be a continuum. Prolonged acute pain through neurodisorganisation may lead on to persistent pain states and chronic pain may be aggravated by further episodes of acute pain. It is thus essential that a detailed understanding of pain progression and of all the treatment modalities is required.

Deficiencies

Pain is often secondary to diagnosis and treatment of the acute condition. This lack of recognition of the damage that pain can cause to the short- and long-term health of the patient has led to unnecessary suffering.

There is now a clear acknowledgement that effective post-operative pain control is an essential part of patient management

Anatomy and physiology

Understanding the anatomy and physiology of the nociceptive and associated neural pathways permits identification of possible interventions to reduce the impact of pain.

Afferent sensory nerve impulses enter the central nervous system via the dorsal root ganglion. These first-order neurones synapse in the dorsal horn and are conducted to the higher centres by second- and then third-order neurones.

Innocuous sensations, touch, pressure, etc. are mediated by specific sensory receptors and are conveyed to the central nervous system by low-threshold, fast, myelinated, primary afferent Aα and Aβ nerve fibres, which travel up the ipsilateral side of the spinal cord in the posterior columns.

Nociceptive information is transduced by non-specific receptors and free nerve endings. These are polymodal and respond to a variety of stimuli, chemical, e.g. histamine, prostaglandins, etc.; thermal and mechanical. They are found in all parts of the body except the interior of bones and the brain. In the cornea of the eye, only free nerve endings are found and abrasions of the cornea can be extremely painful. Pain results from prostaglandins, histamine, and peptides, released from damaged tissues, activating receptors located on these free nerve endings.

The nociceptive signals are transported by primary afferent high-threshold afferents, thinly myelinated fast Aδ and unmyelinated slow C nerve fibres. These signals are integrated and modulated within the central nervous system, starting at the dorsal horn of the spinal cord. The information is then carried via second-order neurones, which decussate one to two levels above the point of entry to form the contralateral spinothalamic and reticular tracts. These interact with neurones in the rostral ventral medulla, parabrachial nucleus and peri-aqueductal grey matter, on the way to the thalamus where they synapse with third-order neurones which then represent the information, primarily on the somatosensory cortex, giving the spatial, discriminative, conscious appreciation of pain; with secondary representation on the amygdala, insula cortex, cingula cortex and hypothalamus, leading to the affective components of pain perception and autonomic representation to the nociceptive input.

'Fast pain' sensation from Aδ fibres is described as stabbing, sharp, electric, or bright. The C fibres carry the second type of 'slow pain', typically described as aching, throbbing or dull. Not all of these fibres are nociceptive, some transfer information of low-threshold stimuli such as touching, brushing and warmth: these may be involved in the idiosyncratic responses sometimes seen in persistent pain syndromes, often referred to as allodynia.

The second-order neurones activate anti-nociceptive pathways because of their synaptic activity in the peri-aqueductal grey matter and nucleus raphe, which release endorphins and encephalins. This and other chemical changes at the synapse of the first- and second-order neurones in the dorsal horn of the spinal cord, modulate the nociceptive input and limit the extent of stimulation which can be perceived as pain, commonly called the 'gate' in gate theory.

This site of modulation is actually pre-synaptic and over 70% of endorphin and encephalin receptors are on the membrane of the first-order primary afferent nerve at the axonal pre-synaptic terminal. These neuro transmitters together with others (norepinephrine, serotonin and GABA) reduce the nociceptive transmission by impairing the release of glutamate and substance P. Dynorphin, GABA and serotonin also inhibit the post-synaptic membrane of the second-order neurone's ability to depolarise and transmit impulses centrally.

Thus the dorsal horn of the spinal cord is not just a relay station for sensory information; it has a regulatory function, using local interneurons and supraspinal mechanisms to inhibit the depolarisation of the second-order neurones.

The dorsal horn is divided into six layers called laminae.

Lamina I is the most dorsal and is a thin layer of large neurones whose axons form part of the spinothalamic tract; there are also small inhibitory interneurons within this lamina.

Lamina II (the substantia gelatinosa) controls the connectivity of the other regions of the dorsal horn and is mainly inhibitory. It does not project directly to higher levels but contains many interneurons involved in the modification of pain transmission, generally referred to as the gate control theory of pain (Melzack and Wall, 1965). Rubbing, acupuncture, or TENS (transcutaneous electrical nerve stimulation) may suppress nociceptive input at this level.

Laminae III to VI receive cutaneous non-nociceptive Aβ afferents and respond to low-threshold receptive fields imitating innocuous sensations.

Action potentials on the primary afferent first-order neurones cause the depolarisation of the pre-synaptic terminal membrane causing a calcium-dependent release of glutamate. This is the main central nervous system neurotransmitter playing a major role in nociceptive transmission in the dorsal horn. It acts at several receptors; acute pain activates the α-amino-3-hydroxy-5-methyl-4-isoxazolepropionic acid (AMPA) receptor, causing fast depolarisation; whereas prolonged painful stimuli activate N-methyl-D-aspartate (NMDA) receptors. By a process of long-term potentiation, activation of NMDA receptors may lead to altered responses to acute pain and initiate the process of persistent (chronic) pain. Substance P, originally thought of as the main nociceptive transmitter, has a modulatory role at the post-synaptic neurokinin 1 receptor.

Interneurones control the post-synaptic membrane of the second-order dorsal horn cell by releasing GABA and inhibit axonal depolarisation, preventing transmission of nociceptive signals. These inhibitory interneurons can be activated by dynorphin, which acts at α-adrenoreceptors on its axon. This causes hyperpolarisation of the dorsal horn cell and inhibits further transmission of the pain signal.

These pre-synaptic and interneurone receptor sites are the first central station where analgesics may act by mimicking the intrinsic neurotransmitters.

Table 3.1 Summary of the pain pathway and analgesic strategies

Pathway	Process	Analgesics
Injury ↓	Results in the release of multiple chemical mediators; including histamine, prostaglandins, bradykinin, serotonin, leukotrienes, glutamate, tumour necrosis factor (TNF) and substance P; leading to the depolarisation of free nerve endings.	Local and/or systemic anti-inflammatoy drugs. Injection of steroid. Use NSAID drugs locally and systemically. Systemic and topical antihistamines. Capsaicin depletes glutamate stores and causes stimulation then inhibition of glutamate transmission; it also causes degeneration of capsaicin-sensitive nociceptive nerve endings.
Nociceptor ↓	The free nerve endings have receptors for many of the chemicals mentioned above.	Depolarisation is inhibited by blocking sodium channels by using local analgesic applied topically, e.g. lignocaine plaster or EMLA cream and by antagonists at receptor sites on the nerve endings.
Nerve ↓	Sodium channel-dependent transmission of nociceptive signals.	The use of nerve blocks with local analgesics, e.g. bupivacaine.
Dorsal root ganglion ↓	The primary neurone outside the CNS of the first-order nociceptor nerve.	Local analgesic block (this will also have effects on Aβ sensory nerve fibres). Implanted nerve stimulator.
Dorsal horn Spinal cord ↓	The synapse between first-order and second-order neurones is the primary site for analgesic action, as discussed in the text.	Epidural and intrathecal (spinal) administration of local analgesics, opioids, GABA analogues (benzodiazepines and baclofen), α2 adrenoreceptor agonists (clonidine) and many more, plus other complex techniques used in pain clinics.
Spino-cortical tracts ↓	The transmission route for nociceptive signals, sodium channel-dependent transmission.	Local analgesics delivered via the epidural and intrathecal routes.
Brain stem ↓	Central integration and processing leading to the downward control and modulation of nociceptive input at the spinal dorsal horn level.	This area is responsive to many neurotransmitters including opioids and α2 sympathomimetics.
Cortical representation ↓	After all the modifications to the original stimulus it is now both consciously (somatosensory cortex) producing a considered response and unconsciously (amygdala etc.), resulting in the emotional response and the effect of past memories being integrated into the overall response.	Many drugs not considered as analgesics will have an effect in this area and influence the global reaction to the nociceptive input. Also psycho-behavioural techniques, e.g. mindfulness, etc. have a modifying effect.
Downward control	Many responses routed via the brainstem will produce signals transmitted to the dermatomal level of the spinal dorsal horn nociceptive input, allowing the modulation of the response to the stimulus.	Downward control originates from many CNS sites but all tend to terminate in the laminae of the dorsal horn, the majority at the synapse between first- and second-order neurones.

Table 3.2 Pre- and post-synaptic pain receptors

Type	Endogenous transmitter	Analgesic
Pre-synaptic receptors (analgesia generally by agonism)		
μ opioid	Endorphins	Opioids
δ opioid	Encephalins	Buprenorphine (metabolised to norbuprenorphine)
GABAβ	GABA	Baclofen
α-2 adrenoceptor	Noradrenaline	Clonidine, tizanidine, dexmedetomidine
5-HT_3	Serotonin	Antagonised by mirtazepine
Post-synaptic receptors (analgesia usually by antagonism)		
AMPA	Glutamate	Alcohol
NMDA	Glutamate	Amantadine, ketamine, methadone
GABA α	GABA	Midazolam enhances GABA activity
5-HT_3	Serotonin	Re-uptake blocked by citalopram

Pain induces a stress response

Analgesic response

Pro-opiomelancortin release secondary to the stress response is cleaved into many different peptides including the endogenous opioids, known as encephalins and endorphins. They exist throughout the central nervous system and these substances prevent the release of neurotransmitters glutamate and substance P, thus inhibiting the transmission of pain impulses, producing an analgesic effect.

Reflex escape response

Pain produces activation of the sympathetic nervous system known as the 'fight or flight' response. The sympathetic nervous system and the neuro-endocrine system result in the physiological responses described below, that are many and intrinsically linked.

Sympathetic nervous system

This system supplies the internal organs and is involved in the body's immediate response to severe pain. The early properties of this response allow the survival of an individual; however, prolonged activation can be detrimental. The sympathetic nervous system is responsible for regulating vascular tone and cardiac output, therefore controlling blood flow and blood pressure within the circulation. Also its stimulating effect on the respiratory system causes bronchiolar dilatation, increasing airflow and oxygen intake. The gastro-intestinal system is inhibited by the sympathetic outflow, affecting digestion by reducing or preventing the secretion of digestive enzymes, inhibiting peristaltic action and decreasing splanchnic blood flow by vasoconstriction.

Neuroendocrine system

This system is responsible for maintaining internal homeostasis despite changes in the external environment, the pancreas, thalamus, hypothalamus, kidneys, pituitary, thyroid, parathyroid, pineal, adrenal glands, ovaries and testes work in conjunction with each other to achieve an appropriate biochemical and physiological response to pain. The co-ordinated neuroendocrine stress response produces higher levels of adrenocorticotrophic hormone (ACTH), catecholamines, antidiuretic hormone (ADH), angiotensin and glucagon.

Corticotrophin-releasing hormone (CRH) release is as a consequence of stimulation by noradrenaline. It triggers ACTH biosynthesis and stimulates the sympathetic nervous system. This results in an increase in blood pressure and heart rate. It also produces the behavioural response to stress.

ACTH. Its main function regulates the production of cortisol from the adrenal gland.

Cortisol supports normal cell metabolism, released by the adrenal cortex in response to ACTH. An increased plasma concentration in response to pain controls the adaptive response to stress that, in the short term, is beneficial. However, in the long term it is injurious. It co-ordinates the actions of catecholamines, and maintains blood glucose levels and energy metabolism during periods of stress. It has an adverse effect on the immune system, inhibiting prostaglandin activity and suppressing the inflammatory response.

Adrenaline and noradrenaline are both catecholamines released in response to pain and act directly on blood vessels, causing vasoconstriction and an increase in cardiac output, increasing blood pressure, allowing better perfusion of vital organs. Catecholamines increase metabolism and inhibit the release of insulin, together with an increased glycogenolysis in the liver.

Glucagon rises during the stress response, elevating the metabolic rate, and lowers insulin levels, and together with catecholamines stimulates glycogenolysis and the release of glucose into the circulation for immediate use by critical organs, such as the brain.

Vasopressin or ADH causes sodium and water to be retained by the renal tubules and stored in the extracellular fluid.

Renin and angiotensin II. Renin secretion is increased by sympathetic activity and enables the release of aldosterone from the adrenal gland, promoting sodium re-absorption by the kidney, and is involved in the conversion of enzymes to form angiotensin II, which causes generalised arteriole constriction, resulting in hypertension.

Growth hormone increases cellular activity and metabolism, increasing protein breakdown, which leads to a negative nitrogen balance and poor wound healing.

Interleukin 1 is released from the hypothalamus following tissue damage and its effects are extensive. It initiates the inflammatory effects of the immune system, inducing the release of ACTH, and acts directly on the adrenal cortex, resulting in the release of anti-inflammatory glucocorticoids.

The changes described above have an impact on multiple body systems to support vital organs by increasing cardio-respiratory performance, facilitating the delivery of oxygen and other nutrients.

Adverse effects caused by unrelieved pain

Many of the adverse physiological effects of injury and stress can be abolished or reduced with current analgesic techniques. However, if these are not applied in an appropriate and effective manner, detrimental effects may occur.

Pain (stress) has a detrimental effect on all body systems

Respiratory

Pain causes an impairment of respiratory pump function, reducing vital capacity, tidal volume and functional residual capacity. These together with increased muscle tone in and around the thoracic cage secondary to pain can affect diaphragmatic function. This results in reduced pulmonary compliance, muscle splinting, and the inability to breathe deeply or cough forcefully. The V/Q mismatch is increased (maximal at three days post-op) and causes hypoxaemia, retention of secretions and alveolar collapse. Hypoxaemia can cause cardiac dysfunction, confusion and delayed wound healing.

Cardiovascular

The stress of unrelieved pain acts as a sympathomimetic causing the release of endogenous adrenaline, and other hormones described above. Together with central stimulation of the heart it leads to tachycardia, increased stroke volume and thus increased cardiac work and myocardial oxygen consumption, risking myocardial ischaemia or infarction, especially if hypoxaemia is present.

The fear of pain reduces physical activity causing venous stasis, increased platelet aggregation and reduced fibrinolysis, and raises the risk of deep vein thrombosis.

Gastrointestinal and urinary

Gastroparesis results from increased sympathetic activity together with nociceptive impulses from viscera and somatic structures. It is one of the reasons for ileus, as well as nausea and vomiting following surgery. It may also result in hypomotility of the bladder and urethra leading to an unpleasant patient experience. The release of hormones described above result in the dysregulation of renal function, leading to salt and water retention, hypokalaemia and intracellular fluid overload.

Neuroendocrine and metabolic

Pain causes a reflex increased sympathetic tone and hypothalamic stimulation. This results in the release of catabolic hormones (catecholamines, cortisol, ACTH, ADH and growth hormones, with glucagon, aldosterone, renin, angiotensin II) and the concomitant reduction in anabolic hormones (insulin and testosterone). This catabolic process leads to increased metabolism and oxygen consumption, sodium and water retention, increased blood glucose, free fatty acids, ketone bodies, lactate and, if it continues, a negative nitrogen balance.

Musculoskeletal system

Noxious stimuli can cause reflex muscle spasm at the site of tissue damage. Muscle dysfunction limits thoracic and abdominal movement in an attempt to reduce muscle pain, a phenomenon known as 'splinting'.

Immune system

Unrelieved pain may result in wound infection, pneumonia and, ultimately, sepsis because of suppression of immune function.

Psychological and cognitive effects

Pain is a major cause of anxiety and fear. Individuals who express high anxiety levels tend also to have higher levels of stress-induced hormones that can, if prolonged, interfere with diet, activity and sleep patterns. Pain plus the residual effects of anaesthesia can affect sleep to the point of insomnia, resulting in further anxiety, depression and anger. A consequence of this cognitive dysfunction may be a confrontational relationship with the medical profession.

Nausea and vomiting

Pain causes nausea and vomiting by two mechanisms:

1. Pain stimulates the vomiting centre in the brain.
2. Disturbance of the gastrointestinal tract activates the release of the neurotransmitter 5-hydroxytryptamine (5-HT3), which causes nausea and vomiting via the chemoreceptor trigger zone in the brainstem.

Persistent (chronic) pain

It is possible that poor pain control leads to persistent pain syndromes; appropriate and effective pain management is crucial to prevent this.

Appropriate and effective analgesia create an optimal environment for recovery

Modifying factors on post-operative pain

There are many factors that influence the course of post-operative pain. Pre-operative treatment of painful conditions, optimising therapy and preparing the patient both physiologically and psychologically will help in improving the post-operative experience the patient has. The site, nature and duration of surgery together with the type and extent of the surgical incision plus other components of surgical trauma have a dramatic effect on the pain and analgesic narrative (e.g. cholecystectomy: open compared to laparoscopic). Not only are these surgical aspects and their complications important in the course of post-operative pain but the conduct of anaesthesia before, during and after surgery can have a significant impact on the pain experienced. If we endeavour to minimise these insults plus improve the quality of post-operative care we can have a major influence on the recovery of the patient.

Assessment and measurement

If you cannot measure it, you cannot improve it! (Lord Kelvin)

Pain is modulated by physiological and environmental factors (not forgetting psychosocial and cultural effects) leading to an individual and subjective experience.

Taking a history of the pain (together with a detailed past medical history) is important not only in the process of diagnosis, but in assessing whether any therapy is making an improvement; however, charting the intensity of the pain is but one facet of an evolving story. The question 'Tell me about your pain?' can be structured by using the word PAIN as a mnemonic.

P.

Place and pattern of pain (SOCRATES)

Using the mnemonic SOCRATES is a recursion on the mnemonic PAIN but is helpful in enabling a complete history of the patient's current and past pain symptoms.

Site

- Where does it hurt?

Onset

- When did it start?
- Sudden (seconds to minutes)?
- Gradual (hours to days)?

Character

- Heavy, burning, stabbing, aching?
- Constant, intermittent, related to time of day/activity?
- Like anything else you have felt before?

Radiation

- Does it go anywhere else?

Associated symptoms

- Depends on type of pain/discomfort

Timing

- Exact sequence of events leading to onset of pain
- The time course of the pain after onset

Exacerbating/relieving factors

- Factors that the patients have noted make the pain worse/better
- Exercise, movement, breathing, analgesia, position

Severity

- You should ask patients to quantify their pain, although this is very subjective
- On a scale of 1 to 10, if 10 is the worst pain ever, how would you rate your pain

A.

Aggravating factors

These can be related to position, movement, eating, light, temperature, etc.

Associated symptoms

Can be in the painful area or elsewhere and characterised by numbness, tingling, allodynia (pain from a non-painful stimulus), and hyperalgesia (pain out of proportion to the stimulus).

I.

Intensity

Usually measured on a categorical (none, mild, moderate, severe), numerical or visual analogue scale (1–10) and performed as existing, within the last hour and as the best and worst in the day (use NIPS: Neonatal Infant Pain Scale or FLACC: Face, Legs, Activity, Cry, Consolability scales in children).

Impact

How is the pain affecting your activity, appetite, sleep, mood, relationships and work?

N.

Nature

Characteristic description: aching, throbbing, sharp, dull, burning, shooting, stabbing, deep, pressure – there are many adjectives based on culture, age and educational achievement.

Neutralising factors: what makes it better?

To ensure safe and effective personal pain management requires consistent, correct and documented measurement of the pain intensity experienced, on a suitable scale

Obviously, this detail is not measured on a regular basis and intensity is used as a surrogate for temporal changes resulting from therapy and recovery, and indicates the need for a further detailed assessment. Intensity should be measured using a scale appropriate to the developmental, cognitive and emotional state. Self-reporting should be used wherever possible as pain is a subjective experience. It should be done in a static (at rest) and dynamic (moving, sitting and/or coughing) style and the score documented on the patient's chart. In the young, cognitively impaired and unconscious (e.g. those in critical care units) the observer-reported scores should be documented. These are based on behavioural and physiological observations and we should be mindful of their shortcomings.

Therapy

Pre-emptive

Analgesia prior to surgery may have advantages in reducing post-operative pain and other neuropathic states such as phantom limb pain. Pre-operative pain should be fully controlled before the onset of surgical-induced pain. If it is not, the prior pain state may amplify the post-operative acute pain experienced.

This scenario occurs when the central nervous system has been sensitised by intense or chronic stimulation, e.g. ischaemic leg. The following surgical stimulus may lead to functional changes, often called 'windup' such that the pain following surgery is perceived as more intense than it would have otherwise been.

This will also occur in those about to undergo surgery that will damage nerve fibres. There is evidence that an immunological component to pain may also lead to chronic post-operative pain states, e.g. complex regional pain syndromes type I (sympathetic reflex dystrophy) and type II (causalgia). Effective analgesia prior to the surgical insult will obtund or prevent these developing.

Pre-emptive analgesia may consist of a simple regimen of analgesics or, if required, more complex techniques such as central neuraxial blockade with local analgesics, opioids, or a central α_2 adrenergic agonist (clonidine). It may also be achieved with systemic administration of opioids, a NMDA receptor antagonist (ketamine, methadone or buprenorphine) or clonidine. Current medication for pain may need to be increased prior to surgery, e.g. the anticonvulsants like carbamazepine, gabapentin and pregabalin, which may be taken for diverse conditions from pancreatitis to migraine.

Be cognisant of the possibility of modifying post-operative pain by using pre-emptive techniques of analgesia

Methods

Pain/analgesic ladder (adapted from WHO recommendation)

If pain persists or increases, move up the ladder until under control.

					STEP FOUR
				STEP THREE	+ Interventional techniques e.g. nerve block, epidural, intrathecal drug administration
			STEP TWO	+ Strong opioid	+ Strong opioid
		STEP ONE	+ Weak opioid	+ Weak opioid	+ Weak opioid
Analgesia		Non-opioid +/− Adjuvant	Non-opioid +/− Adjuvant	Non-opioid +/− Adjuvant	Non-opioid +/− Adjuvant
Description of Pain	No pain	Mild pain	Moderate pain	Severe pain	Worst possible pain
Pain Score	0	1–3	4–6	7–9	10

Pain/analgesic ladder (adapted from WHO recommendation)

Tips and tricks

Muscle spasm – Orthopaedic procedures may produce sites of increased tension in muscle groups, leading to intrinsic and reflex muscle spasm. This can be alleviated by either direct muscle relaxants (e.g. dantrolene) or by suppressing the spinal reflex arc (e.g. baclofen). Diazepam is commonly used because of its anxiolytic, spinal GABA and sedative effects; however, care should be exercised because of its synergistic and idiosyncratic activity with opioids.

Magnesium is an NMDA antagonist, thus acting as an analgesic cofactor; it also has a direct effect on opioid receptor affinity.

Patient groups

Paediatric – children present problems of measurement, depending on developmental age. There are many psychosocial and family aspects of pain that make paediatric pain relief a skill that is rarely achieved.

Elderly – Start low, go slow; the elderly present pathological (ageing organs) processes that affect both the pharmacodynamics and pharmacokinetics of drug action. This leads to difficulty in assessing dose, and drugs can produce idiosyncratic effects that are unexpected.

Pain management services

Pain services are an important resource for the surgical team, enabling the education of ward staff and effecting a safety-conscious environment.

There are organisational benefits with enhanced recovery programmes that rely on appropriate and effective analgesia.

Conclusion

Appropriate and effective analgesia preventing any stress caused by pain will have a positive effect on patient outcome.

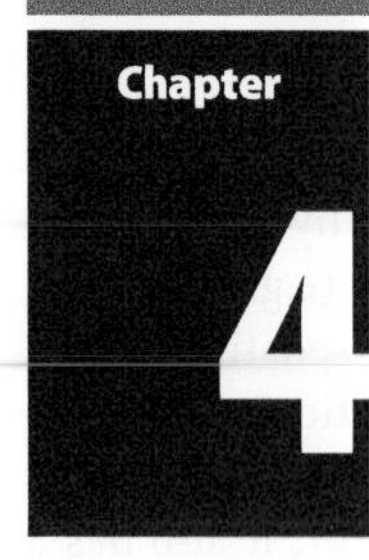

Local anaesthetics

David Tew

In Genesis 2:21, God caused Adam to fall into a deep sleep; and while he was sleeping, he removed one of his ribs and closed up the place with flesh – so it would appear that anaesthesia is the oldest profession (just ahead of thoracic surgery!).

We had to wait from then until 1846 for a publication heralding the arrival of ether, 'Insensibility during surgical operations produced by inhalation' (recently voted as the most influential paper ever published in the 200-year history of the *New England Journal of Medicine*), administered by a dentist (Dr Morton) and written up by a surgeon (Dr H.J. Bigelow).

Early inhalational anaesthesia was both astonishing and flawed (imperfect operating conditions and a high mortality rate) so alternatives to general anaesthesia were continually sought.

Local anaesthesia began when Karl Koller introduced topical cocaine for eye surgery (1884) and a surgeon (August Bier) described cocaine-based spinal anaesthesia in 1898 for ankle surgery in a patient who had endured 'severe reactions' to general anaesthesia. Bier and his assistant Hilldebrandt had developed the technique by performing spinal anaesthesia on each other, testing their blocks with numerous kicks to the shins. Both endured very severe spinal headaches and they celebrated with large cigars! Bier described intravenous regional anaesthesia (IVRA) in 1908.

Local anaesthetic techniques are now an indispensible anaesthetic tool, used as a sole technique or as an analgesic adjunct to general anaesthesia, and they play a crucial role in enhanced recovery programmes for a number of surgical specialties. They offer the best possible analgesia with almost none of the side effects associated with opioids. They are, however, not without risk and patients have either died or been seriously injured as a consequence of these techniques, so a judgement of risk versus benefit is required every time they are employed.

Local anaesthetic drugs are delivered using several different techniques. Local infiltration analgesia (LIA) is usually placed by the surgeon at the time of surgery, peripheral nerve blocks (PNB) are usually performed by anaesthetists and occasionally surgeons; central neuraxial blocks (CNB) such as spinals or epidurals are placed by anaesthetists.

Pharmacology of local anaesthetic drugs and safe dosing

Local anaesthetic drugs exist as a mixture of ionised and non-ionised forms. The balance of each form is dependent on prevailing pH. Local anaesthetics work by blocking sodium

A Surgeon's Guide to Anaesthesia and Peri-operative Care, ed. Jane Sturgess, Justin Davies and Kamen Valchanov. Published by Cambridge University Press.

Table 4.1 Types of local anaesthetics

First-generation drugs (cocaine, procaine, tetracaine)	Ester linkage	High risk of anaphylaxis
Second-generation drugs (lidocaine, prilocaine, ropivacaine, bupivacaine)	Amide linkage	Reduced risk of anaphylaxis

Table 4.2 'Safe maximum dose' of local anaesthetic drug

Bupivacaine	2 mg/kg
Lidocaine	3 mg/kg
Prilocaine	6 mg/kg
Ropivacaine	3–4 mg/kg

channels in nervous tissue but the block occurs on the inside of the cell. It is the unionised (lipophilic) fraction that is able to cross the cell membrane but it is the ionised fraction that exerts the pharmacological activity inside the neuron.

This explains the variations in speed of onset and duration of action of different local anaesthetic drugs. The common structure for all local anaesthetic drugs is an aromatic end and an amine end joined by an intermediate chain.

The duration of action is largely determined by the degree to which a drug is lipophilic. This is governed by the length of the carbon chain on the amine end. The two drugs with the longest chains, and duration of action, are bupivacaine and etidocaine. These highly lipophilic drugs (if given systemically) are the most toxic to the heart and have been responsible for cases of patient death.

Most local anaesthetic drugs are presented as a racemic mixture of the two isomeric forms of the same drug. Ropivacaine and *l*-bupivacaine are however single isomer preparations. Levo-bupivacaine was developed when it became apparent that one isomer was less cardiotoxic than the other. Using a single isomer offers the same anaesthetic action with less cardiotoxicity. This does not mean the drug is safe – about 25% more *l*-bupivacaine is required to produce an equivalent cardiotoxic effect compared to the racemic mixture – so it remains possible to produce catastrophic cardiovascular collapse. Ropivacaine was developed because it appeared less cardiotoxic than bupivacaine, and gained popularity with a reputation for producing more sensory block than motor block.

The 'safe maximum dose' of local anaesthetic drug is designed to minimise the risks associated with systemic toxicity caused by absorption of the drug from the tissues into which it has been correctly injected (Table 4.2). It is not the safe dose to give intravenously. This concept is not without criticism since the absorption rate from different sites is not uniform. The conditions under which an injection is carried out also have an influence.

Complications

Systemic toxicity

If large doses of local anaesthetic drugs are inadvertently administered systemically to an awake subject, clinical deterioration follows a common pattern:

1. The patient will feel different and describe feeling lightheaded or dizzy, associated with tingling usually in the face and especially the lips. They may report feeling very anxious or jittery or have a strong feeling of impending doom – the experience is usually unpleasant.
2. Loss of consciousness or fitting, usually of short duration (minutes rather than hours, and self-limiting) which will almost certainly be accompanied by apnoea.
3. Cardiovascular instability, most commonly in the form of hypotension, but rarely (with the long-acting lipophilic drugs) they will have a cardiac arrest, exhibiting malignant ventricular dysrhythmias. These are notoriously difficult to treat and require resuscitative efforts to continue for up to 90 minutes (the amount of time required for the lipophilic drugs to exit the cardiac myocytes).

The conscious patient should be encouraged to report such feelings as a marker of systemic absorption which would prompt the injection to be stopped.

Intravenous access should be secured prior to injection of local anaesthetic. It has become apparent in the last decade that intravenous lipid given while performing resuscitation is almost always rapidly life-saving in these circumstances. 'Lipid rescue' is so effective that a supply of 10% intralipid should be immediately available in any clinical area where local anaesthetic drugs are administered in doses sufficient to cause this very serious complication. Guidelines for 'Management of Severe Local Anaesthetic Toxicity' are available (www.aagbi.org) and the website www.lipidrescue.org is a forum for continuous evaluation of lipid rescue.

Nerve damage

Nerve damage is sometimes seen following surgery (see also Chapter 30). In cases where regional anaesthesia has been involved it is generally accepted that at most around 50% may be attributable to the regional technique while the remaining 50% will be attributed to other factors.

Temporary nerve dysfunction is not uncommon following any form of local anaesthetic technique and is usually manifest as a numb or dysaesthetic area of skin, which will usually resolve within four to eight weeks after surgery. Motor weakness is less common and will have a more protracted course (up to six months) before recovery.

Permanent nerve damage is rare but very serious and needs to be considered under the headings of peripheral nerve (PNB) or central neuraxial blockade (CNB). Epidural and spinal anaesthesia constitute CNB.

Permanent PNB damage is so rare that it is difficult to get reliable, accurate estimates for any individual block although rates of 1:5,000 to 1:10,000 are widely quoted. Blocks that target (unprotected) nerve roots, e.g. interscalene brachial plexus or lumbar plexus, are thought more likely to cause damage. Studies looking at legal claims for damage characterise the number of patients damaged (numerator) but offer no data in respect of the total number of blocks performed (denominator), so do not permit any calculation of incidence or risk. There have been a number of such studies. The American Closed Claims analysis has reported since 1988, and UK authors have reported on claims made against the NHS litigation authority (NHSLA) between 1995 and 2007.

The following are thought to be a mechanism of injury to nerves:

- needle to nerve contact
- intraneural injection
- ischaemic disruption of the neural blood supply
- chemical toxicity of local anaesthetic drugs.

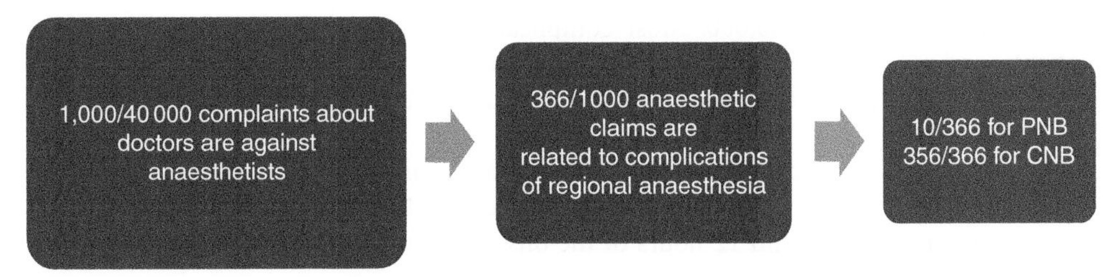

Figure 4.1 Claims to the NHS Litigation Authority (NHSLA) between 1995–2007 relating to regional anaesthesia.

Ultrasound studies have shown that intraneural injections are far more common than previously realised but rarely lead to complications because they involve the connective tissue rather than being injections into the nerve fasicules.

Permanent damage following central neuraxial blockade (CNB)

Central neuraxial blockade (spinals, epidurals and combined spinal and epidural) are very powerful tools for providing safe anaesthesia and analgesia but also carry some of the greatest potential risks. The damage can be to neural tissue or cardiovascular collapse.

In the early 1990s it became apparent that relying on intermittent intramuscular injections of opiates for post-operative pain relief produced poor outcomes for patients, particularly after major surgery. This led to the introduction of acute pain teams, patient-controlled analgesia (PCA), an increase in the uses of PNB, and an explosion in the use of epidural techniques for pain relief following abdominal surgery.

The Australian MASTER study in 2002 randomised 941 surgical patients to receive epidural analgesia or systemic opioids. Findings suggested that epidural provided better analgesia for the first three days, and a reduction in respiratory failure but overall was equal to controls with respect to major peri-operative morbidity. This led to a reduction in epidural use in Australia and beyond.

The UK NHSLA data showed us that one of the most common reasons for an anaesthetist to be sued was for complications related to central neuraxial block (see Figure 4.1).

Two themes for complaint emerged:

1. Inadequate analgesia in fit, young (obstetric), awake patients having brief epidurals (less than 24 hours)
2. Serious nerve damage in sicker, older patients having laparotomies with epidural analgesia extended for up to five days.

In 2009 the UK Anaesthetic community attempted to quantify these risks (National Audit Project 3) by monitoring the complications of all central neuraxial blocks for one year (numerator data) and measuring the total number of neuraxial blocks in a two-week period to estimate the total number of blocks given over that year (denominator data). There were 52 complications in 707, 000 CNB. It is worth noting that fully two-thirds of cases where damage was initially judged to be severe subsequently recovered over the following six months.

The authors of the subsequently published paper assessed complications as definitely, very likely, possibly or unlikely to have been caused by CNB. The estimates of risk were calculated as pessimistic (definitely caused by CNB) and optimistic (unlikely to be caused by CNB). The risk of permanent injury was 2.0 per 100,000, and catastrophic injury (death or paraplegia) was 0.7 per 100,000. Most complications occured in surgical peri-operative patients, and risk was lower with spinal than epidural CNB (see Chapter 4).

If a patient has post operative nerve damage it may not be caused by any CNB the patient has received.

Early recognition and treatment of epidural haematoma or infection can significantly improve the prognosis for recovery of nerve function. The best prognosis occurs when decompression occurs within 12 hours of the onset of symptoms.

The most useful red flags are:

- Severe increasing back pain
- Loss of motor power or dense sensory block

Both symptoms should be looked for, and anaesthetic/pain team opinion sought as soon as possible. Epidural techniques are now focused on patients most likely to benefit from them – related to the nature of their surgery (e.g. upper abdominal incisions/thoracic incisions).

Nerve location techniques

Central neuraxial blockade

Central neuraxial blockade is one of the most powerful techniques and is performed as either a spinal or epidural injection. These techniques can be used as a sole technique, as a combined technique (CSE) or with a general anaesthetic.

Table 4.3 The incidence of complications from peri-operative central neuraxial blockade (CNB)

Regional technique	Complication	'Optimistic Risk' (per 100,000)
Spinal	Permanent nerve damage	1.6
	Death or paraplegia	1.1
Epidural	Permanent nerve damage	8.2
	Death or paraplegia	1.0

N.B. Note the much higher risk of permanent nerve damage with epidural CNB in this population.

Table 4.4 The different techniques available to locate peripheral nerves, and their uses

Technique	Operator	Uses
Direct vision	Surgeon at time of operation	Wound infiltration catheters High-volume local infiltration analgesia (with/without elastomeric pump)
Paraesthesia	Emergency department physicians	Femoral nerve block (largely historical in anaesthesia)
Peripheral nerve stimulators	Anaesthetist	Peripheral nerve blocks (largely superseded by or in conjunction with ultrasound)
Ultrasound	Anaesthetist	Peripheral nerve blockade and central neuraxial blockade Pain blocks Thought to be safer but no evidence to support this

Table 4.5 Comparison of spinal and epidural blockade

	Spinal	Epidural
Technique	Subarachnoid injection into the CSF	Injection into the space between the ligamentum flavum and the meninges
Surgery	Any below umbilicus, but time limited	Any below umbilicus, top up of local anaesthesia permits extended use
Speed of onset	Rapid 3–5 min	Slower up to 30 min, but some techniques allow faster onset for emergency surgery
Duration of action – anaesthesia	Limited to 2–3 hours, unless a spinal catheter is inserted. This is uncommon	Can be extended up to 5 days
Duration of action – analgesia	2–3 hours if local anaesthetic only used, analgesia can be extended by injection of adjuncts, e.g. opioids, ketamine, clonidine	Usually advised to remove after 3 days, but can be used for 5 days Low-dose local anaesthetic with low-dose opioid allows best analgesia while maintaining minimal motor block
Selectivity	Use of hyperbaric solutions can 'fix' the local anaesthetic more quickly and limit spread of block. Positioning the patient can permit a more unilateral block	Using high-volume local anaesthetic can allow caudad spread
Type of block	Profound motor/sensory block	Can be more selective to sensory rather than motor block
Insertion point	Safe to insert below L2 (below the terminal end of the spinal cord)	Can be used throughout the entire spinal column. Cervical epidurals are performed for chronic pain patients
Complications (for nerve damage and death see Table 4.3)	Intra-operative hypotension Respiratory depression if opioids are used	Post-operative hypotension Unilateral or inadequate block
	Post-dural puncture headache, unable to perform block, urinary retention, itch if opioids used	
Relative contra-indications	Severe aortic stenosis or patients with cardiac disease dependent on a fixed peripheral vascular resistance, systemic sepsis, sepsis at the site of injection, anticoagulation/anti-platelet therapy, coagulopathy, thrombocytopaenia, previous spinal injury/surgery, raised intracranial pressure, current central nervous system disease	
Pre-requisites	Patient consent, if used without general anaesthesia the patient must be able to lie still for the duration of the procedure (some COPD/cardiac patients will be unable to lie flat for any period of time, some elderly patients will become confused and disoriented)	

It is commonly assumed, incorrectly, that central neuraxial blockade is always safer than general anaesthesia. In a 1988 report, 13 out of 14 patients had a catastrophic outcome (death or severe neurological damage) following spinal-related cardiac arrest. This has improved. Currently around one in four patients suffering a spinal-related peri-operative cardiac arrest is likely to suffer a poor outcome.

Anticoagulation deserves special mention. When a patient has deranged clotting for any reason the risk of epidural haematoma increases. There have been particular issues around the timing of prophylactic doses of low molecular weight heparins (LMWH) and spinal or epidural manipulation. Current advice is that no CNB needle should be advanced unless 10–12 hours have elapsed since the last dose of LMWH. Many units prescribe LMWH at 18.00 h to allow regular administration (protecting the patient from developing a DVT) while permitting safe CNB on the following day's theatre list. Once a CNB has been performed then at least two hours should elapse until LMWH are administered. These rules apply to the removal of spinal/epidural catheters as well.

Complications you may be called about:

1. Block failure – if possible discuss with an anaesthetist and be prepared to start a different analgesic plan.
2. Post-dural puncture headaches – worse when a patient is upright and improves if they lie flat, owing to low CSF pressure. They are usually self-limiting with good analgesia and intravenous hydration. Occasionally it will be necessary to use an epidural blood patch. The patient should be informed of all options. It is worth getting an anaesthetist involved in discussions with the patient from the start.
3. Hypotension – most central neuraxial block induces a sympathetic block (one or two dermatomal levels higher than the measured sensory level), which can lead to peripheral vasodilatation.
4. Generalised itch will sometimes require treatment with chlorpheniramine. It is usually self-limiting.
5. Urinary retention.
6. Loss of lower limb motor power following thoracic epidurals would not normally be expected. This requires emergency assessment to exclude the possibility of epidural haematoma.

Peripheral nerve blocks

Upper limb blocks

Interscalene block

- Can be used for anaesthesia or post-operative analgesia
- Most often used for orthopaedic, plastic and vascular surgery around the shoulder
- Needle inserted at the interscalene groove
- Often causes temporary ipsilateral diaphragmatic paresis (not suitable for bilateral blocks, and needs careful consideration in the patient with severe limiting respiratory disease)
- Commonly causes a Horner's syndrome, with ipsilateral ptosis and miosis
- Temporary nerve dysfunction in up to 15% of patients, but permanent damage is rare
- Most frequently performed with ultrasound guidance in the awake patient
- Serious complications include injection of local anaesthetic into CSF, damage to vertebral artery, intravascular injection of local anaesthetic, pneumothorax.

Supraclavicular block

- Can be used for anaesthesia or post-operative analgesia
- Most often used for orthopaedic, plastic and vascular surgery
- Needle inserted behind the subclavian artery just above the first rib
- Most frequently performed with ultrasound guidance in the awake patient, allowing the operator to block C8 and T1 elements that were often missed previously
- Useful for surgery to the elbow, forearm and hand
- Block dense enough to allow the awake patient to tolerate the use of a tourniquet
- Ipsilateral diaphragmatic paresis in up to 40% of patients
- Serious complications include damage to vertebral artery, intravascular injection of local anaesthetic, pneumothorax.

Both techniques allow catheters to be sited next to the plexus, and a continuous infusion of local anaesthetic. Catheter tip migration away from the nerve can occur. This leads to failure of analgesia. Tunnelling the catheter helps to prevent this and also reduces the infection risk.

Other upper limb blocks

Infra-clavicular blocking is technically challenging owing to the depth of the nerves around the axillary artery but the risk of diaphragmatic paresis is reduced and it offers a lower chance of catheter migration if one is being used.

The axillary brachial plexus block (performed in the axilla around the axillary artery) blocks four peripheral nerves (musculocutaneous, radial, median and ulnar nerves). It is a good alternative in patients not suited for supraclavicular block. The risks of pneumothorax and diaphragmatic paresis are less. The patient is unlikely to tolerate an upper limb tourniquet and will require a supplemental block.

All the major nerves of the arm (radial, median and ulnar) can be blocked individually at a variety of locations in the upper and lower arm, either as rescue blocks for failed plexus analgesia or as discrete blocks combined with general anaesthesia.

Lower limb blocks

The lower limb differs from the upper limb principally because it has two plexi supplying predominantly the ventral (lumbar plexus) and dorsal (sacral plexus) aspects of the limb. This makes it more difficult to block the lower limb for awake surgery using peripheral nerve blockade as two injections will be needed. For awake surgery on the lower limb – spinal anaesthesia is usually the first-choice technique.

Lumbar plexus blockade

- Useful for any surgery involving the femur
- Targets the L2, L3 and L4 nerve roots as they form the femoral, lateral cutaneous nerve of leg and obturator nerve within the body of psoas muscle
- Commonly performed using a peripheral nerve stimulator (although increasingly some operators use ultrasound to guide some aspects of the block)
- Reputation for increased risks of complications, particularly when using landmarks technique and high volumes of local anaesthetic. Using a nerve stimulator and

smaller volume injections of local anaesthetic (or the use of catheter techniques) may mitigate these risks.

Femoral nerve blocks

- Useful for surgery involving the femur
- Needle inserted in the groin
- Commonly performed with ultrasound guidance
- Were most frequently used for major knee surgery but are becoming used less frequently with the introduction of enhanced recovery programmes that have a focus on early mobilisation
- Modified low-dose femoral nerve blocks are used in some centres.

Sciatic blocks

- Can be performed at any level from the buttock to the popliteal fossa
- Their use in major knee surgery is increasingly contentious
- Useful in major foot and ankle surgery, particularly of the hindfoot
- Foot drop for the duration of the block, which can impede mobilisation following midfoot and forefoot surgery
- Useful for patients undergoing below-knee amputation to provide prolonged analgesia in combination with spinal or general anaesthesia
- For above-knee amputation it is common practice for the surgeons to place a catheter alongside the cut sciatic nerve to allow infusion of local anaesthetic in the post-operative period.

Ankle blocks

- Used for foot surgery, although it is now common for surgeons to infiltrate as they operate
- An ultrasound-guided posterior tibial nerve block will cover the majority of structures within the foot (except the skin) without producing foot drop
- It is technically possible to use ultrasound to display and block all the other nerves supplying the foot – saphenous, superficial and deep peroneal and sural.

Prolonging the block

1. Use a long-acting drug (experimentally, liposomal-encased drugs offer the prospect of blocks lasting for days).
2. Infuse the drug continuously using a catheter.

Truncal blocks

Intercostal blocks

- Used to block the T6 to T11 dermatomes
- Provide wound analgesia, but are less reliable for deep pain (autonomic innervation)

- Useful for open cholecystectomy, thoracotamy. Mid-line wounds require bilateral blocks
- Needle inserted at the lower margin of selected ribs in the mid-axillary line and injecting
- 3–4 ml of local anaesthetic is injected close to the neurovascular bundle;
- Complications include pneumothorax, damage to the neurovascular bundle and rapid uptake of local anaesthetic into the systemic circulation.

Transversus abdominus plane blocks (TAP blocks)

- Analgesia for lower abdominal wounds, at or below the T10 dermatomal level;
- Large-volume local anaesthetic is placed between the transversus abdominus and internal oblique muscles using ultrasound guidance;
- Can be performed bilaterally;
- Most commonly used for lower abdominal surgery in enhanced recovery programmes or where CNB is contra-indicated.

Intravenous regional anaesthesia (IVRA or Bier's block)

- Technique for blocking the extremities often used outside of the theatre environment;
- Requires distal intravenous access in the operative limb and intravenous access in the non-operative limb;
- A meticulous technique to avoid systemic migration of local anaesthetic drug is required;
- Produces a rapid-onset, dense block of up to one hour duration;
- Prilocaine is considered the drug of choice;
- Complications include systemic migration of local anaesthetic and methaemoglobinaemia. Bupivacaine is contra-indicated.

Summary

Local anaesthetic techniques can be used to provide anaesthesia (awake surgery) and very effective peri-operative analgesia with little or no systemic side effects in suitable patients. Opiate-sparing analgesic techniques feature prominently in enhanced recovery programmes.

An understanding of the pharmacology, use and complications of local anaesthetics will help the surgeon to be safe and confident in their practice.

Further reading

Albright GA. Cardiac arrest following regional anesthesia with etidocaine or bupivacaine *Anesthesiology* 1979; **51**: 285–7.

Bigeleisen PE. Nerve puncture and apparent intraneural injection during ultrasound-guided axillary block does not invariably result in neurologic injury. *Anesthesiology* 2006; **105**: 779–83

Bigelow HJ. Insensibility during surgical operations produced by inhalation. *The Boston Medical and Surgical Journal* 1846; **XXXV** (160): 309–17.

Borgeat A. Acute and nonacute complications associated with interscalene block and shoulder surgery: prospective study: a prospective study. *Anesthesiology* 2001: **95**; 875–80.

Caplan RA. Unexpected cardiac arrest during spinal anesthesia: A closed claims analysis of predisposing factors. *Anesthesiology* 1988; **68**: 5–11.

Covino BG. Systemic toxicity of local anaesthetic agents. *Anesth Analg* 1978; **57** (4): 387–8.

Horloker TT. Regional anesthesia in the patient receiving antithrombotic or thrombolytic therapy. *Reg Anesth Pain Med* 2010; **35**(1): 64–101.

Major complications of central neuraxial blocks. The 3rd National Audit Project of the Royal College of Anaesthetists' Lead Investigator Dr T Cook. Also published in the *Brit J Anaesth* 2009; **102**: 179–90.

Rigg JRA. Epidural anaesthesia and analgesia and outcome of major surgery: a randomised trial. *Lancet* 2002; **359**: 1276–82.

Rosenblatt MA. Successful use of a 20% lipid emulsion to resuscitate a patient after a presumed bupivacaine-related cardiac arrest. *Anesthesiology* 2006; **105**: 217–18.

Weinberg G. Lipid emulsion infusion rescues dogs from bupivacaine-induced cardiac toxicity. *Reg Anesth Pain Med* 2003; **28**(3): 198–202.

Wulf HFW. The centennial of spinal anesthesia. *Anesthesiology* 1998; **89**(2): 500–6.

Basic sciences

Sedation

Justin Davies and Jane Sturgess

Definition

Sedation is the term used to describe a continuum of a drug-induced state from normal alert consciousness to complete unresponsiveness. Surgeons may be exposed to sedated patients in the operating theatre, on the ward, in the emergency department and in the endoscopy suite (where procedures include upper and lower GI tract endoscopy, bronchoscopy and cystoscopy). In addition, there may not be an anaesthetist present when a patient under the care of a surgical team is sedated. Therefore, an understanding of this topic is essential to minimise risk and maintain patient safety.

Levels of sedation have been defined by the American Society of Anesthesiologists (ASA), and are often referred to as levels 1 to 4:

1. **Minimal sedation (or anxiolysis).** This is a drug-induced state during which patients respond normally to verbal commands. Cognitive function and co-ordination may be impaired, but cardiovascular and respiratory function will be unaffected.
2. **Moderate sedation/analgesia (or 'conscious sedation').** This is a drug-induced state that results in reduced consciousness. Patients will respond to verbal commands and no interventions are required to maintain a patent airway. Cardiovascular function is usually maintained.
3. **Deep sedation/analgesia.** This is a drug-induced depression of consciousness during which time patients cannot be easily roused but do respond purposefully following repeated or painful stimulation. There may be impairment of independent ability to maintain ventilation and patients may need assistance in maintenance of a patent airway with spontaneous ventilation being potentially inadequate. Cardiovascular function is maintained.
4. **General Anaesthesia.** This is a drug-induced loss of consciousness. Patients are not rousable, even with painful stimulation. Patients will generally require assistance maintaining patent airway and positive-pressure ventilation may be required. Cardiovascular function may be impaired. General anaesthesia also requires amnesia, unlike the previous three levels where it is optional. Additionally general anaesthesia concerns itself with analgesia too.

Which drugs are used?

This decision is affected by factors relating to the procedure, and factors relating to the patient.

A Surgeon's Guide to Anaesthesia and Peri-operative Care, ed. Jane Sturgess, Justin Davies and Kamen Valchanov. Published by Cambridge University Press.

The main procedural factors are the duration of the procedure, the level of sedation required, the amount of assistance available, the location sedation is being administered in, and the level of training in sedation that the responsible person has received.

Patient factors need to include the degree of anxiolysis and analgesia required, the drug history (looking specifically for drug interactions or potential tolerance to sedative agents) and the co-morbidity and age of the patient.

Sedation can be achieved with inhalational agents, oral agents or intravenous agents.

In general, level 1 may be achieved with Entonox® (50% nitrous oxide and 50% oxygen) alone, level 2 with opioids (such as fentanyl or pethidine) and benzodiazepines (such as midazolam or diazepam) and level 3 may require ketamine or propofol. See Section III, Chapter 27 'Common Drugs and Doses' for further details of these drugs. Levels 3 and 4 will not be discussed in detail as they lie outside the remit of this chapter.

Safety first

There are many working groups that issue guidance on conscious sedation. Most agree that, for intravenous sedation, a titrated dose (repeated small incremental doses) of a single agent is the safest and most reliable method to choose. Again, published guidance suggests the use of midazolam as the agent of choice. It is fast onset, reasonably fast offset and maintains cardiovascular stability when given in low doses (less than 10 mg). A safe rule of thumb is to administer no more than 1 mg/minute.

Many healthcare providers are choosing to use dual-agent sedation (most frequently an opioid and a benzodiazepine). This has the advantage that very small doses of each agent can be given as they act synergistically to provide safe sedation. Opioids provide analgesia and sedation, but also cause dose-dependent respiratory depression. Some patients can be very sensitive to benzodiazepines or opioids, as a part of their pharmacogenetics, and hence smaller doses are required. Using more than one drug to provide sedation has the disadvantage that should the patient become over-sedated it is difficult to diagnose whether the opiate or the benzodiazepine is responsible.

Drug antagonists/reversal agents

Flumazenil is used to reverse the effects of benzodiazepines. There are reported cases of status epilepticus being induced in patients given flumazenil who were either epileptic or chronic users of benzodiazepines.

Naloxone is used to reverse opiates and has a short half-life (30 to 80 minutes), whereas opiates have longer terminal half-lives (fentanyl 3.5 h, pethidine 4 h, morphine 3 h). Patients recover from the sedative effects of low-dose opiates as the drug is redistributed within the body, lowering the plasma concentration. Fast recovery is not owing to drug metabolism. In high doses some drug metabolism is required to permit recovery. When naloxone is given for opiate overdose it should be remembered that the antagonism may wear off before the opiate has been metabolised. This is pertinent in the outpatient setting. If naloxone is given the patient must have an extended period of observation for re-sedation.

Special patient groups

The elderly present a number of pharmacological problems that can result in over-sedation. They usually require a reduced dose.

1. Polypharmacy with likely drug interactions.
2. Reduced circulating volume. This means a given dose reaches a higher intravascular concentration than it would in a young fit healthy person.
3. Increased circulation time. This means it takes longer for the drug to produce its effect. Patience is required when sedating the elderly.
4. Reduced liver mass and altered metabolism. The drug will be present for a longer period of time.
5. Undiagnosed confusion/dementia. This may be worsened with sedation, leading to an inexperienced practitioner over-sedating the patient to continue with the procedure.

The pregnant patient has altered physiology, dependent on the trimester. She also presents as two individuals.

1. In the first trimester teratogenic drugs must be avoided. There are reported cases of benzodiazepines causing teratogenicity. Fentanyl and pethidine appear to be safe.
2. In the second and third trimester the patient will need to have the gravid uterus displaced from her major abdominal vessels when lying supine. This is most easily done with a wedge under the left hip or a 15 degree left tilt on an operating table. Failure to do this can result in cardiovascular collapse and cardiac arrest.
3. In all trimesters the pregnant patient will have altered circulating volume and haemodynamic status. Cautious titration of sedative drugs is required.
4. In the third trimester patients are at risk of aspiration.

Children

1. NICE have issued specific guidance on sedation in children and young people for diagnostic and therapeutic procedures (Guidance CG112).
2. For children having moderate sedation there is a requirement for at least one member of staff to have intermediate life support training.
3. For children having deep sedation there is a requirement for at least one member of staff to have advanced life support training.
4. Midazolam and fentanyl are considered safe to use for moderate sedation for endoscopy and painful procedures.
5. It is sensible to discuss complicated cases with a paediatric anaesthetist.

Monitoring

Surgeons will regularly be exposed to patients requiring minimal (level 1) and moderate (level 2) sedation. Pulse oximetry should always be used for level 1 sedation, but no other particular monitoring is required. However, level 2 sedation requires a much greater degree of training, monitoring and equipment.

Requirements for safe level 2 sedation

- Medical and nursing staff trained in the principles and practice of sedation and a minimum of basic life support
- ASA grade recording
- Appropriate fasting (which will vary according to local guidelines)
- Informed consent
- Selection of the appropriate drug(s) at the appropriate and safe dose
- Dedicated intravenous access

- Availability of suction
- Patient monitoring, including pulse oximetry, heart rate, ECG trace, non-invasive BP recording and capnography (if available)
- A dedicated trained member of staff to observe the sedated patient and highlight any concerns to the 'operator'
- Oxygen delivery (2l via a nasal cannula is often adequate)
- Availability of reversal agents (for example, flumazenil for bendodiazepines, naloxone for opioids)
- Availability of resuscitation facilities
- Availability of facilities and appropriately trained staff to monitor the patient following sedation, until the vital signs and conscious level have returned to pre-procedure levels

If the procedure or patient requires a very deep level of sedation, or sedation plus analgesia, it may be prudent to abandon and consider requesting general anaesthesia.

Complications: may include central nervous system depression with loss of consciousness, respiratory depression, airway obstruction, hypoxia, tracheal aspiration, allergic reaction, hypotension, tachycardia, angina/myocardial infarction, cardiac arrest and death.

Audit: It is essential that all clinicians performing sedation carry out regular audit of their work within a clinical governance framework.

Further reading

Continuum of depth of sedation: definition of general anaesthesia and levels of sedation/analgesia. USA: American Society of Anesthesiologists, 2009.

Practice guidelines for sedation and analgesia by non-anesthesiologists. *Anesthesiology* 2002; **96**: 1004–17.

Guidelines on Safety and Sedation for Endoscopic Procedures. London: British Society of Gastroenterology, 2003.

Guidelines for Provision of Services for Anaesthesia in the Non-theatre Environment. London: Royal College of Anaesthetists, 2011.

http://publications.nice.org.uk/sedation-in-children-and-young-people-cg112/guidance.

Safe Sedation of Adults in the Emergency Department. *Report and Recommendations by The Royal College of Anaesthetists and The College of Emergency Medicine Working Party on Sedation, Anaesthesia and Airway Management in the Emergency Department, 2012*; London. https://www.rcoa.ac.uk/system/files/CSQ-SEDATION-ED2012.pdf.

Physics and measurement

Ari Ercole

Heat and temperature

Temperature control is clinically important. Peri-operative hypothermia, in particular, carries a significant morbidity and surgical patients are at particular risk from operative heat loss combined with impaired heat conservation caused by anaesthesia. Furthermore, effective re-warming of patients that have been allowed to become cold can be very difficult. Careful pre-operative and intra-operative management can avoid this if the mechanisms of heat loss and redistribution within the body are appreciated.

Measuring heat and temperature

Heat is a form of energy. It arises from the random jostling motion of the particles that make up the matter from which everything is made. The amount of thermal movement is measured by the concept of temperature; objects with little thermal energy having a low temperature. The Celsius/centigrade scale is commonly used in clinical practice and is defined in terms of the freezing (0°C) and boiling (100°C) points of water at standard atmospheric pressure. The SI unit of temperature, however, is the kelvin where 0 K is defined as the temperature at which thermal disorder ceases (absolute zero). A change in temperature of 1°C and 1 K are defined to be the same magnitude so that absolute zero turns out to be equal to -273.15°C.

There are numerous ways of measuring temperature but in current clinical practice the following methods are most commonly exploited.

- *Mercury thermometers* rely on the thermal expansion of this liquid metal in a glass capillary but are no longer popular owing to potential toxicity if broken.
- *Thermistors* are components whose electrical resistance changes with temperature. They are typically made from semiconductor materials. These devices are cheap, compact and reliable and have a wide range of medical applications in disposable temperature sensors, for example nasopharyngeal probes, skin surface probes and in thermodilution cardiac output measuring equipment such as the pulmonary artery catheter.
- *Thermocouples* consist of a combination of two dissimilar metals in electrical contact, which generates a voltage in response to heating (this is known as the Seebeck effect). These can be physically small, rugged and cheap but require a second junction at a fixed temperature as a reference. The voltages generated are small and require amplification.

A Surgeon's Guide to Anaesthesia and Peri-operative Care, ed. Jane Sturgess, Justin Davies and Kamen Valchanov. Published by Cambridge University Press.

- *Thermopiles* are constructed from arrays of miniaturised thermocouples in series and are used to detect the heating effect of far infrared radiation emitted from warm surfaces. Thermopiles are used in applications such as tympanic membrane thermometers. These have the advantage of measuring core temperatures minimally invasively (non-contact) but require an unobstructed optical path (i.e. unreliable in the presence of significant ear wax or if not properly inserted).

Heat as energy

Body temperature disturbances are a direct result of changes in the amount of heat energy in the tissues. The total energy is a balance between heat production by metabolism and heat loss. The distribution of heat energy within the body is carefully regulated. However, both general and regional anaesthesia may disturb thermoregulation and heat loss may be increased because of open body cavities, irrigation, etc.

The human body may be considered as having two thermal compartments: the core and the periphery. Although the core is usually well perfused and has a uniform well-regulated temperature, anaesthesia leads to vasodilation, which very quickly redistributes core heat through mixing with the peripheral volume. If the patient is peripherally cold pre-operatively, this redistribution may lead to a rapid drop in core temperature after induction of anaesthesia.

Subsequently, heat energy may be lost from the patient to their surroundings by a number of processes: conduction, convection, evaporation and radiation. Once the patient becomes hypothermic, the normal thermogenesis caused by shivering cannot occur in the presence of intra-operative neuromuscular blockade. Worse still, the large heat capacity of the mixed core and peripheral compartments means that once a patient has been allowed to become cold, re-warming is very difficult and therefore care should be taken to avoid this situation.

Radiation may account for around 60% of intra-operative heat loss. Infrared radiation is emitted by any warm object in proportion to the fourth power of its temperature. Since objects may also absorb infrared radiation from the environment, radiative loss can be minimised by maintaining a warm theatre environment.

Thermal *conduction* occurs when two materials of different temperatures, such as a patient and warming device, are placed in direct contact causing heat to diffuse from hot to cold. The amount of energy (in joules) required to increase the temperature of an object is a property of the material and is known as the heat capacity (or specific heat capacity if measured per kilogram of material). Water has a much higher specific heat capacity than air, for example. This is one reason that forced hot air heating (e.g. Bair Hugger® or Warm Touch® systems) in theatres is slow to warm a patient since the air carries little thermal energy, whereas the body requires a lot of energy to increase its temperature. Conversely, cold irrigation fluid is effective at causing patient cooling since it has a relatively high heat capacity. Similarly, under-patient warming mattresses can carry a large amount of heat energy; however, their effectiveness is diminished by any insulating material between them and the patient such as sheets and canvases.

Not all materials conduct heat to the same extent. Wrapping or covering patients prevents heat loss since trapped air is a good thermal insulator. It also prevents heat loss by *convection* where air that has been warmed around the patient rises causing this heat to be lost.

As heat is transferred to a material it heats up by an amount governed by its heat capacity, as described above. However, additional energy is required to convert a solid to a liquid (latent heat of melting) or from a liquid to a gas (latent heat of vaporisation). This energy can be considerable and has important clinical implications. For example, *evaporation* of sweat or water from a patient causes a considerable cooling effect, as heat is lost from the body in converting the liquid to a gas. As an example of the reverse process, steam at 100°C has a higher specific energy content than liquid water at the same temperature. Although evaporative losses are usually small, unless the patient is sweating, they may be significant from large surgical incisions. Large heat losses may also occur from the evaporation of surgical antiseptic solutions, particularly those that are alcohol-based. Respiratory evaporative heat loss may also occur; however, modern anaesthetic circuits incorporate heat and moisture exchange filters that minimise this.

Properties of gases and liquids

Gases and liquids are *fluids*. They share the property that they can deform. This has two important implications. Firstly, if subjected to a pressure difference, fluids will flow. The amount of flow depends on the pressure difference and the amount of friction. This has important consequences in haemodynamics and resuscitation. Secondly, they can be made to fill a space and transmit *pressure* to their surroundings. This has important clinical implications. For example, in a pneumoperitoneum, the gas pressure is transmitted to all intra-peritoneal structures with implications for perfusion (owing to pressure on vasculature) and ventilation (pressure on the diaphragm). Understanding pressure has important safety implications too, since the storage and use of gases at potentially dangerously high pressures is common in clinical practice.

Properties of gases

Where does pressure come from? Thermal energy means that all particles of matter are constantly moving. The constituent particles of a gas do not interact to any great extent and may be thought of as being constantly in collision with any container in which they are constrained. Every time such a collision takes place, tiny forces are exchanged so that the container constrains the gas and, simultaneously, the gas exerts a force on the container. The total force on the container depends on the number of collisions per unit time. This in turn depends on the number of gas particles per unit volume (the density of the gas) and the speed at which they are moving on average, which is determined by the temperature. This force per unit area pushing on the container wall is called the *pressure*.

The SI unit of pressure is the pascal (1 newton force/square metre of area) although the kilopascal (kPa) is more useful in clinical practice. The weight of the air above the earth causes a pressure around us to which we are all exposed known as atmospheric pressure. Atmospheric pressure reduces with height but standard atmospheric pressure at sea level is approximately 101 kPa. Pressure can also be expressed in terms of the height of a column of fluid that it can support which leads to two other common units: the millimetre of mercury ($1\ \text{kPa} \approx 7.50\ \text{mmHg}$) and centimetre of water ($1\text{kPa} \approx 10.2\ \text{cmH}_2\text{O}$).

The pressure, volume and temperature of a gas are all related. For a given number (n) of moles of an ideal gas (one in which the particles do not interact with each other) there are relationships between pressure (P), volume (V) and temperature (T, measured in kelvin)

$$PV = nRT$$

where R is the universal gas constant (8.31 J $K^{-1}mol^{-1}$). From this law, we can reach several important conclusions. If we hold everything else constant then:

1. Pressure increases as the volume of a gas is compressed (Boyle's Law).
2. Pressure increases with increasing temperature (Gay–Lussac's Law).
3. The volume of a gas expands as temperature increases (Charles' Law).
4. Pressure increases as more gas molecules are introduced into a fixed volume.

In reality, gas particles do interact slightly but the above relationships are a good approximation for many gases. However, at low temperatures the thermal motion energy becomes less significant and eventually even previously insignificant intermolecular interactions may come to dominate and the gas will liquefy. The temperature at which this happens is called the boiling point of the substance. The boiling point itself depends on pressure; at high pressures the gas particles are forced closer together so the boiling point increases because the liquid state is stable at higher temperatures.

Conversely, there is a critical temperature below which liquefaction can be brought about by forcing the gas particles together through pressure alone. Gases such as oxygen, nitrogen, air and argon have a critical temperature much below room temperature so cannot be liquefied simply by pressurisation. This has important practical implications. Typically, medical gases such as these are stored at room temperature as highly pressurised gas in cylinders. However, gases such as carbon dioxide or nitrous oxide have a critical temperature above room temperature and therefore will liquefy once pressurised. The pressure at which liquefaction occurs at the critical temperature is called the critical pressure but will be less at lower temperatures. Such gases are in fact stored in cylinders as liquids. As gas is withdrawn from the cylinder, liquid evaporates maintaining the pressure at the critical pressure until no liquid remains. Furthermore, this critical pressure is itself a function of temperature. For these reasons, cylinder pressure cannot be used to measure how full such a cylinder is; it must instead be weighed. Furthermore, if such cylinders are heated to above the critical temperature of their contents, the liquid must become a gas and this could lead to a large increase in pressure, although some room for expansion is deliberately allowed when the cylinders are filled.

A further consequence of gas particle interactions is that sudden expansion of a gas leads to cooling as heat is used to break intermolecular attractive forces. This effect can be considerable and is used practically to cool some cryosurgical instruments. The same effect can lead to cooling of carbon dioxide cylinders for laparoscopic procedures or nitrous oxide cylinders and pipework during use with the potential to cause frostbite.

Conversely, sudden pressurisation of a gas may lead to the generation of high temperatures. Opening of oxygen cylinder valves quickly leads to rapid pressurisation of the gas within the pressure regulator and the potential generation of large amounts of heat. When combined with the combustion supporting properties of oxygen, this has resulted in fires and explosions.

Partial pressure

Consider a mixture of several ideal gases. Since they do not interact, the collisions of each of the constituent parts with the container may be thought of as being an independent contribution to the total pressure within the container. Thus, if the total pressure that we measure as a result of all the collisions is P_{tot} then this may be thought of as the sum of partial pressures (by convention denoted by lower case p) from each constituent.

$$P_{tot} = p_1 + p_2 + p_3 \ \ldots \ \text{(Dalton's Law)}$$

Air, for example, contains 21% oxygen by volume. It stands to reason that we would therefore expect the same fraction of the collisions with the container walls to be caused by oxygen molecules. This means that the partial pressure of oxygen is 21% of the total pressure.

Therefore, at one atmosphere barometric pressure (101 kPa), the partial pressure of oxygen is 21% × 101 = 21 kPa. As an example, air at the summit of Mount Everest, although still 21% oxygen, has a barometric pressure now of 30 kPa so the partial pressure of oxygen would now only be 21% × 30 = 6.3 kPa.

Partial pressure is an important concept since it is differences in partial pressures of gases that determine diffusion, as we shall see when we consider gas solubility.

Fluid flow

Laminar flow and viscosity

In contrast to solids, fluids (gases or liquids) deform readily when subjected to forces. As a result, fluids can flow when subjected to pressure. Understanding the factors affecting fluid flow is important in understanding perfusion and ventilation.

Figure 6.1 (upper panel) depicts fluid flow in a tube with circular cross section. In this example, the fluid is moving uniformly with the streamlines being parallel. Such flow is said to be *laminar*. However, the velocity is not the same everywhere. Fluid at the edge travels more slowly because of the influence of the tube wall. This velocity gradient means that fluid near the centre must slip past fluid moving more slowly towards the edge. This leads to friction forces that tend to resist flow. The amount of friction depends on the velocity gradient (which depends on the tube) and the viscosity of the fluid.

As a result of viscosity, the flow rate Q (volume per unit time) along a tube of length L with circular cross-section of radius r depends on the pressure difference ΔP, determined by the Hagen-Poisseuille relation, which can be written as:

$$Q = \frac{\pi r^4}{8\,\mu L}\Delta P$$

where μ is the viscosity. We see that for a given pressure difference, flow *decreases linearly with length* of tube (L) but *increases as the fourth power of tube radius* (r^4). This has important implications in medicine, in particular for vascular access. The maximum flow rate that can be obtained decreases rapidly with smaller diameter vascular access devices (because of the fourth-power dependence). Therefore cannulas for rapid infusion must be short and have a large diameter, particularly if blood (which has a higher viscosity than saline) is to be transfused. 'Daisy-chained' infusion adaptors and tubing may contribute considerably to the total resistance to flow and should be avoided if high flow rates are to be achieved.

Turbulence

Strictly speaking, the Hagen-Poisseulle equation is only valid for the laminar flow of an incompressible fluid and is only approximately accurate, for example, in the airway,

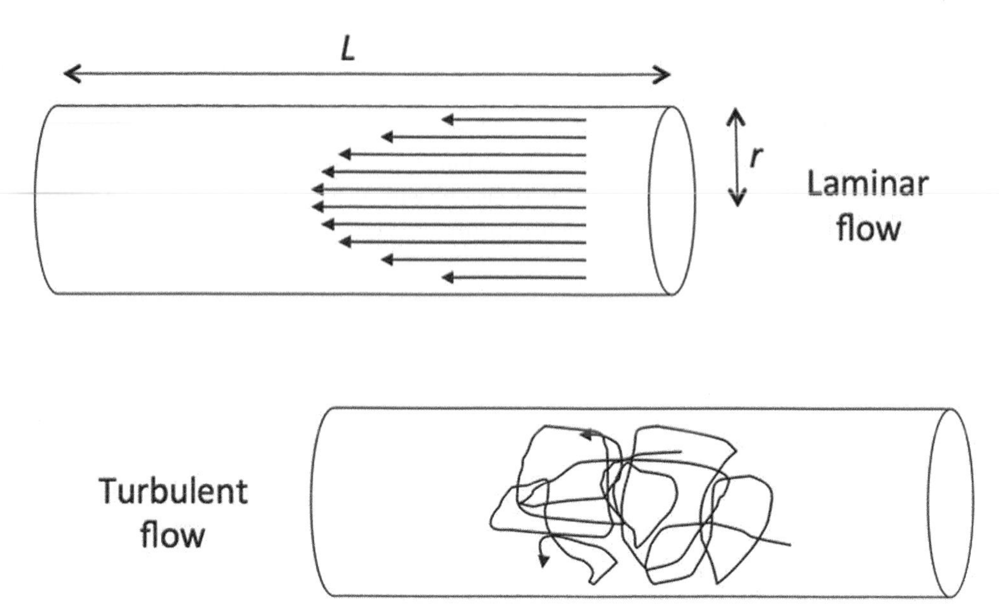

Figure 6.1 Flow through a circular tube. In laminar flow (upper panel), the streamlines, which represent the direction and speed of fluid travel, are parallel and ordered. Flow velocity is highest in the centre of the tube and decreases in a parabola towards the walls. Friction occurs as fluid slips past adjacent fluid moving at a different speed and tends to resist flow. In turbulent flow (lower panel) the streamlines are disordered and unpredictable. The large velocity gradients cause substantial friction and consequent resistance to flow.

although other empirical laws exist to describe the flow of gases. Figure 6.1 (lower panel) shows a different kind of flow in which the streamlines are disordered and unpredictable called *turbulent* flow. Turbulence *tends* to arise at high flow velocity and in larger tubes, where the ordering effect of the vessel walls is less pronounced. Turbulent flow is also favoured when the density of the fluid is high, or if the viscosity is low. Turbulence may also occur when there is a sharp discontinuity or kink in a fluid-containing conduit.

Turbulent flow is wasteful of energy and usually avoided in nature. Turbulence may occur in pathological situations, however. Normally, the airway is smoothly tapered and branched. However, partial airway obstruction such as is seen with laryngeal tumour pathology leads to turbulent gas flow. As well as giving rise to the characteristic stridor or wheeze, turbulence increases the resistance to flow and consequently increases the work of breathing significantly, in addition to the extra resistance from the obstruction. Oxygen–helium mixtures (Heliox) can be helpful in such circumstances as the reduced density promotes laminar flow and reduces the resistance to turbulent flow.

The vascular tree is similarly smoothly tapered and branched to limit turbulence. However, turbulent blood flow is also sometimes seen with pathology such as aneurysms and arterial atheroma, and indeed may contribute to their development through abnormal shear stresses at the vessel wall. Turbulent blood flow may also lead to thrombus formation.

The presence of cells and proteins increases the viscosity of blood. At a haematocrit of 40, blood has approximately three times the viscosity of water. This is reflected in the larger lumen (and shorter length) of blood-giving sets. The effect is also appreciable in the vasculature and improved flow can be obtained by deliberate hypervolaemic haemodilution and this is often employed to improve perfusion after microvascular surgery. However, the

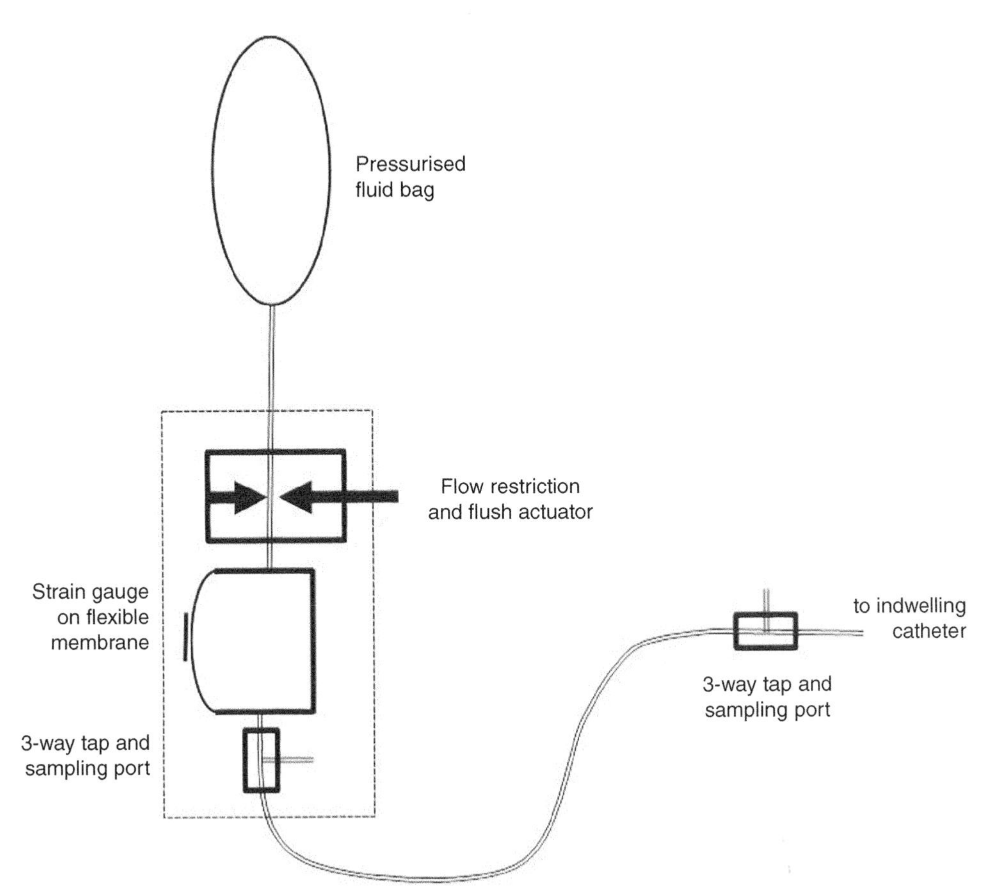

Figure 6.2 Schematic diagram of a fluid-filled invasive blood pressure measurement system. The pressure transducer/flush and sampling port arrangement are connected to the indwelling catheter by a short length of semi-rigid tubing. The fluid column transmits the pressure signal to the diaphragm, whose deformation is converted to an electrical signal by a strain gauge.

improved flow must be balanced against reduction in oxygen-carrying capacity with lower haematocrit. Blood flow in the microcirculation is more complex still. In small blood vessels laminar blood flow tends to be maintained because of the influence of the vessel walls. In vessels smaller than 200–300 microns in diameter, the influence of erythrocytes on the flow becomes appreciable. Providing there is sufficient flow velocity, red cells occupy the centre of the stream forming a column of cells surrounded by plasma. This has the result of flattening the parabolic flow profile of Figure 6.1, reducing velocity gradients and therefore *reducing* the effective viscosity of the blood (Fåræus–Lindqvist effect), thereby improving flow.

Equipment for invasive blood pressure measurement

Invasive blood pressures such as arterial pressure, central venous pressure or pulmonary artery pressure are usually measured by connecting a suitable indwelling catheter to a fluid-filled tube (Figure 6.2). This tubing transmits the pressure in the blood vessel to a pressure transducer mounted at an appropriate height relative to the patient's body.

The pressure transducer itself consists of a membrane, which is arranged in such a way as to deform in response to the applied pressure. Attached to the membrane are strain gauges, which alter their electrical resistance in response to the change in membrane shape. The strain gauges, which are positioned so as to be differentially stretched or compressed, are arranged in a circuit known as a Wheatstone bridge that converts the resistance change into an electrical voltage, as well as providing a degree of compensation for changes in the ambient temperature. In this way, pressure changes in the blood vessel are transduced into an electrical signal that can be recorded or displayed as a pressure or pressure waveform.

The tubing system is fed from a pressurised fluid bag via a flow restriction so that a continuous steady flow of approximately 5 ml/h of fluid keeps the system patent. A 0.9% saline solution is normally used. Glucose-containing solutions must be avoided since contamination may give rise to falsely high sampled blood glucose measurements and this has led to cases of harm resulting from inappropriate treatment. The system may also be used for blood sampling and a flush valve that bypasses the restriction allows the system to be cleared of blood afterwards. The pressure tubing is more rigid than that used for the administration of intravenous fluids. Use of the correct tubing, which should also be as short as possible, is important in ensuring the system has the correct resonant properties (see below). The transducer must be positioned at the same vertical height as the heart to record an accurate blood pressure. Unlike non-invasive blood pressure measurement, the position of the limb used does not affect the measured pressure.

Fluid-filled pressure transducer systems exhibit the property of resonance: if a sudden change in pressure is applied then the fluid will oscillate back and forth at a characteristic frequency which is designed to be much higher than the pressure waveform of interest. This makes the system very responsive, but can distort the signal. The system is with some damping to reduce these oscillations to a level for optimal fidelity. An optimally damped system gives a fast response, at the expense of a small amount of overshoot in the pressure signal. The waveform recorded from an under-damped system will overshoot unacceptably, leading to over-estimation of the systolic pressure and under-estimation of the diastolic. The reverse is true of an over-damped system although in both cases the mean pressure is accurate. Over-damping is recognised by a featureless, smooth, low pulse–volume waveform. The presence of an obstruction (e.g. thrombus or a 'positional' line) in the blood vessel may replicate this waveform. This is known as attenuation rather than damping and tends to underestimate both systolic and diastolic pressures. In this situation, the mean pressure is also underestimated.

Solubility

In contrast to what happens at the walls of a gas-filled container, gas molecules colliding with a fluid interface (Figure 6.3) may chemically associate with the fluid and become *dissolved*. At the same time, dissolved gas particles may also happen to escape back into the gas phase.

The concentration of dissolved gas C is determined by the partial pressure p such that:

$$p = kC \qquad \text{(Henry's Law)}$$

where k is a constant which depends on the solubility of the gas in the particular solvent of interest, which is also a function of temperature. Differences in partial pressure between the solution and the surroundings are the determinant of diffusion in and out of solution – gas molecules move in or out of solution until the partial pressures in the two phases equalise.

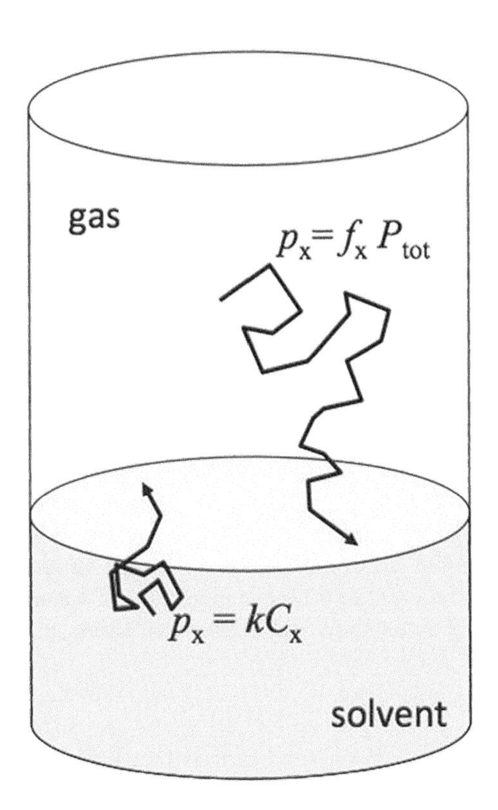

Figure 6.3 Particles of gas 'x' move randomly, exerting a partial pressure p_x, which depends on the volume fraction of x, f_x and the total pressure in the container P_{tot}. Some of these particles may enter the solvent. As the concentration of dissolved particles C_x rises, molecules increasingly are able to escape back to the gas phase. How easy this is depends on the solubility of the gas. At equilibrium, partial pressure of dissolved and free gases is equal.

Blood gas transport is an important application of Henry's law. Alveolar gas is in equilibrium with pulmonary capillary blood. Oxygen, for example, is rather insoluble in plasma and therefore for a given partial pressure, the concentration would be very low. However, dissolved oxygen is also avidly bound to haemoglobin (some 98% of oxygen is bound). This would reduce the concentration of freely dissolved oxygen and therefore the partial pressure of oxygen in solution would fall. This in turn allows more oxygen to pass from the alveoli into the blood until the partial pressures in the gas and dissolved phases equilibrate again. In this way, the oxygen-carrying capacity of blood for a given partial pressure of oxygen is much greater than that achieved by dissolving alone. In the tissues, where oxygen consumption keeps the partial pressure of oxygen low, oxygen diffuses out of the blood along this reversed concentration gradient. This releases oxygen from the haemoglobin to replace it until the haemoglobin becomes sufficiently desaturated that the partial pressure of oxygen equilibrates with that of the tissues.

Gas solubility is itself a function of temperature. In contrast to solids, gases become increasingly soluble at lower temperatures, i.e. they exert a lower partial pressure. Blood gas analysers measure partial pressures at normal (37°C) body temperature. This is why partial pressures measured at body temperature and pressure must be temperature corrected in hypothermia or pyrexia. For example, if the patient was hypothermic then the gas would be more soluble in the patient and therefore its partial pressure would have been lower than measured. Blood gas analysers also report temperature-corrected values for PO_2, PCO_2 (and therefore pH). These are the partial pressures that would be found if the measurement had been made *in vivo*.

Electricity

Charge, potential and current

Electricity arises from the presence or movement of electrical charges. When an electric field is applied, electrical charges experience a force. The SI unit of electrical charge is the coulomb. It is equivalent to the charge carried by approximately 6×10^{18} electrons. The flow of electrical charge in a conductor is called a *current* and is usually denoted as I. The SI unit of current is the ampere, which is equal to the flow of 1 coulomb per second.

Electrical charges can be either positive or negative in sign. Electrical charges are surrounded by electrical fields in such a way that like charges tend to repel one another whereas opposite charges attract. If the charges are in excess, their repulsion leads to a high potential energy state and, given a conducting pathway, they will move to a region of lower potential energy. The potential difference, V, between two points is measured in volts (energy per unit charge).

Most conductors are not perfect – they possess the property of electrical *resistance*. This is analogous to the resistance to fluid flow caused by a constriction in a pipe. If the constriction is great, then a very high pressure is required to achieve a given flow of water. Similarly, electrical current in a conductor depends on the voltage difference across the conductor and its resistance, R by:

$$I = V/R \qquad \text{(Ohm's law)}$$

The SI unit of resistance is the ohm (symbol Ω). A good conductor is one with low resistance so that only a very small voltage is required to achieve a high current. Conversely, insulators are materials with very high electrical resistance – only a very small current flows when a voltage is applied.

Storing charge: capacitance

A capacitor is an electronic device created by sandwiching an electrical insulator (called a dielectric) between two conductors (Figure 6.4). When a voltage is applied, the resulting electric field causes charges to be attracted and build up on opposite faces of the dielectric. Even though the device is an insulator, there must be a brief flow of current while this happens. As the charge accumulates, an equal and opposite voltage builds up across the capacitor until the flow of current stops. The capacitor is now said to be charged and will retain this charge even when disconnected from the voltage source. The amount of charge stored for a given voltage is called the capacitance and is a property of the size of the dielectric.

Capacitors have several applications in electronics. Firstly, if designed properly, capacitors can be charged to very high voltages. In this case, a great deal of energy can be stored. This energy can be released very quickly. If the capacitor is connected to a conductor with low resistance, the resulting discharge current can be very high. Defibrillators contain a bank of capacitors, which can be charged to high voltage (typically greater than 1000 V). Transthoracic resistance varies but is typically quite low at around 50 Ω so that this voltage causes a pulse of a very high current to flow until the capacitor is discharged. In practical defibrillators, other circuitry is used to modify the shape of this pulse for optimal defibrillation effectiveness.

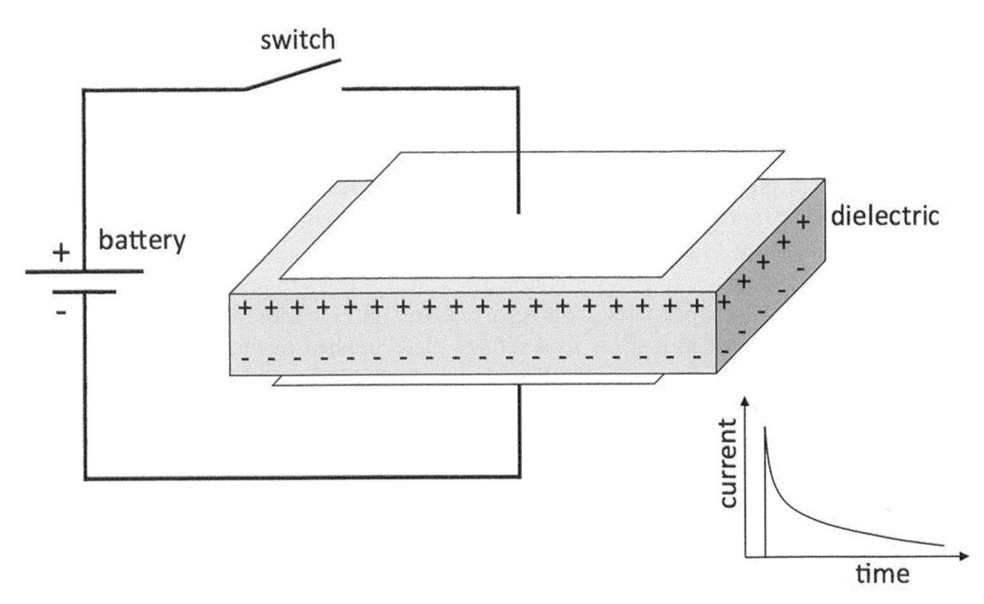

Figure 6.4 A capacitor is formed by sandwiching a thin layer of insulator (called a dielectric) between two conducting plates. Capacitors have a high electrical resistance and do not conduct direct currents. However, when the switch is closed, a brief transient current flows as charges accumulate on the dielectric. The charges cause a voltage to be established, which eventually opposes the voltage of the battery. The capacitor is then charged.

Capacitors also find application in the control of alternating currents, as we shall see below.

Applications of direct and alternating current: sensing and electrosurgery

Direct current (DC) describes the situation where the flow of charge is always in the same direction. By applying a time-varying voltage, it is also possible to make the current change its direction of flow periodically in time. Such a current is called an alternating current (AC) and has a number of useful properties.

The number of reversals of direction of current per second is known as the frequency of the AC current. It is denoted by f and measured in hertz (symbol Hz, equivalent to one cycle per second).

AC can behave differently to DC. Capacitors connected to alternating voltages are repeatedly charged and discharged, a transient current now flowing with each cycle. In other words, although capacitors are electrical insulators for DC, they conduct AC currents. Impedance is an extension of the concept of resistance to AC circuits: capacitors have high resistance to DC but their impedance to AC falls with increasing frequency. Electronic filters exploit this property to only transmit or impede signals of a specified frequency range. An example is in the processing of small-amplitude signals such as the ECG that would otherwise be swamped by interference by electrical noise in the operating theatre from the mains (at 50 Hz) and from electrosurgical equipment (higher frequencies).

The DC voltages applied to a conducting volume, such as the human body, pass through deep tissue along paths of least resistance. Current through the heart may cause arrhythmias; high DC or low-frequency AC voltages are dangerous since even a few milliamps can be fatal. At very high frequencies, however, the current becomes confined largely to the surface of the body ('skin effect'). By using high frequencies (radiofrequency range, 100 kHz to 1 MHz), high voltage currents can be applied to tissues relatively safely and this fact is exploited in electrosurgery. By applying this current in a pulsatile manner, modern diathermy can be adjusted from cutting (lower powers, continuous AC), through blending to coagulation (high power, short pulses of AC). The electrodes used for electrosurgery are small, which leads to a very high current density. This concentrates the energy deposited and consequently leads to localised heating.

While the intracardiac currents generated by electrosurgery are small enough to be safe, surface currents may be appreciable. This is particularly the case with monopolar diathermy where the return current must flow to a return 'plate' applied to the patient, potentially some distance from the surgical site. The return electrode has a large surface area to minimise the current density. It must be applied smoothly, avoiding irregular surfaces or bony prominences, with the longest edge facing the surgical site to avoid high current densities and consequent burns. Modern electrosurgical equipment employs active electrode monitoring to mitigate this and ensure a good contact of the return electrode.

The return electrode should also ideally be positioned to keep current paths as far from ECG electrodes as possible. Despite filtering circuitry, interference from electrosurgery (in particular monopolar) can be significant. The ECG may be uninterpretable during electrosurgery and can lead to erroneous alarms from the anaesthetic monitoring equipment. Similarly, implantable cardiac devices are vulnerable to interference. Inhibition, reprogramming, damage, intracardiac burns or inappropriate discharge of implantable defibrillators are all in principle possible. It is essential to establish the exact function of the implanted device and thought given to whether the device should be reprogrammed to a safe mode before surgery. Ideally, electrosurgery should be avoided although this is usually impossible. Bipolar equipment is preferable as the current paths are much more localised. Where unipolar electrosurgery must be used, the return plate must be positioned to keep current paths away from the implantable device as much as possible. Diagnostic checks should be run on the device after surgery.

It is possible to have unexpected/unwanted return paths, particularly when performing laparoscopic electrosurgery. Although laparoscopic instruments are insulated, we have already seen that high frequency AC can pass through insulators. Thus the electrosurgical electrode can become capacitatively coupled to other metalwork such as the laparoscope even if only the insulation is in contact. This can lead to distant burns.

A number of modifications to basic electrosurgical equipment have been described. Argon beam coagulation involves the coupling of a monopolar source with a jet of argon gas. In this process, the argon becomes ionised creating a plume which produces non-contact coagulation and haemostasis with less smoke production. Argon gas is inert and insoluble and may lead to overpressure and embolism when employed in laparoscopic surgery.

The LigaSure® is a modified bipolar device consisting of a grasper that applies a controlled pressure and a power source that delivers a precise amount of energy by adjusting for the tissue electrical impedance. In this way charring is avoided and the device is able to cause optimal fusion and haemostasis of even relatively large vessels.

The harmonic scalpel employs a different method of heat generation. A piezoelectric element in the hand piece delivers ultrasonic energy via an acoustic drive chain to the cutting element. When applied to the tissues, friction from the intense vibration leads to very localised heating, protein denaturation, coagulation and cutting with relatively little smoke generation.

Further reading

Davey A, Diba A. *Ward's Anaesthetic Equipment*, 5th edn. Elsevier Saunders, 2005.

Ercole A. Attenuation in invasive blood pressure measurement systems. *Br J Anaesth* 2006; **96(5)**: 560–2.

Ercole A. Combined flow rates of venous access devices and attachments. *Resuscitation* 2007; **74(2)**: 394–5.

Macdonald DJ. Anaesthesia for microvascular surgery. A physiological approach. *Br J Anaesth* 1985; **57(9)**: 904–12.

Sessler D. Peri-operative heat balance. *Anesthesiology* 2000; **92(2)**: 578–96.

Chapter 7

Cardiothoracic cases

Kamen Valchanov and Pedro Catarino

Why is the relationship between cardiothoracic surgeons and anaesthetists closer than other specialties?

First of all the anaesthetist has to induce the patient in anaesthesia, and keep them safe until the cardiac or pulmonary operation has improved the cardio-respiratory status. The patients subjected to this type of surgery traditionally have very advanced disease, necessitating surgical intervention.

Both surgeons and anaesthetists manipulate the cardio-respiratory variables at the same time and therefore it is paramount the team working has solid foundations. The surgeon will also manipulate the very organs which are maintaining cardio-respiratory homeostasis. Therefore each must have awareness of what the other is doing.

In this chapter we will focus on the foundations of cardiothoracic surgery interactions with anaesthesia and explain basic concepts and reasons for disagreement between the specialties in the hope of providing the knowledge basis for a harmonious relationship and the best surgical outcomes.

What are the most important requirements from the cardiothoracic anaesthetist?

It has to be remembered that cardiothoracic surgery commonly involves risk of higher magnitude than other surgical specialties. With this in mind, and patient safety and best outcomes remaining paramount, we have to focus on the anaesthetic interventions required. It is commonly believed that major cardiac or thoracic surgery cannot be conducted without general anaesthetic. While this is true of most cases, almost all of these procedures can be done under epidural anaesthesia.

Does the type of anaesthesia matter? It cannot be denied that the magnitude of impact on patient outcome is different between surgery and anaesthesia. Poor myocardial protection during cardiopulmonary bypass (CPB) carries a much worse prognosis compared to poor analgesia or awareness under anaesthesia. While the type and conduct of anaesthesia and analgesia for cardiac and thoracic surgery do matter indeed, it is difficult to measure in the context of changing patients, surgeons and surgical techniques. The impact could possibly be measured in very large randomised controlled trials addressing primarily anaesthesia, none of which exist.

A Surgeon's Guide to Anaesthesia and Peri-operative Care, ed. Jane Sturgess, Justin Davies and Kamen Valchanov. Published by Cambridge University Press.

The question of an ideal anaesthetic for cardiac or thoracic surgery has been asked by many researchers, but unfortunately the evidence is conflicting on whether intravenous anaesthetic agents are better than inhaled ones, whether regional analgesia is better than intravenous, whether post-operative care is better managed by anaesthetists or surgeons. Could a particular anaesthetist be better than another? As in all walks of life teamwork is likely to produce the best results for the patient.

Team working in cardiothoracic surgery?

Team working in cardiothoracic surgery starts from pre-operative assessment. The difference in this specialty is that advanced cardiac or respiratory disease need to be present for us to operate on and hence are not normally a reason for postponing surgery and seeking optimisation. The following few examples will illustrate the point:

Case 1: 56-year-old male lifelong smoker presents with left main stem coronary disease, ischaemic changes on ECG and intermittent angina at night. On physical examination the surgical team finds no murmurs, obesity or fine end-expiratory crackles indicating pulmonary oedema. During the anaesthetic assessment, history of intermittent claudication after 50 metres is elicited; mild expiratory wheeze found; and poor mandibular protrusion, indicative of possible difficult intubation. Pre-operative CXR reveals a mass in the right pulmonary hilus leading to a CT indicative of inoperable tumour involving the right main bronchus. From a surgical point of view the question is: should the patient have coronary grafting, given left main stem disease and angina? A separate question is: will the patient survive coronary surgery and what is the longevity of inoperable right main bronchus tumour. Clearly a case like this should be discussed at the multi-disciplinary team meeting (MDT), and the fact the patient's airway management could be challenging becomes the lowest priority.

Case 2: 88-year-old patient with no coronary disease, but severe aortic stenosis and poor left ventricular (LV) systolic function, and severe COPD, diabetes and chronic renal failure, who presents with shortness of breath. The pre-operative assessment reveals signs of pulmonary congestion. The predicted surgical mortality for open aortic valve replacement is clearly very high. However, they may be suitable for transcutaneous aortic valve implantation (TAVI). While the anaesthetic management of this patient is likely to be challenging, the temptation to cancel surgery must be resisted and the case discussed at MDT. It is conceivable that such a patient can benefit from a TAVI procedure and improvement in their quality of life.

Cardio-respiratory physiology

Cardio-respiratory physiology in the patient remains the same regardless of whether the physician interpreting and treating it stands at the chest or the head end. The basic concepts hold true for both surgeons and anaesthetists. While the majority of cardiovascular physiological concepts are discussed in the first section of the book, there are a few facts important to remember in the context of cardiothoracic surgery.

Cardiac output (CO) provides circulation of blood, oxygen delivery and CO_2 removal from the tissues. Low cardiac output could be a result of pump failure or low blood volume. Lower than usual cardiac output could be temporarily sufficient in a patient who has less than a resting state metabolism, i.e. receives muscle relaxation and no nutrition in intensive care post-operatively.

Systemic blood pressure can be measured as systolic, diastolic or mean. Mean arterial pressure (MAP) is the more accurate variable when invasively monitored (via arterial line) and hence more reliable to guide patient management. The MAP is governed by CO and systemic vascular resistance (SVR). It has to be remembered that the heart produces higher CO when SVR is low. Hence, paradoxically, sometimes use of vasodilators like intravenous nitrates (GTN) could in fact increase MAP because of increased CO. The mechanism of this effect is by reducing venous congestion, i.e. pre-load, and improving the Frank–Starling curve position of overstretched myocardial fibres and improving contractility; but also importantly by reducing supraphysiological peripheral vasoconstriction, hence the resistance against which the heart pumps (afterload). The CO is also a result of production of stroke volume (SV) and heart rate (HR).

$$CO = SV \times HR$$

Therefore, faster HR is likely to produce better SV, unless it is fast enough to compromise diastolic filling of the ventricles. In practice, heart rates of 90–100 bpm are frequently used in the peri-operative setting, but also increase the myocardial oxygen demand. As such, the goals of slow HR prior to myocardial vascularisation (prior to CPB) and faster HR after the surgical intervention are desirable. In some cases, a higher HR may be desirable prior to CPB, such as aortic regurgitation, where the higher HR reduces the diastolic time in which the regurgitation occurs. After a period of myocardial ischaemia the heart is stiffer and less able to adapt its SV to a low HR and maintain CO.

Cardio-respiratory pharmacology

It is beyond the scope of this book to teach detailed anaesthetic pharmacology. However, general considerations of anaesthetic medication in the cardio-respiratory settings have to be discussed.

1. Inotropic and vasopressor agents used in management of heart failure and vasoplegic states are discussed in chapter 27.
2. General anaesthetics: General anaesthesia is provided by an induction agent and anaesthetic maintenance. Both volatile and intravenous anaesthetics have been used and there is no evidence that one is better than the other in either cardiac or thoracic surgery. However:
   a. Intravenous induction agents produce faster induction than the inhalational. Propofol or benzodiazepines are most commonly used in the modern world. Propofol bolus produces cardiodepression and peripheral vasodilatation and hence low MAP. Therefore, smaller doses of propofol are often used during induction of very ill cardiac patients.
   b. Maintenance anaesthesia is most easily achieved by intravenous infusion (commonly of propofol), but volatile anaesthetics can be used during CPB too, via a vaporiser mounted on the CPB machine. Volatile anaesthetics (isoflurane, sevoflurane, desflurane) are more frequently used in thoracic surgery, but it has to be remembered that while they are bronchodilators and may improve oxygenation, they may leak in the atmosphere if a bronchus is open, or not be delivered to the patient if there is critical airway stenosis.
   c. Volatile anaesthetics may provide ischaemic preconditioning in cardiac surgery, and are more reliable in ensuring depth of anaesthesia.
   d. Intravenous anaesthetics are more convenient for transferring a sedated patient post-operatively to intensive care units (ITU), but are less reliable in ensuring depth of anaesthesia.
   e. Propofol overload syndrome has also been described during prolonged use of large quantities in ITU.

3. Analgesia can be provided by intravenous or regional anaesthetic techniques.
   a. Pain after sternotomy is seldom problematic, and easily managed by means of intravenous analgesics. However, thoracotomy pain is known to be one of the most severe, therefore regional analgesia is often needed.
   b. The conventional analgesia for sternotomy is oral mild opioids (e.g. codeine) and paracetamol, or morphine patient-controlled analgesia (PCA) but this varies in different centres. Epidural analgesia is also used, but less frequently as it has shown only analgesic superiority, yet there is a risk of epidural haematoma and paraplegia because of anticoagulation for CPB.
   c. Epidural and extrapleural (paravertebral) analgesia is used for thoracotomy patients. Epidural analgesia has higher complication and hypotension rates, but could provide better analgesia in the first 24 hours.
   d. Minimally invasive thoracoscopic surgery is increasingly popular, and the need for epidural analgesia may be reduced.
   e. A very important role of intravenous opioids during cardiac surgery is blunting the sympathetic response to surgery in a patient with reduced coronary blood flow prior to CPB. Large doses of fentanyl or morphine can be used, or in recent years the short-acting and more potent remifentanil is used as an infusion.
4. Muscle relaxation is not essential for cardiothoracic surgery. However, it has three important roles:
   a. It facilitates tracheal intubation, and reduces trauma to the airway.
   b. Muscle relaxation reduces the oxygen demand from the muscles reducing the body's metabolic demands to lower than resting state.

Case 3: A 25-year-old patient presents to a local hospital for cholecystectomy, but is declined by the local anaesthetic team because of severe left ventricular impairment. The condition is investigated, and because of congestive cardiomyopathy the patient is listed for heart transplantation. The question is how to administer safe anaesthesia for the patient during cardiac surgery prior to CPB, which could take up to two to three hours? In the absence of any myocardial contractility reserve, the best chance for such a patient is to use careful monitoring, judicious anaesthetic induction, and profound muscle relaxation, which will reduce oxygen demand to a minimum.

   c. Muscle relaxation during thoracic surgery abolishes the movement of the diaphragm and facilitates surgical access.

What happens in the cardio-respiratory anaesthetic room?

Invasive monitoring and lung isolation

Occasionally, anaesthetic induction and preparation could take longer for cardiac and thoracic surgical patients. This does produce some friction between teams but is best resolved by working together. When the patient is difficult for the anaesthetist, they could also be difficult for the surgeon.

a. Cardiac surgical patients universally require invasive monitoring. Placing arterial lines, central venous pressure (CVP) lines, and pulmonary artery flotation catheters (PAFC) in the current era of infection control guidelines and ultrasound guidance could be a time- consuming process. In addition, most cardiac patients require placement of a transoesophageal echocardiography (TOE) probe for intra-operative diagnosis and monitoring. Large bore venous access preparing for extensive blood loss during aortic surgery is also essential.

b. Thoracic surgical patients sometimes require awake placement of epidural catheters, lung isolation by endobronchial intubation (double-lumen tubes) or bronchial blockers, and careful positioning. The time spent in this preparation could be shortened by team work of all practitioners, i.e. turning the patient, urinary catheteriation, etc.
c. Use of an anaesthetic room is a luxury in the UK. In other countries all preparation procedures are done in the operating theatre, and this may be conducive to improved team working.

How does the anaesthetic change during cardiac surgery?

The concept of a cardiac anaesthetic is not real. Patients undergoing cardiac surgery need anaesthesia. Commonly, this is general anaesthesia. The important principles of anaesthesia should still be maintained:

a. Monitoring is usually invasive with a minimum of an arterial line and a central line, as well as TOE. Additional monitoring such as pulmonary artery pressure with PAFC, cerebral oxymetry, depth of anaesthesia monitoring, core temperature monitoring, cerebrospinal fluid pressure monitoring could also be necessary.
b. The patient must be anaesthetised at all times, and there must not be any recall. The estimated awareness under anaesthesia for cardiac surgery is no different than for any other surgery and is likely to be in the range of 0.05%.
c. During CPB, the lungs are deflated. This facilitates surgical access, but is not mandatory.
d. During CPB traditionally intravenous infusion of propofol is maintained (although volatile agents can be administered via the CPB machine), and if the CVP line lies in the right atrium (RA) which is open for the purposes of surgery, the anaesthetic will enter the CPB circuit through the suction channels, and hence return to the patient with considerable delay. It is simplest to use CVP lines placed in the superior vena cava (SVC) rather than the RA.
e. Temperature. Procedures performed with CPB commonly involve systemic cooling of the patient, typically to 30–34°C for straightforward cardiac surgery and down to 18–20°C for procedures involving the aortic arch. Attention to re-warming at the end is vital.
f. Maintaining good oxygenation is important in pre- and post-CPB stages as hypoxia, hypercarbia and acidosis impair both left and right ventricular function.
g. Maintaining adequate perfusion of the brain reduces the risk of cognitive injury, although the pathophysiology of this is complex.
h. Maintaining optimal MAP, HR and rhythm are important, although no specific figure can be used as guidance.
i. Anaesthesia must not be discontinued until surgery is completed and haemostasis ensured.
j. Satisfactory positioning of the patient to facilitate exposure is important and to maintain cardiac filling despite distortion of the heart. The right pleura may need to be opened to allow space for the heart while the left lateral surface of the heart is exposed.

Anaesthetic consideration for cardiac surgery without CPB

Not all cardiac cases require CPB. When the heart chambers need not be open (e.g. coronary artery grafting) the surgery could be carried out on a beating heart 'off pump'. The anaesthesia for such cases is no different but there are important considerations:

a. There is no CPB circuit to cool or warm the patient, hence temperature control is important. Usually a warmer temperature than usual is required in theatre.
b. As the heart does not stop it may need to be manipulated in different positions to allow for surgery in different regions. This requires meticulous attention to MAP, pre-load, HR and rhythm. Attention to electrolytes such as K^+ and Mg^{2+} is also important.
c. Full anticoagulation is not always necessary and this could reduce the risk of post-operative bleeding.
d. Minimally invasive techniques could be employed, hence reducing post-operative pain and speeding up recovery.

Case 4: 76-year-old patient is undergoing 'off-pump' coronary bypass grafting. For one of the grafts the heart needs to be stabilised in a position distorting the great veins and hence venous return is compromised. The MAP is reduced to 40 mm Hg for more than ten minutes and the rhythm changes to ventricular fibrillation. What can be done?

First thing is to return the heart to an anatomical position and defibrillate it. Secondly, the anaesthetist must ensure adequate perfusion to the myocardial zone grafted, and the surgeon can use a shunt. Optimal pre-load could be achieved with judicious fluid bolus; if the HR is slow, temporary epicardial pacing can be used; potassium levels should be adequate (usually 5 mmol/l or more), as well as magnesium to be considered; vasopression with metaraminol or phenylephrine could temporarily improve myocardial perfusion; inotropic support with adrenaline or dopamine could be used at the price of temporarily increasing myocardial oxygen demand; insertion of intra-aortic balloon counterpulsation (IABP) will also augment coronary perfusion. If all these manoeuvres fail, prompt institution of CPB will be safest.

Coagulation management

There is nothing more contentious in cardiac surgery than coagulation management. The science of it is poorly understood, yet practised millions of times every year, and most doctors seem to have strong views on the subject.

a. To establish CPB the blood needs to be anticoagulated. This is normally achieved by a bolus of heparin (e.g. 300 U/kg). Then activated clotting time (ACT) or activated partial thromboplastin time (APTT) need to be measured. Once adequately high the CPB can commence. If the blood clots, the patient dies. ACT $>$ 400 is deemed safe for CPB.
b. At the end of CPB the heparin effects should be reversed. Traditionally the anaesthetist administers protamine. It is scientifically documented that protamine reduces MAP. It is not (other than anecdotally) documented that in vivo protamine increases the pulmonary arterial pressure, or affects RV performance directly.
c. A sufficient amount of protamine is needed to reverse anticoagulation. As the half-life of protamine is shorter than the half-life of 300 U/kg heparin, further doses are often required.
d. If other coagulation parameters are deranged these need to be corrected promptly to avoid excessive bleeding. Blood products may need to be summoned without delay.
e. Fibrinolysis is always present to a degree. To reduce it antifibrinolytic agents like tranexamic acid are administered.

Transoesophageal electrocardiogram (TOE)

TOE is now recommended in both the USA and Europe for routine use in all cardiac operations

a. The reasons for use of intra-operative TOE are: to confirm the pre-operative diagnosis; exclude new diagnoses (which could be found in up to 13% of the patients); and to monitor cardiac function.
b. There is evidence that for surgery on the mitral valve, and congenital heart problems, TOE could lead to a change of management.
c. All cardiac anaesthetists in the 21st century have some expertise in peri-operative TOE. However, it has to be remembered that there should be a separate anaesthetist and echocardiographer.
d. TOE carries a risk of oesophageal perforation (0.05%), which carries an estimated mortality of 50%.
e. There is 2-D and 3-D TOE (with a few minor advantages in the latter relating to mitral valve imaging).

Post-operative care for cardiac patients

All cardiac surgical patients need to be cared for in a specialised area. This has different names, staffing and level of care in different hospitals.

a. The patient can be woken up and trachea extubated in the operating theatre at the end of surgery, or transferred to ITU sedated, ventilated and intubated.
b. Haemostasis and adequate cardiac function need to be ensured prior to discontinuing anaesthesia and sedation.
c. Normal temperature avoids the risks of shivering, and the accompanying increased oxygen demand.
d. Haemodynamic management needs to be maintained according to patient needs.
e. In some units the post-surgical management is guided by surgeons, in others by anaesthetists, and in some by a team. There is no evidence to suggest one mode is superior to another.

Case 5. A 78-year-old patient is recovering in the cardiac ITU following CABG and AVR. Surgery was uneventful. The AV was replaced because of moderate stenosis, and the previously moderately impaired LV systolic function is now improved. The patient is extubated two hours post-operatively: there is no bleeding, but the patient complains of moderate pain, yet they are drowsy. The duty intensive care team decides to avoid further opioid analgesia and instead administer single dose NSAID. The pain improves but in an hour's time the urine output stops. The surgical team is called as the prescribed urine output of 0.5 ml/kg/h cannot be achieved. The surgeon prescribes a diuretic bolus. This does not improve the situation and the intensivists are called again. They institute a minimally invasive CO monitor and decide that the patient needs volume replenishment instead. The surgeon comes again and prescribes more diuretic as the CVP has climbed. The intensivist arrives and there is a conflict at the bedside. The patient is anuric, and needs haemofiltration in a few hours.

Lessons: Communication and team working benefit patients. NSAID in cardiac peri-operative patients can readily exacerbate the acute tubular necrosis following CPB. Conflict benefits nobody.

Heart failure management

Heart failure patients often require cardiac surgery and intensive care. Without exception these have to be managed by an MDT.

a. Some heart failure patients need merely volume reduction by diuretics or haemofiltration in ITU.
b. Some patients need support with an IABP. Placement needs to be guided by fluoroscopy or TOE. Adequate positioning is important to ensure maximal benefit.
c. Some patients need ventricular assist devices (VAD). The anaesthesia for these patients is no different from other cardiac operations, but an experienced practitioner is often involved.
d. Some heart failure patients need temporary extracorporeal membrane oxygenation (ECMO) as a bridge to heart transplantation, VAD, or recovery.

Heart and lung transplantation anaesthesia

Heart transplantation anaesthesia is the same as any other cardiac operation. The specific considerations include:

a. The ventricular function is very poor, and meticulous balance between oxygen demand and delivery must be catered for.
b. Immunosuppression must be administered according to institution protocols.
c. TOE monitoring is essential.

Case 6: A 28-year-old patient with post-partum cardiomyopathy is undergoing heart transplantation. After the graft is implanted and re-perfused, the anaesthetist/echocardiographer reports that the organ is not contracting. What are the options for further management?

The heart could be re-perfused for longer for recovery; an IABP could be used to reduce afterload and optimise coronary perfusion; or inotropic support could be started. If the graft still does not contract, ECMO could be continued in ITU with the hope that the graft will improve, or while awaiting a re-transplant. These are the most stressful times in cardiac surgery, with team working is tested to extremes.

Pulmonary hypertension (PH)

Pulmonary hypertension is often unrecognised pre-operatively, but not infrequently problematic during separation from CPB.

a. PH can result from thromboembolism, congenital heart disease, mitral valve disease, pulmonary disease, or be of mixed aetiology.
b. In the extremes of PH it is a threat to life. In these cases, the RV is larger than LV, poorly contracting, and not very sensitive to inotropic medication.
c. In all cases of PH care must be taken to maintain normal oxygenation, CO_2 and pH, or the pH may be exacerbated/worsened.
d. Mechanical support like IABP and ECMO may be required.

Anaesthesia and aortic surgery, minimally invasive surgery, cathlab procedures, electrophysiology

a. Aortic surgery carries a risk of massive blood loss; coagulopathy, spinal cord damage; and brain insult. The anaesthesia for these operations must incorporate appropriate monitoring, large-bore venous access, and blood product availability.
b. Minimally invasive surgery is more demanding for the anaesthetist compared to conventional cardiac surgery. Mini sternotomy surgery is associated with lower post-operative pain scores, and anaesthesia should be geared for early extubation. Minimally invasive mitral surgery involves peripheral CPB cannulation (and the anaesthetist may need to perform jugular cannulation), as well as lung isolation for surgical access to the heart. Partial CPB operations are used for operations not requiring heart chamber opening, e.g. coronary grafting. The anaesthesia must be focused on early extubation.
c. Interventional procedures like intracardiac shunt percutaneous closures, mitraclips, and TAVI are more challenging for anaesthetists. The team is often out of their comfort zone; the patients could be in extremis; CPB in case of complications may not be immediately available.
d. Anaesthesia for electrophysiology (EP) procedures is simple. It must avoid medication acting on the conduction system as this could impede the results of EP investigations. Particular parts of these procedures require the patient to be very still, and hence muscle relaxation could be advantageous. Fast recovery is the norm. Propofol and remifentanil infusions, as well as muscle relaxation, are very successful in these cases.

Thoracic anaesthesia basics

While thoracic surgery can be done without general anaesthesia, the latter can make it much easier and more successful. Important considerations of thoracic anaesthesia involve the following:

a. This is the area of surgery where the most team working is required.
b. Pre-operative assessment is always by MDT. Thorough investigations avoid many of the intra-operative pitfalls.
c. Deflation of one lung to facilitate surgical access is needed most of the time. This can be achieved by either endobronchial intubation or bronchial blockers.
d. Endobronchial (double lumen) tubes are large and may be traumatic. These can be difficult to place, and placement needs to be bronchoscopically verified. They allow better and faster deflation of the non-ventilated lung.
e. Bronchial blockers are easier to position, and require bronchoscopic guidance. They are slower in deflating the non-ventilated lung.
f. One-lung anaesthesia aims at maintaining normal oxygenation and normocarbia. However, it is of paramount importance to avoid ventilator-induced injury to the contralateral lung. In such cases permissive hypercapnoea and relative hypoxia may have to be tolerated.
g. The operated lung may need to be intermittently inflated if oxygenation cannot be achieved any other way. This disrupts surgical work and can be very stressful.
h. Excessive haemorrhage during thoracic surgery is infrequent but life-threatening. The anaesthetist must provide monitoring and prompt resuscitation for such critical incidents.

Analgesia post-thoracic surgery

Thoracotomy is one of the most painful surgical incisions. Additionally, it can lead to development of chronic post-surgical pain in up to 50% of the patients. Some of the chronic post-thoracoctomy pain is neuropathic (non-nociceptive). Neuropathic pain results from nerve damage (i.e. severed intercostal nerve during thoracotomy) and does not have the propensity for healing with time. It can render patients whose lungs are cured from surgical disease disabled and degrade rather than improve post-surgical quality of life. There is no evidence to support one type of analgesia over another in preventing development of neuropathic pain, but there is evidence to suggest that patients with poorly controlled acute pain are more likely to develop subsequent chronic pain. Particular operations, like surgery on nerve tumours (e.g. schwannomas), are more likely to produce chronic post-thoracotomy pain. Such patients could benefit from early referral to the hospital pain team. Several factors play a major role in management of thoracic surgical patients:

a. Larger surgical incisions are more likely to produce more pain. Video assisted thoracoscopic surgery (VATS) is associated with reduced pain post-operatively and earlier hospital discharge. However, there is no particular analgesic technique, which alone has been documented to change major surgical outcomes like mortality. Surrogate surgical outcomes like respiratory physiology, rate of chest infections, hospitalisation time, can be improved by regional anaesthesia compared to systemic analgesics.
b. Thoracic epidural infusions are the gold standard of analgesia post thoracotomy. They are not normally required after VATS.
c. Thoracic epidural advantages are:
    a. Reliable analgesia, not including post-thoracotomy shoulder pain.
    b. Simple single infusion.
    c. Improvement in post-thoracotomy respiratory volumes.
d. Thoracic epidural disadvantages are:
    a. Could be difficult to place, and can be associated with nerve damage.
    b. Anaesthetises both sides of the chest, which is not needed. It also blocks the sympathetic system in the thoracic and abdominal regions, producing hypotension.
    c. Bleeding can produce epidural haematoma, with a risk of paraplegia.
    d. It is associated with urinary retention, and hence need for catheterisation.
e. Paravertebral (extrapleural) blocks and infusions. These are bolus injections or infusions via percutaneously or VATS-placed catheters, and anaesthetise the thoracic section of paravertebral ganglia.
    i. Advantages of paravertebral infusions are: safer than epidurals; bleeding unlikely to produce paraplegia; anaesthetise only a hemithorax, and less risk of hypotension or urinary retention.
    ii Disadvantages of paravertebral infusions are: less reliable than epidurals; analgesia similar to epidurals only after 24 hours; local anaesthetic infusions often need to be backed up by intravenous opioid PCA, requiring double infusion.
f. Intercostal blocks: These are adequate for less extensive surgical incisions where the pain is expected to subside quickly. These are the safest modality of regional anaesthesia for thoracotomy.
g. Spinal opioid injections: this technique was popular in the past in some centres. It is not commonly used because the safest deposition of spinal opioid is at a lumbar level; the

lumbar CSF opioid then has to be water soluble (morphine) to travel to the higher thoracic regions; this can produce significant late respiratory depression (within 24 hours), when the patient is no longer in the safe environment of the post-anaesthesia recovery area.

h. Systemic analgesics: morphine, diamorphine, fentanyl, and sufentanyl have all been used intravenously, most commonly in a form of patient-controlled analgesia (PCA). This is a safe mode of analgesia, but has a number of disadvantages:
   i. Analgesic efficacy is poorest.
   ii High doses of opioids may be required, and hence the rate and severity of side effects increase.
   iii. All opioids are respiratory depressants, and hence produce worse respiratory physiology parameters post-operatively.
   iv. Nausea and vomiting, itching, delirium, hallucinations are common side effects.

i. Simple analgesics: paracetamol is safe and commonly prescribed post-operatively. However, it lacks analgesic potency and needs to be combined with a mild opioid or another non-steroidal anti-inflammatory drug (NSAID).
   i. Codeine, dihydrocodeine, dextropropoxifen are mild opioids suitable for lower levels of pain, and have similar side effects, including drowsiness, nausea, constipation, delirium. There is a genetic predisposition for some patients to be better suited for one and not another agent.
   ii. Tramadol and tapentadol are opioid agents, but also block n-methyl-d-aspartate (NMDA) receptors. This combines both analgesic routes and may produce similar analgesia with lower side-effect profile. Again patients are differently suited to these agents.
   iii. NSAIDs: these are very efficacious mild analgesics, but have to be used with caution in thoracic patients with reduced intravascular volume and poor renal perfusion pressure. They may also be counterproductive in pleurodesis surgery aiming at producing an inflammatory response.

j. Gabapentinoids: gabapentin and pregabalin are anti-convulsants used in chronic pain states. There is some evidence that they reduce the systemic opioid analgesic requirements and, if given pre-emptively, could reduce the rate of chronic pain post thoracotomy. The evidence for this is still weak, and hence prescribing such agents is best discussed with the hospital pain team.

Extreme organ support

Conventional organ support in ITU entails mechanical ventilation, haemofiltration, inotropic support and simple mechanical support for heart failure (e.g. IABP). In some patients this is not sufficient to maintain life. In those patients in whom there is a need to bridge to recovery, another organ support, or transplantation, there could be a requirement for extracorporeal membrane oxygenation (ECMO). This type of support is only provided in cardiothoracic ITU settings as it employs a modified CPB circuit and specialised expertise is essential. The ECMO is similar to haemofiltration with the difference that it exchanges gases (O_2 and CO_2) rather than electrolytes (creatinine, urea, K, etc.). There are different modes of ECMO depending on the type of cannulation:

a. Central ECMO (Figure 7.1a): The blood is drained from the patient's venae cavae, oxygenated, CO_2 removed, and returned to the patient's ascending aorta. Such a setting

(a)

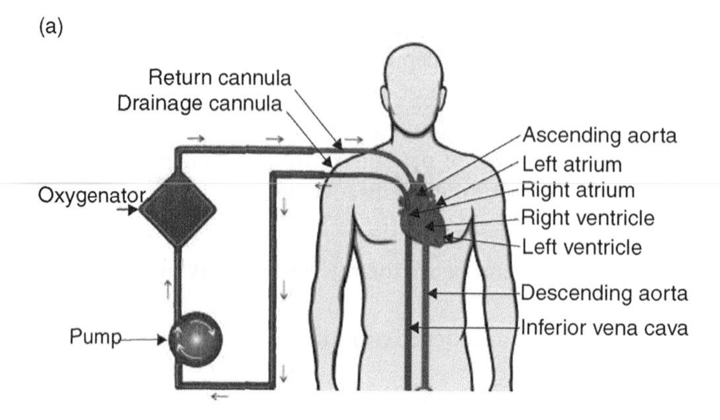

(b)

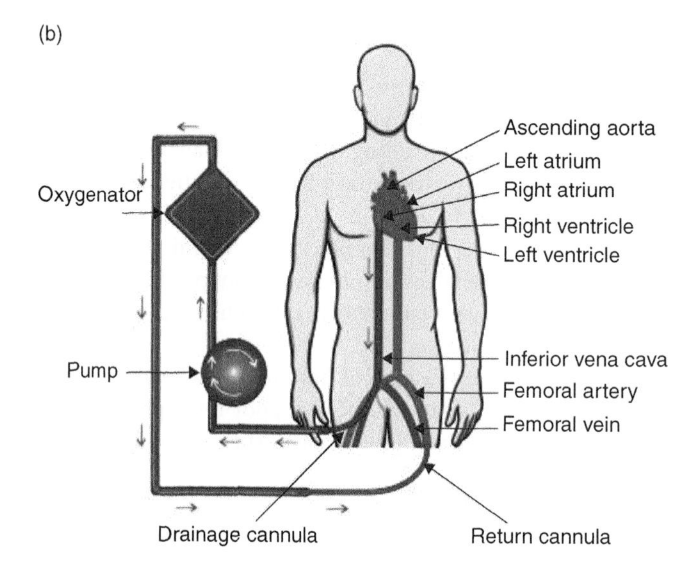

(c)

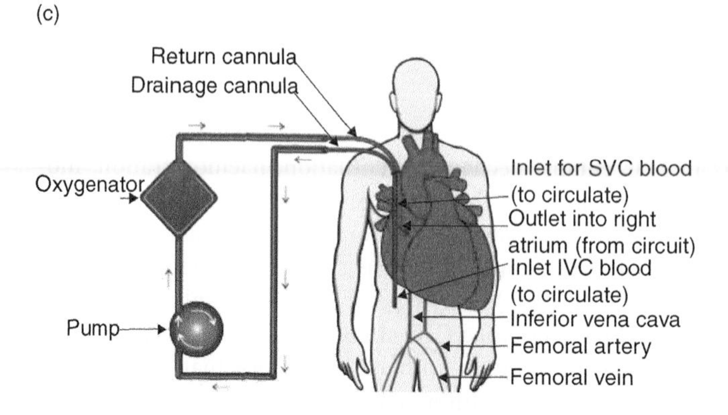

Figure 7.1 (a) Central ECMO. (b) Peripheral veno-arterial ECMO. (c) Periperal veno-venous ECMO. ©Hung, Vuylsteke, Valchanov. Originally published in *JICS* 2012; **13(1)**: 2–9.

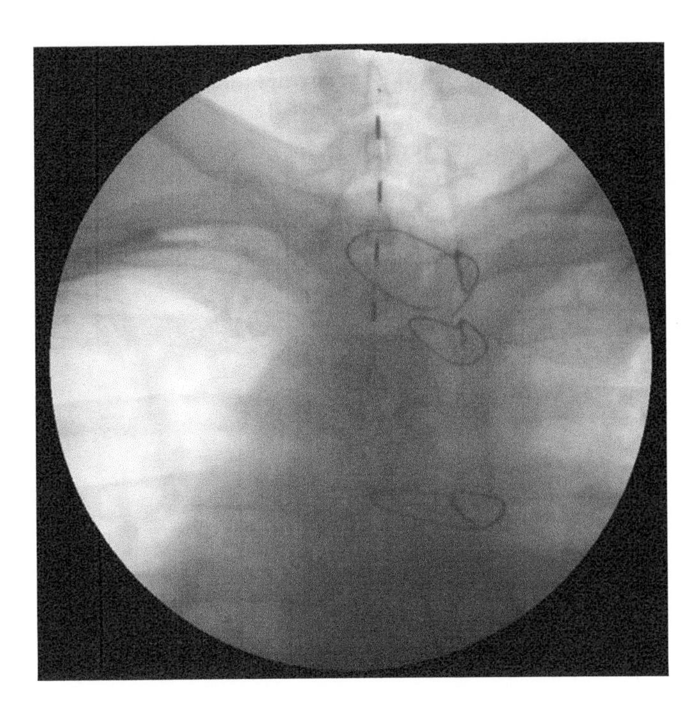

Figure 7.2 Spinal cord stimulator lead placed in high thoracic, low cervical epidural space.

allows high flows and is suitable for support of both cardiac and respiratory failure. However, it necessitates chest opening, and hence the risk of infection and bleeding is high.

b. Peripheral veno-arterial ECMO (Figure 7.1b): The blood is drained from inferior vena cava (IVC) via percutaneously placed cannula, oxygenated, CO_2 removed and returned to the patients's femoral artery via a percutaneously placed cannula. It is suitable for support of circulatory or respiratory failure, but is well suited to allow cardiac recovery. Flows can be limited by size of vessels or cannulae, and there is a mix of oxygenated blood in the aorta because of ECMO flow and native cardiac output. On the other hand cannulation is simple and it has a lower risk of infection and bleeding.
c. Peripheral veno-venous ECMO (Figure 7.1c): The blood is drained from venae cavae through percutaneously placed single or double cannulae, oxygenated, CO_2 removed, and returned to the patient's right atrium via a percutaneously placed cannula. This modality is suited for respiratory failure support only. Risk of infection is low.

Refractory angina

Refractory angina is a type of pain. Angina is called refractory when despite the treatment of coronary artery disease by percutaneous interventions or coronary bypass grafting the patient still experiences ischaemic episodes, presenting with angina. In some patients the risks of further surgery or coronary stenting outweigh the potential benefits. Typical cases are patients with small vessel distal disease, which can still produce ischaemia. These patients need pharmacological management with beta-blockers, nitrates, ranolazine, but when these are not adequately controlling angina episodes, the anaesthetists can help with interventional treatment. As the nerve supply to the heart is via the thoracic sympathetic chain the conduction of these signals can be inhibited by spinal cord stimulation (SCS). These devices consist of a high thoracic or low cervical epidural lead (Figure 7.2) connected to a pulse generator box, which generates paraesthesiae in the anginal area. This treatment is only performed in specialised centres and is successful in up to 80% of the patients, and has been shown to be cost efficient.

Colorectal cases

Jane Sturgess and Justin Davies

There are three main groups of patients presenting for colorectal surgery – those with intractable severe inflammatory bowel disease (IBD), those with malignancy, and those with benign anorectal problems. This chapter will concentrate on the first two patient groups.

Enhanced recovery has become synonymous with improved outcomes, shortened hospital stay, and improved patient satisfaction. The vast majority of research on enhanced recovery started in colorectal surgery. Many of the practices in care pathways, anaesthetic technique and post-operative care have subsequently been adopted by other surgical specialties.

Pre-operative assessment – general considerations

Pneumoperitoneum

The majority of major abdominal and pelvic colorectal surgery is now performed laparoscopically or with laparoscopic assistance. All patients must be assessed to see if they will tolerate:

i. Pressure effects of a pneumoperitoneum
ii. Physiological challenges of a pneumoperitoneum
iii. Physiological effects of steep Trendelenburg position

Nutrition and electrolytes

All patients are at risk of malnutrition and electrolyte imbalance. Specialised dietetics advice, and involvement of gastroenterologists will avoid complications and improve post-operative recovery. The malnutrition can be chronic and requires careful management of the 'starved' individual to prevent re-feeding syndrome or liver failure with nitrogen overload.

Items to consider specifically are:

i. Potassium (diarrhoea and vomiting), causes cardiac rhythm problems
ii. Magnesium (malabsorption), causes cardiac rhythm problems and muscle weakness
iii. Sodium (if on i.v. replacement fluids or sodium-depleting drugs)
iv. Albumin (indicator of liver function, healing problems, infection risk), important when considering whether to restore intestinal continuity with an anastomosis
v. Liver function (alters drug metabolism)

A Surgeon's Guide to Anaesthesia and Peri-operative Care, ed. Jane Sturgess, Justin Davies and Kamen Valchanov. Published by Cambridge University Press.

Haemoglobin

This patient group is commonly anaemic. Early detection of anaemia can guide appropriate pre-operative treatment. Initial diagnosis can be aided by looking at the mean cell haematocrit (MCH) to determine whether the patient is normochromic, and the mean cell volume (MCV) to determine the red cell size.

Transfusion of packed red cells may be immunosuppressive and is often avoided intra-operatively in cases of malignancy if possible. In cases of severe anaemia, the benefits of transfusion outweigh the possible increased risk of local disease recurrence.

i. Hypochromic microcytic – likely iron deficiency from slow, on-going blood loss, common in those with colorectal cancer (particularly right-sided lesions). If chronic, it is cheap and safe to give iron replacement therapy as soon as possible before planned surgery
ii. Normochromic microcytic – anaemia of chronic disease, common in IBD and other medical conditions such as rheumatoid arthritis, chronic renal impairment, etc.
iii. Normochromic normocytic – often the result has been taken after an acute bleed. Transfuse if ongoing acute blood loss
iv. Normochromic macrocytic – either a consequence of malnutrition (check B vitamins), liver failure (check LFTs, possible metastases or alcohol excess) or thyroid dysfunction

Thromboembolic disease

These patients are particularly at risk because of:

i. Malignancy
ii. Pelvic mass effect
iii. Dehydration
iv. Pro-coagulant state
v. Surgery to be performed – positioning head down, pelvic surgery

Fluid balance

Bowel preparation is used less frequently in current colorectal practice. Full oral bowel preparation can cause severe dehydration. Intravenous fluid replacement ought to be considered in those with pre-existing renal impairment, and the anaesthetist informed.

Fluid balance is of greatest concern in acutely unwell patients presenting for emergency surgery. Those with acute inflammatory crises (for example, acute severe ulcerative colitis), and those with large bowel obstruction can have significant third space fluid loss that is not easily detected. Fluid balance charts, patient weight and urine output charts can guide fluid replacement. Induction of anaesthesia in the hypovolaemic patient can cause cardiac arrest. Persistent peri-operative hypotension, and inadequate fluid resuscitation is the leading cause of acute renal injury.

Coronary disease

For patients with malignancy presenting for urgent, potentially curative resection the important questions are:

i. Does the patient have a problem that can be rapidly improved/treated?
ii. Will further cardiac investigations alter the peri-operative and/or post-operative management?
iii. Will the results of the investigations influence the risks discussed with the patient?

Ischaemic heart disease

It is unlikely that patients will be able to wait for coronary artery bypass graft or valvular heart surgery, nor will they be likely to tolerate the anticoagulation required if they have a bleeding malignant lesion.

They will however benefit in some cases from cardiology review and angiography to determine the site and nature of stenotic arterial lesions. Some may be amenable to stenting. If not suitable for a stent, the ventriculogram gives information about ventricular function, and knowledge of the site of the lesion permits the anaesthetist to prepare for adverse cardiac events, and stratify risk.

Drug-eluting stents are high-risk for thrombosis if anti-platelet agents are stopped, even for short periods of time. Current evidence supports the use of lifelong aspirin, and clopidogrel for at least one year after stent insertion.

Many patients will benefit from beta-blockade. This should be started at least two weeks before surgery. A heart rate of 60 beats per minute indicates adequate blockade. Beta blockade may cause increased risk of stroke if given acutely with resultant unmonitored hypotension.

Statins should be continued as much as possible throughout the peri-operative period – recent evidence supports their use to prevent cardiac events and also to reduce the stress response to septic episodes. There is no evidence for commencing therapy acutely.

Left ventricular failure/outflow tract obstruction

The presence of acute left ventricular failure and/or severe aortic stenosis greatly increases the risk of an adverse cardiac event, and increases mortality and morbidity (see Section III Chapter 22 'Scoring systems'). Crescendo angina, acute breathlessness or syncopal attacks are red flag indicators of severe disease. Careful management of systemic vascular resistance is essential for cases of aortic stenosis. A transthoracic echocardiogram (TTE) will allow the anaesthetist to prepare and arrange additional monitoring (CVP/cardiac output/arterial line) and possibly inotropes. An intensive care bed may be required.

Rhythm disturbance

New atrial fibrillation/flutter (AF) should be discussed with a cardiologist for advice on anticoagulation. Fast AF should be referred to cardiology for either cardioversion or rate control. Stable controlled AF needs no further investigation.

Bradyarrhythmias may require intra-operative pacing. Tri-fascicular block should be referred to cardiology, especially if there are syncopal episodes.

Ventricular arrhythmias/prolonged QTc need an implantable cardiac defibrillator that should be turned off during surgery, and restarted in the recovery room.

Respiratory disease

Patients for laparotomy require endotracheal intubation. This can precipitate severe intractable bronchospasm in some patients. Those at risk include:

i. Brittle uncontrolled asthma/COPD
ii. Current chest infection
iii. Recent severe lower respiratory tract infection (< six weeks)
iv. Some smokers

Lung function tests should be considered in those listed for major surgery with severe respiratory disease. A peak flow rate can be assessed easily in clinic. The important questions are:

i. Is there a degree of reversible airway disease that can be improved?
ii. Will the patient require post-operative physiotherapy?
iii. Will the patient require post-operative ventilatory support, invasive or non-invasive?
iv. What SaO_2 is correct for this patient? And what dose of oxygen is it safe to administer?

Surgery-specific questions:

i. Massive hernia repair. Will the patient tolerate less freedom of movement for the abdominal contents? Will respiratory failure ensue when the abdominal defect is repaired and the diaphragm potentially splinted in the patient with restrictive lung disease?
ii. Malignancy and a sudden increase in breathlessness. Have pulmonary embolus and pleural effusion been excluded/treated before proceeding to surgery? If left untreated both contribute significantly to peri-operative morbidity and mortality.

Cardiopulmonary exercise testing (CPET or CPEX)

This is a non-invasive test that is increasingly used to assess cardiac, respiratory and metabolic fitness for major colorectal surgery, permits risk stratification and plan peri-operative anaesthesia and post-operative intensive care. It involves the patient exercising on a cycle ergometer or treadmill against an increasing workload. The patient cycles at a steady rate (60 rpm) for three minutes against no resistance, then the resistance is increased and the patient asked to continue pedalling at a steady rate until either three minutes is completed or they become exhausted. The resistance is removed and the patient cycles slowly to cool down.

Table 8.1 Variables obtained during CPET

Measured	Data collected	Outcome measure
1. 12- lead ECG 2. Blood pressure 3. Spirometry 4. Respiratory gases (0_2, CO_2) 5. Pulse oximetry	1. ECG (rest and exercise) 2. VO_2 (L/min) 3. VCO_2 (L/min) 4. Ventilation (L/min) 5. Heart rate, rest and exercise (BPM) 6. Respiratory exchange ratio (RER) 7. Work rate (W)	1. VO_2 at anaerobic threshold (ml/kg/min) 2. VO_2 peak – the highest O_2 consumed (ml/kg/min) 3. Ventilatory equivalents for O_2 and CO_2 (VE/VO_2 and VE/VCO_2)

Other disease

1. Glaucoma – prolonged head down position may increase intra-ocular pressure further, with the risk of inducing visual loss. All topical ocular medication should be given before surgery and consideration made to returning the patient to supine during surgery every one to two hours for five to ten minutes to allow venous drainage.
2. Dementia/cerebrovascular disease – prolonged head down position in combination with pneumoperitoneum reduces cerebral venous drainage and can lead to cerebral oedema

Table 8.2 CPET terms explained

Term	Explanation
VO_2	Oxygen uptake
VCO_2	Amount of CO_2 exhaled
Anaerobic threshold (AT)	Where metabolism changes from ATP production to lactate production
RER	Ratio of CO_2 elimination to O_2 uptake
Peak VO_2	Highest O_2 uptake during the test, dependent on sex and age
VO_2 max	Maximal O_2 uptake. No volitional component – a physiological endpoint
Ventilatory equivalents	Markers of ventilation/perfusion ratio. Patients with COPD have elevated VE/VCO_2 and VE/VO_2. COPD patients may have a progressive rise in VE/VCO_2 after AT
FVC	Volume of air that can be forcibly expired after full inspiration
FEV1/FVC ratio	Used in the diagnosis of obstructive and restrictive lung disease

and an increase in post-operative confusion. A mini mental state examination can help identify patients with subtle signs of pre-operative confusion.

3. Liver disease – patients with portal hypertension, ascites or cirrhotic liver disease can progress to decompensated liver function during the peri-operative period. This can be induced by anaesthetic drugs, other drugs, sodium overload, sepsis or blood loss.
4. Renal disease – prolonged pneumoperitoneum can cause a compartment-like syndrome and compress the kidney, reducing its blood flow, resulting in 'hypotensive' acute renal injury.
5. Spinal arthritis – Lloyd Davies, lithotomy and supine positions can stress lower back injuries. Prone surgery patients with cervical spine stenosis should have their head and neck placed in the neutral position.

A robust pre-admission and assessment process allows even the most high-risk patients to be admitted on the day of surgery.

Operative management

Pre-medication

Surgical pre-medication includes:

i. bowel preparation (either oral or enema form)
ii. carbohydrate oral supplement, usually taken the preceding night and two hours before surgery. There is a theoretical risk of aspiration on induction of anaesthesia but if the gastro-oesophageal junction functions normally this risk has not been realised.

Anaesthetic pre-medication includes:

i. analgesia – if the surgery is of short duration
ii. anxiolysis – given only to the very anxious
iii. anti-emesis – given only to patients with high risk of vomiting
iv. antacid/gastric pro-kinetics – given to those at risk of aspiration, usually ranitidine and metoclopramide.

Induction

Standard intravenous anaesthesia, endotracheal intubation and intravenous fluids.

Maintenance

Anaesthesia can be maintained with volatile agents or total intravenous anaesthesia. Whichever agent is chosen a crisp awakening with minimal 'hangover' is the technique of choice to permit early mobilisation.

There are a few key areas that require close attention to enable enhanced recovery:

i. Anti-emesis. Two agents are often used in combination to prevent post-operative vomiting, allowing the patient to eat and drink as soon as possible post-operatively. An NG tube is often placed for surgery. It is aspirated to ensure an empty stomach and removed at the end of surgery
ii. Thermoregulation. The patient is actively warmed to ensure normothermia throughout, and certainly by the end of surgery. This reduces coagulopathy and shivering (increased metabolic activity and oxygen demand)
iii. Normoglycaemia
iv. Careful fluid balance – see 'Monitoring' below
v. Use of opioid sparing analgesic techniques – see 'Analgesia' below
vi. Electrolyte balance – patients should have close management of sodium, potassium and magnesium. A short period of ileus with fluid and electrolyte loss should be anticipated
vii. Transfusion. Transfusion trigger is generally 80 g/l, and transfusion is avoided where possible (see earlier in this chapter). The transfusion trigger for patients with IHD is higher at 100 g/l to maintain oxygen delivery to the myocardium

Monitoring

The advent of enhanced recovery came almost hand-in-hand with the concept of restricted fluid therapy for colorectal surgery. Henrik Kehlet was at the forefront of developments in these areas for major surgery. He has been instrumental in developing enhanced recovery programmes (see later). Current advice is that fluid replacement should be goal directed, especially in high-risk patients.

Many cardiac output monitors are available to the anaesthetist, but non-invasive monitors have found preference in this group of patients. The oesophageal Doppler has been studied most frequently in colorectal patients. Many of the studies have small patient numbers but demonstrate reduced length of stay for patients given goal-directed therapy. Some anaesthetists question the reproducibility and reliability of the numbers generated by the monitor. Nevertheless, NICE have supported the use of the oesophageal Doppler in high-risk patients undergoing major surgery. Other non-invasive monitors that could be used are technologies that interpret an arterial waveform and require the insertion of an arterial line (e.g. Lidco®).

Analgesia

Opiate-sparing techniques are frequently adopted. This can be with local anaesthetic techniques, or with oral/intravenous analgesics.

Table 8.3 Summary of analgesic techniques for abdominal surgery

Local anaesthetic technique	Epidural	Considered by many as the gold standard for analgesia and recommended in national enhanced recovery documents. Can cause problems with hypotension and reduced mobility. Recent studies for enhanced recovery have found no outcome/length of stay benefit from epidural analgesia. Still considered appropriate for open laparotomy. Used much less frequently for laparoscopic-assisted surgery.
	Spinal	Can be used with local anaesthetic alone, providing anaesthesia for up to 2 hours. Most commonly used with added ultra-low dose opiate to prolong analgesia. Obtunds the physiological response to pneumoperitoneum. Lasts from 12–24 hours depending on opiate. Once local anaesthetic has worn off the patient has analgesia and full motor power. Studies have shown no outcome/length of stay benefit when compared to PCA. Can be used in combination with PCA.
	TAP (transversus abdominis plane) Blocks	Can be used as sole analgesic technique. Sited by either anatomical landmarks or more commonly under ultrasound guidance. Require large volumes of local anaesthetic (approaching maximum dose). Can be especially useful for patients that cannot be offered or refuse a central neuraxial block. Becoming used more frequently but no evidence to show it as a superior technique.
	Pain busters/ elastomeric pumps	Insertion of a catheter into the rectus sheath by the surgeon that is attached to a local anaesthetic delivery device that the patient squeezes to administer analgesia on demand. Gives the patient some control. No evidence of benefit but good levels of patient satisfaction.
	Rectus sheath block	Sited by the surgeon at the end of surgery under direct vision. Requires large volume of local anaesthetic. Lasts up to 12 hours depending on local anaesthetic chosen. Often useful to supplement other analgesic choices.
	Caudal block	Considered 'essential' in TEMS surgery to permit surgical access by paralysing anal sphincter muscles. Not suitable for abdominal surgery in adults.
Intravenous analgesia	PCA	Evidence shows no difference in outcome/length of stay between spinal and PCA. PCA can be morphine, fentanyl or oxycodone. A fentanyl PCA may cause less nausea and vomiting, and is the authors' preference.

Table 8.3 *(cont.)*

Opiate-sparing analgesics	Lidocaine	Studies have shown the use of intravenous lidocaine by infusion can 'enhance recovery' by reducing opiate requirements. Patients require less opiate, and tolerate diet sooner.
	Magnesium	A recent large meta-analysis considering all abdominal and pelvic surgical specialties showed opiate-sparing effects. It is difficult to say if this makes any difference to clinical outcome. Colorectal patients may be magnesium depleted.
	Ketamine	Can be given as a bolus or infusion.
	Gabapentin	Evidence shows gabapentin to be opiate-sparing, and suggests that it may decrease long-term pain problems. It can be given for acute as well as chronic pain. Short courses are acceptable and can be started pre- or post-operatively.
	Clonidine	Alpha antagonism. Useful for pain and control of agitation.
	NSAIDs	COX inhibitor, should be considered in patients with difficult to control pain. Not suitable in inflammatory bowel disease. Recent concern over possible higher rates of anastomotic leakage with some NSAIDs.
	Paracetamol	Regular prescription should be considered in all, given intravenously or orally.

Anaesthetic considerations during major colorectal surgery

Major colorectal resection, whether carried out open or laparoscopically, requires close communication between surgeon and anaesthetist. The main issues to consider are:

i. **Position.** The physiological effects of the steep head-down Lloyd–Davis and lithotomy positions have been discussed above. However, lower-limb compartment syndrome is a rare but catastrophic complication that can occur when surgery is performed in steep Trendelenburg and Lloyd–Davis positions with the legs elevated. A number of simple measures can reduce this risk:
   - Limit the duration of elevated legs up to a maximum of 90 minutes before they are rested in the neutral position for 5 minutes
   - Physical movement of the legs to prevent continuous pressure of the posterior muscle compartments
   - Avoiding the use of compression stockings in those with peripheral vascular disease
   - Care must be given to padding the legs when they are placed in stirrups, in order to avoid subsequent neurological injury because of pressure-effects (e.g. common peroneal nerve injury, leading to foot drop, walking problems and lower limb sensory loss)

- The patient must be well supported on the operating table, for example with the use of a beanbag and straps, so that the patient does not slip or fall during times of extreme head-down positioning and sidewards tilt (often required to allow movement of the small bowel in order to improve the surgical view during laparoscopic cases)

ii. **Pelvic bleeding.** Rectal surgery, particularly total mesorectal excision (TME) for rectal cancer and surgery for other pelvic malignancies, risks significant, rapid bleeding. This may be from the iliac vessels, pelvic side wall vessels or pre-sacral venous plexus. If encountered, immediate notification to the anaesthetist is mandatory, such that blood and other blood products may be arranged, with initial packing of the pelvis to provide control. Pre-sacral venous bleeding may be controlled with a suture ligation, sterile drawing-pin ('thumbtack'), coagulation of a section of muscle (often rectus abdominis) over the bleeding vessel or packing with subsequent pack removal 24 to 48 hours later.

iii. **Transanal endoscopic microsurgery (TEM).** This minimally invasive technique for the resection of rectal neoplasms via the anus has become increasingly popular. The operative position of the patient will be determined by the tumour location, and the patient may need to be in the supine, prone, right lateral or left lateral position. Although a general anaesthetic is required, this is often supplemented with a caudal block for pain relief but also to permit instrument access (see analgesia). Analgesic requirements are low after this type of surgery, and caudal, paracetamol and PRN tramadol often suffice. Paralysis until the end of the procedure is necessary to avoid the patient straining or moving, with the risk of bowel perforation.

Post-operative management

Recovery room

The only considerations are to return the patient to normal as soon as possible. As many lines and tubes should be removed as possible. The patient should be warm, pain free as far as possible, and encouraged to drink (assuming nausea is controlled). The enhanced recovery programme, and many UK centres, advocate observation on the high dependency unit post-operatively. This will facilitate haemodynamic monitoring/manipulation and careful fluid balance, but the authors feel that it is not necessary for the majority of patients.

Intensive care

Intensive care is required for patients that were recognised as high-risk, those that require elective ventilation post-operatively, haemodynamic support or renal replacement therapy.

Patients that have had emergency laparotomy for intra-peritoneal faecal contamination are very likely to need post-operative intensive care. They may need more than one organ support.

Enhanced recovery

Table 8.4 The elements of a good enhanced recovery programme

Pre-operative	Peri-operative	Post-operative
Optimisation of chronic health problems	Goal-directed fluid therapy	Eat and drink as soon as possible
Managing patient expectations, patient information, start discharge planning process	Minimally invasive surgery	Mobilise as soon as possible, with daily target distances to walk
Informed consent	Minimal use of drains and nasogastric tubes	Early removal of urinary catheter, drains, etc.
Anaesthetic and surgical planning/risk stratification	Short-acting anaesthetic	Procedure-specific goals
'Pre-habilitation'	Normal physiology	Early (appropriate) discharge
Carbohydrate loading	Opiate-sparing analgesia	Physiotherapy
Day of surgery admission		

Cardiac risk post-operatively

Anaesthesia disrupts normal sleep and rapid eye movement (REM) patterns for at least three days after surgery. Patients with ischaemic heart disease remain at risk for acute coronary events from relative hypoxia, especially overnight, if they obstruct their airway (snoring) during abnormal sleep. Chest pain at this time should be taken seriously. It is worth considering supplemental low-dose oxygen overnight for those at highest risk.

Tachycardias should be avoided in high-risk cardiac patients. Oxygen supply to the endocardium occurs during diastole, which is shortened to a greater degree than systole in tachycardic patients. It is important to ensure adequate pain relief, normal plasma electrolytes (especially potassium) and anti-emesis. Intravenous cyclizine can cause a tachycardia, and reduced doses should be considered.

Beta blockers have been suggested for high-risk patients undergoing major non-cardiac surgery. This is currently a controversial area, with one of the main investigators of the landmark paper having his research discredited. Nonetheless, European cardiac guidelines still recommend considering beta-blockade electively in the post-operative period. What does seem clear is that they should not be started in the acutely ill patient. New onset tachyarrhythmias in the post-operative period should trigger abdominal examination and radiological investigation to look for the signs of anastomotic breakdown.

Conclusion

General surgical patients make up the largest cohort of elective surgical practice, with colorectal surgeons providing a large proportion of emergency cover in this setting. Those patients undergoing elective major colorectal resection are likely to require specific pre-operative and intra-operative preparation. Major co-morbidities and diabetes are common in this patient group and special consideration should be given to cardio-respiratory monitoring and optimisation. Enhanced recovery programmes aim to achieve early mobilisation and return to normality, as well as accelerated discharge from hospital. This has led to improved short-term surgical outcomes, particularly when combined with a laparoscopic approach.

Further reading

Gustafsson UO, *et al.* Guidelines for peri-operative care in elective colonic surgery: Enhanced Recovery After Surgery (ERAS®) Society recommendations. *World J Surg* 2013; **37**: 259–84.

Levy BF, *et al.* Randomized clinical trial of epidural, spinal or patient-controlled analgesia for patients undergoing laparoscopic colorectal surgery. *Br J Surg* 2011; **98**: 1068–78.

Upper gastrointestinal cases

Mark Abrahams and Richard Hardwick

Introduction

The range of surgical procedures, the potential anatomical hazards, and the problems associated with patient co-morbidities make upper gastrointestinal surgery a stimulating specialty for surgeon and anaesthetist. In recent years, the near-universal move towards minimally invasive surgery and early ambulation have been mirrored in upper GI surgery, providing further challenges for the surgical team.

The cases demonstrated here are not meant to reflect the vast range of upper GI surgical procedures, but highlight particular anaesthetic challenges associated with this type of surgery. Case 1 discusses the anaesthetic management of laparoscopic surgery, with specific concerns relating to the management of analgesia and post-operative nausea and vomiting. Case 2 discusses upper GI surgery in the morbidly obese, an increasingly common problem for surgeons generally, particularly in the developed world, and especially relevant to the upper GI surgeon practising bariatric surgical techniques. The final case focuses on the management of the patient undergoing oesophagectomy, and discusses the practical management, physiology and evidence-based rationale for treatment; from pre-operative anaesthetic assessment of the patient to post-surgical care in the high-dependency or intensive care setting.

Case history 1: Laparoscopic oesophageal fundoplication

Case history

A 24-year-old woman with a history of hiatus hernia and severe gastro-oesophageal reflux disease is booked for an elective Nissen fundoplication procedure using a laparoscopic approach.

Past medical history

Mild asthma

History of post-operative nausea and vomiting with previous anaesthetics

Clinical examination

Weight 72 kg. BP 130/75. HR 78 bpm regular.

Patient complains of reflux symptoms on lying flat.

Introduction

As well as the routine difficulties encountered with laparoscopic surgery, the patient with oesophageal reflux disease is at risk of regurgitation and aspiration of gastric contents on induction of anaesthesia. In addition, sudden increases in intra-abdominal pressure because of straining, retching or vomiting in the post-operative period could potentially result in breakdown of the cruroplasty and herniation of the fundal wrap. Laparoscopic surgery is associated with increased risk of post-operative nausea and vomiting (PONV), and prevention of PONV in this group of patients, while continuing to provide good post-operative analgesia, is a particular challenge.

Pre-operative assessment

The anaesthetist is advised to pay particular attention to assessing the degree of reflux, as well as a thorough examination of the respiratory system. A proportion of patients with gastro-oesophageal reflux disease (GORD) suffer from intermittent or continuous subclinical aspiration of gastric secretions. This can result in frequent chest infections, bronchoconstriction or pneumonitis.

The history of mild asthma is unlikely to cause significant anaesthetic problems and should not necessarily preclude the use of non-steroidal anti-inflammatory drugs (NSAIDs) in the peri-operative period, as severe bronchoconstriction with NSAIDs will occur in only a small proportion of asthmatics.

Because of the risk of aspiration with anaesthesia and the requirement for a rapid-sequence induction, an assessment of the risk of difficult intubation is essential. In the 'at-risk' patient, strategies for managing a difficult or failed intubation should be discussed with the anaesthetic team prior to induction. The anaesthetist may consider an awake fibre-optic tracheal intubation in the high-risk patient.

Induction and maintenance of anaesthesia

Because of the risk of aspiration, the patient is anaesthetised in a 30° head-up position. Following pre-oxygenation, a rapid-sequence induction (RSI) is performed using a fast-acting depolarising neuromuscular blocking agent such as suxamethonium, or high-dose non-depolarising drug such as rocuronium. In the latter, as muscle relaxation is slower in onset, there may be a short delay before ideal intubating conditions. Gentle ventilation of the lungs is possible at this stage, but the anaesthetist must be careful to avoid inflation of the stomach with gas as this greatly increases the risk of regurgitation and post-operative nausea. Unless there is a suspicion that gas has entered the stomach, insertion of a nasogastric tube is rarely necessary and, if used to deflate the stomach, should be removed afterwards.

With the less emetic modern volatile agents such as sevoflurane or desflurane, the choice of anaesthetic agent is less important than a balanced anaesthetic technique; avoiding high doses of anaesthetic agent, opioid analgesics or other pro-emetic drugs, and maintaining cardiovascular stability; in particular, avoiding episodes of hypotension. The intravenous anaesthetic agent, propofol, has inherent anti-emetic properties and total intravenous anaesthesia (TIVA) using a propofol infusion is the anaesthetic technique of choice for fundoplication surgery. Anaesthesia may be supplemented with an infusion of a short-acting potent synthetic opioid, such as remifentanil (0.1–0.2 mcg/kg/min). The use of nitrous oxide should be avoided and ventilation can be maintained with a mixture of oxygen and air.

Optimal ventilation in laparoscopic surgery depends upon individual lung anatomy and physiology as well as surgical factors such as the degree of table tilt and intra-abdominal pressure. Volume-controlled ventilation has the advantage of maintaining stable lung tidal volumes during the different phases of surgery, but may produce higher airway pressures. Pressure-controlled ventilation can provide lower peak and mean airway pressures, but tidal volumes delivered to the patient will increase when the pneumoperitoneum is released, risking volume-trauma to the lung if ventilator pressure settings are not reduced. Good communication between surgeon and anaesthetist is essential.

Anaesthetic considerations with pneumoperitoneum

Modern insufflators control gas flow very carefully and extreme cardiovascular reactions to gas insufflation are uncommon. The threshold abdominal pressure leading to haemodynamic changes is around 12 mmHg in healthy patients and, in general, the use of a slow insufflation rate and the lowest practical inflation pressure is preferable. Most surgical procedures will require pressures below 15 mmHg, and intra-abdominal pressures above 20 mmHg for prolonged periods are unsafe.

Very rarely, patients may develop a transient bradycardia or asystole during insufflation, possibly because of a direct pressure effect on the vagus nerve. This may require treatment with an anticholinergic drug such as glycopyrrolate.

The normal reaction to pneumoperitoneum is tachycardia and hypertension. A transient increase in venous return and cardiac filling pressure on insufflation is followed by continuous pressure on the inferior vena cava and splanchnic vessels, resulting in reduced venous return to the heart and a reduction in cardiac output, with a simultaneous increase in systemic vascular resistance and arterial pressure. The reverse Trendelenburg position can magnify this response by decreasing venous return further because of the effect of gravity. Hypercapnia associated with CO_2 systemic absorption results in tachycardia and hypertension.

Increased intra-abdominal pressure may also cause a reduction in renal blood flow, producing oliguria and causing stimulation of the renin–angiotensin system. In prolonged pneumoperitoneum, the release of hormones such as angiotensin, antidiuretic hormone and aldosterone can result in hypertension and fluid retention.

The temptation, in the patient who becomes tachycardic and hypertensive during the pneumoperitoneum phase, is to increase anaesthetic concentrations or to treat with opioid analgesics. This physiological response, however, is transient, and returns to normal upon release of the pneumoperitoneum. Over-treatment with anaesthetics or analgesics during the pneumoperitoneum phase can lead to hypotension when the abdominal pressure is released and an increased risk of post-operative nausea and vomiting.

Post-operative nausea and vomiting

Eliminating post-operative nausea and vomiting is a clinical priority in fundoplication surgery, because of the risk that retching or straining in the recovery period may disrupt the cruroplasty. The causes of PONV are multifactorial and include patient factors (e.g. female sex, history of previous PONV, anxiety), surgical factors such as the presence of pneumoperitoneum, and a number of anaesthetic factors, including intra-operative hypotension, the type and dose of anaesthetic agent, and the administration of peri-operative opioids.

Because of the multiple causes of PONV, a single anti-emetic agent is unlikely to be effective as a sole pharmacological therapy and a multimodal approach to the prevention and treatment of PONV by combining anti-emetic therapies with different modes of action is recommended. Glucocorticoids (e.g. dexamethasone 6.6 mg iv) have central anti-emetic effects acting at the medulla and are best given at induction. The 5-HT_3 antagonist drugs such as ondansetron have potent anti-emetic effects. A dose of 8 mg iv can be given towards the end of surgery and may be continued (ondansetron 4–8 mg iv tid) for 24–48 hours post-operatively. The H_1-antagonist drugs such as the antihistamines/anticholinergics, and cyclizine (50 mg po/im tid), may also be given routinely but can produce sedative effects. There is less robust evidence for the effectiveness of the anti-dopaminergic drugs, metoclopramide and prochlorperazine, especially in prevention of nausea, but they can be effective as a treatment of established nausea in individual responders.

The emetic effect of opioid analgesics is dose-related and, in general, occurs at a lower dose than the drugs' analgesic actions. Individual titration of opioid dose to analgesic levels is prudent. The use of opioid-sparing analgesic adjuvants such as paracetamol and NSAIDs, is recommended.

Epidural analgesia is not normally necessary for laparoscopic fundoplication surgery and, indeed, may delay ambulation. Local anaesthetic infiltration of port site wounds (preferably prior to the skin incisions) provides effective post-operative analgesia for most patients in the immediate post-operative period. The use of patient-controlled opioid analgesia (morphine or fentanyl PCA) is also not recommended for routine use because of the potential for provoking nausea and vomiting. The majority of patients will achieve good post-operative pain control using regular paracetamol/NSAIDs and 'as required' administration of small doses of oral morphine or equivalent opioid. Referred pain from the diaphragm to the shoulders and neck is often experienced by these patients and does not generally respond to standard analgesics. It is self-limiting and patients should be reassured that it will settle spontaneously within a few hours. Finally, the importance of non-pharmacological techniques such as transcutaneous nerve stimulation (TENS), physiotherapy, promotion of ambulation and, above all, reassurance and management of patient expectations, cannot be underestimated.

Case history 2: Upper GI surgery in the obese patient

Case history

A 42-year-old obese woman with recurrent episodes of cholecystitis is booked for an elective laparoscopic cholecystectomy.

Past medical history

Morbid obesity
Type II diabetes mellitus, well-controlled with oral diabetic medication
Moderate hypertension
Obstructive sleep apnoea (OSA)

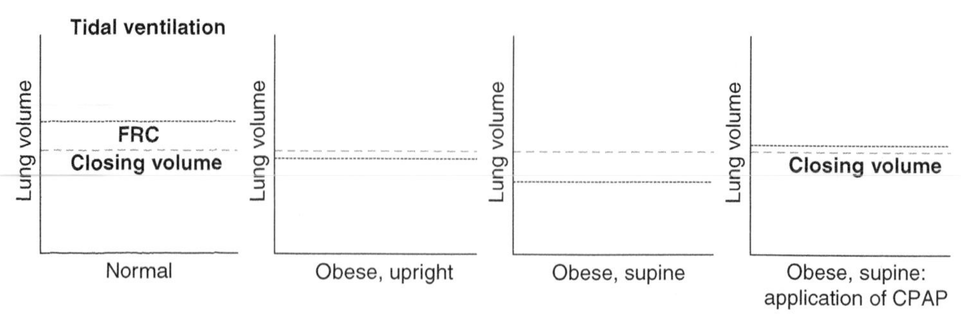

Figure 9.1 The use of CPAP in the obese patient: small airways in the lung tend to collapse at very low lung volumes. The volume at which this occurs is known as the closing volume. In young, fit patients, normal tidal ventilation occurs at a volume above this level. In the obese patient, the weight of the chest wall and abdomen compresses the lung, causing tidal ventilation to encroach upon the closing volume. The CPAP restores the FRC above the closing volume. Key: FRC (functional residual capacity): The residual volume in the lung at the end of normal tidal expiration. Closing volume: The volume of the lung at which smaller airways start to collapse and are no longer ventilated. CPAP: Continuous positive airway pressure.

Clinical examination

Weight 165 kg. Height 164 cm. BMI 61 kg/m^2. BP 155/85. HR 82 bpm regular.

Shortness of breath on moderate exercise (<one flight stairs). No shortness of breath at rest.

Introduction

The prevalence of obesity is increasing, especially in the developed world, and it is becoming increasingly common for morbidly obese patients to present for elective surgery. Upper GI surgeons may also be involved in bariatric surgical treatments for obesity.

Pre-operative assessment

Co-morbidities in the obese patient, such as cardiovascular disease and diabetes mellitus, may influence anaesthetic and surgical risk, and should be assessed thoroughly pre-operatively. Examination should also include an assessment of the airway as intubation and ventilation can be difficult in very obese patients.

The presence of obstructive sleep apnoea (OSA) is a significant risk factor in obesity surgery and the surgeon should consider pre-operative treatment with CPAP in patients with moderate or severe OSA, as this has been shown to reduce peri-operative complications (Figure 9.1). The patient must stop smoking at least six weeks prior to surgery and if this has not been achieved, surgery should be delayed until it has. Veno-thrombotic event (VTE) prophylaxis is essential and will usually be provided by peri-operative low-molecular weight heparin given subcutaneously.

Induction and maintenance of anaesthesia

The patient should be pre-oxygenated in a sitting or 30° head-up position as this increases functional residual capacity (FRC) and delays deoxygenation on induction. Obese patients have a lowered FRC because the lungs are compressed by the weight of the chest and abdominal contents. Oxygen stored in the lungs is depleted quickly and obese patients desaturate very quickly. During ventilation, the anaesthetist may employ ventilator strategies, such as lung recruitment manoeuvres and the addition of PEEP of 5–15 cmH_2O, to restore FRC and improve oxygenation. Airway pressures tend to be higher as the ventilator is forced to lift the weight of the chest wall and pressure-controlled ventilation may help to reduce peak and mean airway pressures.

Correct positioning of a morbidly obese patient on the operating table is a critical step in successful laparoscopic surgery. The table should be designed for heavy patients and allow a range of options including the beach chair (sitting) and standing position. Both these allow a steeply reverse Trendelenburg position (head up), and encourage abdominal wall fat and intra-abdominal omentum to move away from the operative field under gravity. This also makes ventilation easier. Careful attention to pressure areas is important. The combination of graduated compression stockings, pneumatic calf compression, leg elevation and protracted operation time can lead to compartment syndrome and should be avoided.

In general, drug doses are calculated according to ideal body weight. As propofol is redistributed to body fat, the calculation for target-controlled infusion should use total body weight.

The use of opioid-sparing multimodal analgesia may reduce the risk of respiratory complications associated with opioids, and the risk of post-operative nausea and vomiting. Obese patients are at risk of respiratory compromise following anaesthesia and the use of techniques such as CPAP or non-invasive positive pressure ventilation (NIV) may improve respiratory function and eliminate the need for re-intubation (Figure 9.1). Even morbidly obese patients can have laparoscopic cholecystectomy done as a day case, but this will be dependent upon the severity of co-morbidities, patient expectations and social support, avoidance of surgical complications and PONV, good analgesia and early mobilisation.

Case history 3: Oesophagectomy

Case history

A 59-year-old gentleman is diagnosed with a squamous cell carcinoma of the oesophagus, situated at 30 cm from the oral margin on oesophagoscopy. After neoadjuvant chemotherapy, the patient is booked for excision of the tumour using a classical Ivor–Lewis approach.

Past medical history

Ex-smoker (30 cigarettes per day for 30 years)
Chronic obstructive pulmonary disease
Hypertension

Clinical examination

Weight 62 kg. BP 172/85. HR 84 bpm regular.

Shortness of breath on exercise climbing two flights stairs or walking >200 m. No dyspnoea at rest. No central or peripheral cyanosis.

Investigations

PFTs	FEV_1	1.8 L (51% predicted)
	FVC	3.1 L (72% predicted)
	FEV_1/FVC	58%

Introduction

The management of the patient undergoing oesophagectomy provides a significant challenge for surgeon and anaesthetist. Centralisation of oesophago-gastric surgery in the UK has created a limited number of high-volume hospitals which has reduced 90-day post--operative mortality from >10% to <5%. This success is multifactorial: patients are better staged (advanced disease is palliated non-surgically), malnutrition is corrected early on, patients are better prepared generally, and when surgeons, anaesthetists and nurses do the same operation together frequently their performance improves. However, complications are still common but less often result in mortality than before because of improvements in ICU management and the use of early surgical re-intervention when appropriate.

Morbidity following oesophagectomy remains high at 30–40% with median length of stay around 14 days. As mortality has fallen, the focus of anaesthetic and surgical management has moved towards reducing both morbidity and length of stay using techniques such as minimally invasive surgery and active anaesthetic management to reduce pulmonary complications, improve the blood supply to the anastomosis, and optimise fluid management. Enhanced recovery protocols are increasingly being used to good effect. They all aim to deliver appropriate fluid replacement, good analgesia, early mobilisation and enteral nutrition.

Pre-operative assessment

Respiratory and cardiovascular complications occur in ~25% and ~12% respectively in patients undergoing oesophagectomy. A comprehensive pre-operative assessment is essential in order to assess the ability of the patient to cope with such demanding surgery, to estimate the likelihood of the patient developing problems (particularly pulmonary) in the post-operative period, and to optimise the patient's physiological state prior to surgery. In particular, patients must not smoke for at least six weeks before their operation.

The nutritional status of patients is often compromised because of swallowing difficulties or the anorexic and emetic effects of neoadjuvant chemotherapy and this, in turn, can increase risk of post-operative complications such as anastomosis breakdown or infection. Any patient assessed by the upper gastrointestinal dietician to be unable to safely nourish themselves should have a fine-bore feeding tube placed early on for enteral feeding.

A general examination of the patient at the 'bedside' can be extremely informative in determining cardiovascular and pulmonary risk. The presence of dyspnoea at rest or with minimal exercise (<one flight of stairs) indicates significant cardiovascular compromise and will probably preclude an oesophagectomy. Symptoms such as orthopnoea or pulmonary oedema, suggesting a degree of cardiac failure, would also constitute a significant anaesthetic risk and may indicate that the patient should be referred to a cardiologist for further investigations such as pre-operative cardiopulmonary exercise testing or thallium

perfusion imaging. Patients with a maximum oxygen uptake (VO_{2max}) <50% predicted have a significantly increased risk of pulmonary complications.

Peri-operative cardiac arrhythmias may cause CVS instability and this, in turn, increases the risk of pulmonary complications and anastomotic leak. Prophylactic use of the antiarrhythmic agent, amiodarone, reduces the risk of peri-operative arrhythmia, but studies show no change in the rate of complications.

All patients undergoing a thoracotomy should have lung function testing using spirometry. In addition, patients with a history of chronic pulmonary disease or cough/dyspnoea should also have arterial blood gases taken for baseline measurement of oxygenation, acid–base status and degree of metabolic compensation. An arterial oxygen saturation (SaO_2) of <90% on air, a PaO_2 <9 kPa with dyspnoea at rest, and a $PaCO_2$ >6.7 kPa, is associated with an increased risk of pulmonary complications.

In the patient above, the FEV_1 <60% and FEV_1/FVC ratio <80% is suggestive of moderate obstructive lung disease. An FEV_1 <1.2 L or <61% predicted is a predictor of pulmonary risk.

Pre-operative optimisation of the patient includes treatment of any acute or unstable underlying medical conditions, electrolyte or metabolic disturbance, and maximising lung function. Patients should be encouraged to take moderate aerobic exercise for at least 30 minutes three times a week (brisk walking, cycling, swimming etc.). Pre-operative physiotherapy in at-risk patients should be considered as this has been shown to reduce pulmonary complications in abdominal surgery.

Induction and maintenance of anaesthesia

The anaesthetic techniques employed depend upon the type of surgery performed, but will be influenced by patient factors, and individual surgical considerations (e.g. expected length of surgery, blood loss and high-dependency care pathways). In general, oesophagectomy can be approached by either a left or right transthoracic, or a transhiatal incision. Transthoracic approaches involving thoracotomy give good visualisation of the oesophagus and surrounding lymph nodes, but require one-lung ventilation during the thoracotomy phase.

The particular surgical technique depends upon a number of factors, including the size and site of the tumour. In general, a laparotomy and right thoracotomy (Ivor–Lewis approach) is suitable for tumours within the middle and distal third of the oesophagus, a left thoraco-abdominal approach is suitable for tumours in the distal third and a three-phase McKeown type resection with laparotomy, right thoracotomy and cervical incision is used for more proximal tumours. In addition, either abdominal or thoracic stages may be performed using minimally invasive techniques. When these are combined with open surgery they are called hybrid operations and when the whole procedure is done laparoscopically/thoracoscopically it is referred to as a minimally invasive oesophagectomy.

Peri-operative pain management

Acute post-operative pain is a major contributing risk factor for pulmonary complications because of reduced sputum clearance and ventilator capacity. Up to 18% of patients develop atelectasis or pneumonia, and most will experience a 30% reduction in vital capacity that can last for one to two weeks following surgery. This reduction is considerably greater if the patient has moderate or severe post-operative pain.

Thoracic epidural anaesthesia is the gold standard analgesic technique in oesophagectomy and has been shown to reduce the incidence of pulmonary complications and respiratory failure, as well as improving microvascular perfusion at the anastomosis. The epidural is sited before surgery and may be established intra-operatively. Alternatively, an infusion of the highly potent, but ultra-short-acting, synthetic opioid, remifentanil (0.1–0.2 mcg/kg/min), may be used during the surgical procedure to stabilise autonomic responses, and the epidural established towards the end of surgery when there is a lower risk of sudden shifts in blood volume. If the latter technique is used, the possibility of opioid-related hyperalgesia following remifentanil infusion should be taken into account, and a dose of morphine (5 mg iv) can be given at least 30 minutes prior to discontinuation of the infusion in order to compensate for this.

Epidural techniques and infusion regimes vary greatly in different centres and many techniques provide the desired outcome of good analgesia, combined with minimal motor blockade and cardiovascular stability. In our centre, the epidural is placed in the awake, sitting patient, prior to induction at the T8/9 level. Following 'top-up' with local anaesthetic agent, the epidural is run as an infusion of 0.1% chirocaine with fentanyl 2 mcg/ml at 0–20 ml/hr. The epidural is continued for around three days postoperatively or until the patient is stable, with good respiratory function, and is likely to step down effectively to alternative analgesics.

Diaphragmatic shoulder pain may not be covered by a single site epidural and treatment of this often requires multimodal analgesia. Paracetamol 1 g qid i.v. or via the jejunostomy can often be effective. The use of NSAIDs may also provide good analgesia but, generally, are avoided because of the risk of renal impairment in the hypovolaemic patient. Similarly, opioids should be used with caution because of the risk of reducing respiratory function further, especially if opioids are already being employed via the epidural.

The anti-neuropathic agents, gabapentin and pregabalin, have not been demonstrated to reduce the incidence of shoulder pain following thoracic surgery, but doses of 1200 mg daily of gabapentin (and 300 mg daily of pregabalin) may reduce the incidence of persistent post-surgical neuropathic pain (incidence ~20% after thoracotomy).

In fact, physical therapy and the use of a TENS machine are often highly effective in treating post-oesophagectomy shoulder pain, and should be considered first-line therapies. Studies have also demonstrated that suprascapular nerve block reduces post-thoracotomy shoulder pain in 85% of patients.

Given the potential consequences of inadequate post-operative analgesia, every effort must be employed to establish effective thoracic epidural anaesthesia. If this proves technically impossible, there are alternative analgesic techniques. Thoracic paravertebral catheters can be placed under direct vision during surgery and have been shown to provide similar analgesia to thoracic epidural, but with less haemodynamic instability. Intrapleural local anaesthetic is less effective and carries a significant risk of systemic absorption producing local anaesthetic toxicity. Intercostal nerve blocks are not recommended.

Induction and maintenance of anaesthesia

Patients with gastric or oesophageal carcinoma are at risk of regurgitation during anaesthesia. Following pre-oxygenation, the patient is anaesthetised in a 30° head-up position, using a rapid sequence induction technique with suxamethonium or high-dose rocuronium. The airway is protected with a standard endotracheal tube (if the abdominal stage is planned first) and ventilation established. The choice of anaesthetic agent is probably less important than the anaesthetic technique employed, but agents with powerful vasodilatatory effects may potentially compromise hypoxic pulmonary vasoconstriction during one-lung anaesthesia (see below) and should be avoided if possible. The volatile anaesthetic agents sevoflurane and desflurane are appropriate. Again, nitrous oxide should be avoided, and the patient ventilated with a mixture of oxygen and air. Interestingly, a study comparing sevoflurane with propofol (TIVA) demonstrated a reduction in inflammatory mediators and adverse post-operative complications with sevoflurane, suggesting that the inhalational anaesthetic agents may exert an immunomodulatory effect on the pulmonary inflammatory response to one-lung anaesthesia. However, the results may be misleading because the propofol group of patients had longer surgical and one-lung times, both known risk factors.

Intravenous access is established with a large-bore (14 G) intravenous cannula, and arterial line, central venous and urinary catheters inserted. In patients with significant cardiac disease, cardiac output monitoring (e.g. using a pulse contouring system) may be considered. The patient is kept warm and core temperature is monitored throughout the surgery.

The principal of fluid management in oesophagectomy is to replace blood and insensible losses, maintaining normovolaemia or moderate fluid restriction; but avoiding hypervolaemia. Fluid overload can compromise anastomotic structure and is associated with pulmonary interstitial oedema and an increased risk of pulmonary complications. There is no evidence showing an advantage of colloid over crystalloid (although animal studies demonstrate improved microcirculation with colloid) and maintenance with crystalloid (e.g. Hartmann's solution) is appropriate.

Following the abdominal stage, the endotracheal tube is replaced with a double-lumen tube (DLT) in preparation for thoracotomy and one-lung anaesthesia. Larger tubes are less likely to cause bronchial mucosal trauma because of high cuff pressures. In general, size 41 Fr for men and size 39 Fr for women are appropriate. Confirmation of the position of the tube using a fibre-optic scope is helpful. Once positioned correctly, the tracheal lumen is opened to air and the bronchial cuff gently inflated (<2 ml) until the bronchus is sealed and any air leak disappears.

The choice of the double-lumen tube is relatively unimportant as both lungs can be isolated using a left-sided tube. However, placing the tube on the side of the dependent lung may reduce the risk of displacement as a result of inadvertent surgical manipulation. Concerns about obstruction of the right upper lobe bronchus with right-sided tubes are less relevant now with the ability to confirm the position using a fibre-optic scope, and it has been demonstrated that the tube position rarely changes once sited. However, position should routinely be re-checked following a radical change in patient position. A bronchial blocker may be employed as an alternative to a DLT.

A 16 G nasogastric tube is inserted into the proximal oesophagus at the time of re-intubation. This will be positioned under direct vision by the surgeon following creation of the oesophageal anastomosis. The patient is then placed in the left-lateral position for the right thoracotomy procedure.

One-lung anaesthesia

Physiology of one-lung anaesthesia

One-lung ventilation results in a right-to-left shunt as pulmonary blood is directed to lung tissue that is not being ventilated. The shunt fraction is considerably less than 50% because

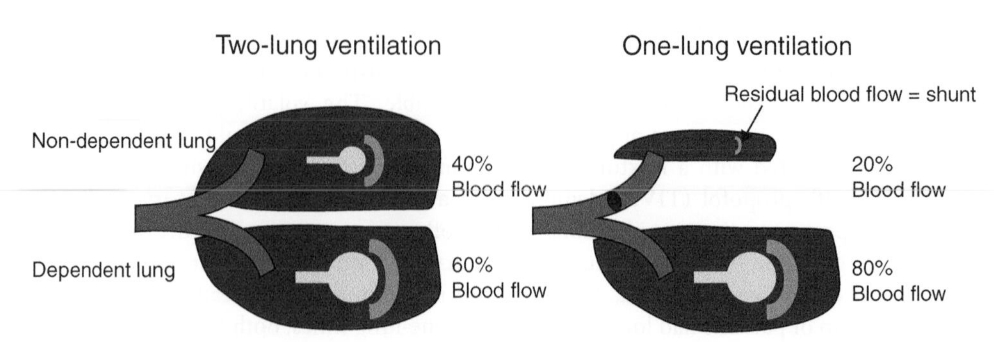

Figure 9.2 The physiology of one-lung ventilation: in the lateral decubitus position, ventilation and blood flow are proportionally greater in the dependent lung because of gravity and anatomical conformational changes. Once one-lung anaesthesia is established, blood flow through the non-ventilated alveoli of the upper lung decreases because of hypoxic pulmonary vasoconstriction, and flow is directed to the ventilated lung. Any residual blood flow to the collapsed lung will return deoxygenated blood to the systemic circulation (shunt).

of a number of physiological factors. In the left lateral position, around 10% of cardiac output is preferentially directed to the dependent lung because of the effect of gravity and anatomical changes in blood vessels. This effect is abolished in the supine position, and makes the risk of hypoxia more likely. In addition, the amount of shunt is reduced because of the effects of hypoxic pulmonary vasoconstriction (HPV). Pulmonary arterial smooth muscle has specialised O_2-sensing cells that are sensitive to small changes in alveolar oxygen (P_AO_2). The HPV is a local response, independent of the autonomic nervous system, which causes progressive pulmonary arteriolar vasoconstriction in the presence of hypoxia. The vasoconstrictive response is proportional with a threshold of <8 kPa. As a result of HPV, widespread vasoconstriction in the non-ventilated lung diverts the majority of the pulmonary blood flow to the dependent (ventilated) lung, and hypoxia (SaO_2 <90%) only occurs in around 8% of patients undergoing one-lung anaesthesia (Figure 9.2).

Ventilatory strategies in one-lung anaesthesia

One-lung ventilation results in an inflammatory response that directly contributes to pulmonary morbidity following oesophagectomy. This inflammatory response varies directly with the duration of one-lung ventilation, and can be increased because of damage to the alveoli as a result of surgical manipulation, over-ventilation of the dependent lung, and re-expansion/reperfusion injuries.

A number of lung-protective strategies are recommended. In general, tidal volumes in the dependent lung should not exceed 4–6 ml/kg with plateau pressures <25 cmH_2O and peak pressures <35 cmH_2O. This can result in a degree of permissive hypercapnia but, as hypercapnia enhances HPV, oxygenation may improve. The relatively low tidal volumes can result in atelectasis in the smaller airways of the dependent lung, and it is recommended that the anaesthetist intermittently carries out alveolar recruitment manoeuvres by providing a sustained positive pressure ventilation. This has to be done carefully, as over-zealous application of pressure could result in baro- and volume-trauma to the dependent lung, as well as reducing venous return to the heart and cardiac output.

A small proportion of patients undergoing one-lung ventilation will become hypoxic (SaO_2 <90%). The reduction in oxygenation can take around ten minutes to occur and is treated by increasing inspired oxygen concentration and optimising ventilation of the dependent lung. Oxygenation of the dependent lung is highly dependent upon PEEP, and

PEEP should be routinely set at an optimal level (above the lower inflection point in the lung compliance curve).

If oxygenation fails to improve, a series of manoeuvres to the collapsed lung may help. The application of oxygen via a CPAP circuit may raise oxygen levels above 90%. The CPAP level can be set under direct vision so that lung inflation is at a level that does not interfere with surgery. If this fails, the application of very small volume ventilation to the collapsed lung, again, under direct vision to ensure minimal interference, can make a significant difference. Alternatively, a pulmonary segment distal to the operating site may be selectively ventilated using bronchoscopic control. Other ventilation strategies include high-frequency jet ventilation and oscillatory ventilation. If all else fails, the lung may have to be ventilated intermittently to restore oxygenation, but this strategy risks re-expansion injury and prolongation of the one-lung ventilation time, and is rarely necessary.

What the surgeon does during the thoracotomy can also help ensure a smooth post-operative recovery. Division of the vagus nerves below the level of the cardiac branches (if oncologically appropriate) helps reduce post-operative dysrhythmias. Gentle retraction of the deflated lung can reduce the degree of lung injury and subsequent interstitial oedema. Preservation of one of the two bronchial arteries can also help to reduce post-operative pulmonary complications. Avoidance of injury to the major airways is of course essential and identification and ligation of the thoracic duct will reduce the incidence of chyle leakage. A well-vascularised gastric conduit anastomosed carefully without tension to the remaining oesophagus using a circular stapler or sutures will ensure a low anastomotic leak rate (currently around 8% in the UK).

Upon completion of the surgical resection, chest drains are inserted and the collapsed lung is re-expanded carefully under direct vision. Once again, over-zealous re-expansion can easily cause barotrauma. The lung segments expand unevenly and localised areas may be exposed to damaging increases in alveolar pressure and volume. Gentle expansion by hand, similar to the alveolar recruitment manoeuvre, is effective, ensuring that pressures do not exceed 20 cmH_2O.

Once surgery is completed and the thoracotomy wound closed, the patient is placed in a supine position and the epidural 'topped up' (if not already established). The nasogastric tube is firmly anchored and protected against inadvertent removal. Providing patient observations remain stable and oxygenation, acid–base status and temperature are within normal limits, anaesthesia is discontinued and the patient woken and extubated. In patients with exceptionally poor cardiovascular or respiratory function, an elective period of post-operative ventilation to allow for optimisation of cardiac and pulmonary function may be planned. The majority of patients are extubated and transferred to a high-dependency area for post-operative care and observations.

Post-operative care of the oesophagectomy patient

Immediate post-operative care

The priorities in early post-operative care are to ensure cardiovascular stability and maintenance of the anastomotic blood supply; and to protect against pulmonary complications by encouraging deep breathing, coughing, and by initiating early physiotherapy and pulmonary toilet. Thoracic epidural analgesia is associated with improved pulmonary function and anastomotic perfusion, but epidural 'top ups' must be carried out cautiously as episodes of profound hypotension can compromise the anastomotic blood supply.

The patient should be moderately fluid restricted and intravenous fluid management with crystalloid at 100 ml/h is adequate for most patients. Approximate therapeutic goals would include maintaining an arterial mean pressure roughly equivalent to pre-operative levels (>70 mmHg for most patients) and urine output >30 ml/h. Abdominal and thoracic drains must be monitored and blood replaced if losses are excessive, maintaining Hb > 8 g.dl^{-1}. Periods of hypotension should be treated promptly, in view of the risk to the anastomosis, but great care must be taken to avoid fluid overload. A single fluid challenge of 250–500 ml colloid can be given but, if hypotension or low urine output continues in the absence of obvious blood loss or haemodynamic instability, consider inotropic support with an α_1-agonist drug (e.g. metaraminol). The goal is to achieve normal arterial pressures, avoiding overdose as excessive vasoconstriction might compromise anastomotic blood flow.

Jejunostomy feeding is normally started on the first post-operative day and i.v. fluids may be reduced as the feed volume is increased. Chest physiotherapy should continue daily and the patient is encouraged to ambulate from post-operative day 1.

Patients are at risk of reflux and tracheal aspiration because of excision of the lower oesophageal sphincter, denervation of the stomach and possible paralysis of the recurrent laryngeal nerve. Patients are nursed in a 30° head-up position with low-level continuous or intermittent nasogastric suction.

Post-operative complications

The most serious complications following oesophagectomy include pulmonary complications such as pneumonia and acute respiratory distress syndrome (ARDS), and surgical problems such as anastomotic leak or gastric conduit necrosis, but any complication can quickly deteriorate to multi-organ failure. Complications can be delayed and respiratory and anastomotic problems often present at three to ten days post-operatively. Approximately 10% of patients require re-intubation for respiratory failure. Early flexible endoscopy to check the viability of the gastric conduit in a sick patient is particularly useful and will also allow the integrity of the anastomosis to be assessed. Small anastomotic leaks are often successfully managed conservatively but major disruptions or necrosis of the proximal part of the gastric conduit will require urgent re-exploration and damage limitation surgery. Patients with anastomotic leaks should receive long courses of broad spectrum antibiotics and anti-fungal agents. Effective and prompt drainage of infected collections in the pleural spaces and mediastinum is important; an experienced interventional radiologist is an essential member of a modern oesophago-gastric team.

Recognition of complications and early involvement of the critical care team is the key to effective management, and communication between the surgical and critical care teams, and established care pathways, can help ensure that patients at risk are treated as efficiently and effectively as possible.

Further reading

Blencowe NS, Strong S, *et al.* Reporting of short-term clinical outcomes after esophagectomy: a systematic review. *Annals of Surgery* 2012; **255**(4): 658–66.

Fischer L. Thoracic anesthesia. *Current Opinion in Anaesthesiology* 2011; **24**: 1–48.

Martin RF (ed). Contemporary management of esophageal malignancy. *Surgical Clinics of North America* 2012; **92**(5): 1077–353.

National oesophago-gastric cancer audit – 2012 annual report. http://www.hqip.org.uk/assets/NCAPOP-Library/NCAPOP-2012-13/Oesophago-Gastric-Cancer-National-Audit-INTERACTIVE-pub-2012.pdf.

Schumann R. Anaesthesia for bariatric surgery. Best practice and research. *Clinical Anaesthesiology* 2011; **25**(1): 83–93.

Schumann R, Jones SB, *et al.* Update on best practice recommendations for anesthetic peri-operative care and pain management in weight loss surgery, 2004–2007. *Obesity* 2009; **17**(5): 889–994.

Chapter 10

Hepatobiliary and pancreatic cases

Hemantha Alawattegama and Paul Gibbs

Anaesthesia for hepatobiliary surgery is complicated by both the complex nature of the surgery and by the underlying condition of the patient that may have contributed to the need for surgery. A liver resection on an otherwise fit and healthy individual with an isolated adenoma is very different to that on a cirrhotic patient. Therefore it is important not only to optimise these patients prior to surgery, but also to take into account the potential risk of post-operative liver dysfunction as a consequence of anaesthesia or surgery.

Pre-operative factors

Assessment of the patient

As with any field of medicine, a thorough history and examination is important. Patients undergoing any type of surgery have to be individually assessed, taking into account their co-morbidities. Pre-existing liver dysfunction needs not only greater assessment but also considerable multi-disciplinary input to ensure a favourable outcome. This group of patients are at significant risk of multi-organ failure and post-operative liver failure. The advent of pre-operative assessment clinics which are nurse-led with anaesthetic support has meant that potential problems can be identified and dealt with prior to day of surgery admission. All patients with chronic liver disease or undergoing a hepatectomy should have the standard pre-operative work-up including full blood count, urea and electrolytes, glucose, liver function tests and prothrombin time performed. Patients with portal hypertension undergoing hepatic resection should have their portal pressures measured (see below).

Portal hypertension can cause problems during even minor procedures such as laparoscopic cholecystectomy or para-umbilical hernia repair because of the presence of a re-canalised umbilical vein at the umbilicus, making laparoscopic port insertion hazardous. Unfortunately complications such as significant bleeding on port insertion still occur because of inadequate examination or history taking in either the surgical clinic or at the pre-operative assessment. It is important to remember that a patient can have significant portal hypertension without ascites or the ascites may be well controlled with diuretics.

Pre-existing liver disease

The liver is responsible for a number of homeostatic functions. As a result, the ability to sustain and recover from surgery can be greatly affected by the presence of hepatic

A Surgeon's Guide to Anaesthesia and Peri-operative Care, ed. Jane Sturgess, Justin Davies and Kamen Valchanov. Published by Cambridge University Press.

dysfunction. Impairment of gluconeogenesis, coagulation, clearance of toxins and handling of drugs (because of abnormal protein synthesis and volumes of distribution) have significant implications both peri- and post-operatively. Assessing the degree of liver dysfunction is still difficult. Function is best assessed by a combination of parameters, as with the Child–Pugh scoring system (Table 10.1). Each value on its own can be a result of a number of conditions but, collectively, their specificity and sensitivity in assessing liver dysfunction has been validated. The classic liver function tests, which include serum alanine aminotransferase (ALT) and serum aspartate aminotransferase (AST) are indicators of hepatic cellular injury rather than poor function, although serial measurements are more meaningful. The ALT measurement is more specific to the liver than AST (the latter being present in other tissues including brain, heart and skeletal muscle). Measurements of lactate and pro-thrombin time are more useful in assessing hepatocyte function during and immediately after surgery.

Child–Pugh scoring system

Table 10.1 Child–Pugh scoring system

Measure	1 point	2 points	3 points
Total bilirubin μmol/l	<34	34–50	>50
Serum albumin g/l	>35	28–35	<28
PT INR	<1.7	1.71–2.30	>2.30
Ascites	None	Mild	Moderate–severe
Hepatic encephalopathy	None	Grade I–II	Grade III–IV

Various studies exist which quantify risk of mortality with Child–Pugh score. Although there is some variation in values quoted they are in the region of:

Childs A	(5–6 points)	10%
Childs B	(7–9 points)	16%
Childs C	(10–15 points)	63%

The MELD (model for end-stage liver disease) score has been used, although the primary function of this system is for patients being assessed for potential liver transplantation. It includes measurements of serum bilirubin, creatinine and INR. Modifications have included sodium levels (MELD-Na and UKELD). The formulae for these are complex.

MELD
$[(0.957 \times \ln \text{creatinine}) + (0.378 \times \ln \text{bilirubin}) + (1.12 \times \ln \text{INR}) + 0.643] \times 10$

UKELD (UK model for end-stage liver disease)
$(5.395 \times \ln \text{INR}) + (1.485 \times \ln \text{creatinine}) + (3.13 \times \ln \text{bilirubin}) - (81.565 \times \ln \text{Na}) + 435$

Table 10.2 Interpretation of the MELD score

Score	Predicted mortality
>40	70%
30–39	50%
20–29	20%
10–19	6%
<9	2%

Morbidity associated with liver disease

Coagulation defects

The liver is responsible for production of fibrinogen and factors II, V, VII, IX, X and XI, as well as protein C, protein S and anti-thrombin. It therefore follows that in patients with liver disease, coagulation defects are common and these can also involve abnormalities in platelets and hyperfibrinolysis, in addition to reduced synthesis of the above clotting factors. The liver produces these factors in excess and in advance, so that a reduction in synthesis and inability to maintain normal haemostasis is usually a late and severe sign of hepatic impairment.

Ascites

Ascites develops as a result of advanced liver disease (low albumin and abnormalities in sodium handling) and portal hypertension. The fluid is a transudate being low in protein in comparison to malignant or inflammatory ascites, which is an exudate. The presence of ascites not only indicates severity of disease, but also poses a risk to post-operative healing, which can lead to the development of bowel herniation. Ascitic fluid results in an increased risk of sepsis, fluid shifts, abdominal wall splinting and in extreme untreated cases, compartment syndrome. Judicious use of diuretics pre-operatively and paracentesis, with appropriate intravascular replacement using 20% human albumin solution (HAS) needs to be instigated prior to surgery. Diuretics need to be given cautiously as their use in patients with liver disease can lead to renal dysfunction. Spironolactone is used as this inhibits aldosterone which contributes to sodium reabsorption and hence water retention. A measurement of portal pressure should be performed prior to undertaking surgery in patients with cirrhosis as this is an accurate predictor of post-operative liver dysfunction. Normal pressure is <10 mmHg. Most units will not operate on patients with pressures in excess of 20 mmHg as the incidence of acute hepatic dysfunction is >50% with a risk of death as a result of acute on chronic liver failure.

Encephalopathy

Encephalopathy arises as a result of the inability of the liver to metabolise and excrete waste products. The main culprits appear to be products such as ammonia, mercaptopurines and GABA. Encephalopathy can be worsened by procedures such as trans-jugular intra-hepatic porto-systemic shunt (TIPSS), which results in hepatic portal vein blood bypassing the liver with little clearance of waste products from the gut. Management includes antibiotics (recently the use of rifaximine has improved the success rate of both treatment and prophylaxis) and laxatives to reduce intestinal ammonia production and absorption, reduced protein intake and the use of probiotics to alter colonic flora. Patients who have a history of encephalopathy pre-operatively need a minimum of HDU care in the immediate post-operative period. The development of encephalopathy in the immediate post-operative phase is concerning as it may indicate the development of acute on chronic liver failure.

Obstructive jaundice

This is associated with an increase in peri-operative complications primarily because of endotoxaemia resulting from translocation of gut pathogens. The complications include renal failure, infection, coagulation defects and poor wound healing. Predictive indicators of post-operative mortality have been shown to be a pre-operative serum bilirubin >11 mg/dl, haematocrit less than 30% and a malignant cause of obstruction. Patients who are jaundiced should if at all possible have the biliary system decompressed prior to surgery, usually by percutaneous transhepatic cholangiographic (PTC) insertion of drains into the biliary tree.

One of the reasons for deranged clotting is that biliary obstruction results in vitamin K deficiency owing to it being a fat-soluble vitamin, which requires the presence of bile salts for absorption. Vitamin K deficiency results in reduced production of factors II, VII, IX and X. All patients who are jaundiced at the time of surgery must have a pro-thrombin time (PT) checked and be given intravenous vitamin K, and fresh frozen plasma if the PT is deranged.

Severely jaundiced patients are also at risk of renal dysfunction (see below) and consideration should be given to ensuring adequate hydration prior to surgery. Pre-operative fasting can be detrimental in such patients, who should have intravenous access established and background crystalloid infusion commenced prior to being made nil by mouth. Previously there was widespread use of intra-operative mannitol to induce a diuresis but it is now reserved for patients whose urine output falls during the surgical procedure.

Anaesthesia and hepatic insult

Anaesthetic volatile gases have been shown to induce or contribute to post-operative liver dysfunction. There is a correlation with incidence and degree of hepatic metabolism of these agents; halothane has the greatest degree of hepatic metabolism and the highest incidence of induced hepatitis (>500 cases in the USA). Desflurane, with the least hepatic metabolism, has the lowest incidence (<1), although caution needs to be applied given its relatively recent introduction in comparison to the other volatile agents. Overall, anaesthetic agents are a rare cause of hepatic dysfunction post-surgery and other more common causes should always be excluded.

Vasodilation and hyperdynamic circulation

Patients with advanced cirrhosis often have a hyperdynamic circulation with bounding pulses and flushed extremities. Peripheral vasodilation occurs because of a variety of vasodilators including nitrous oxide being released and leads to raised cardiac output, increased blood flow in the limbs and reduced flow to the kidneys and brain. The reduced renal blood flow and effective reduced blood volume leads to sodium and water retention by activation of the renin–angiotensin system and contributes to the development of ascites (see above). Anaesthesia needs to take account of the relative low intravascular fluid volumes; CVP measurements may be helpful to guide fluid replacement and the use of invasive monitoring for patients with liver disease is more frequently employed, even in procedures in which it would not be usually considered necessary (for healthy patients).

Hepato-pulmonary syndrome

This occurs in patients with advanced chronic liver disease and results in arterial hypoxaemia in the absence of primary cardiopulmonary disease. It is characterised by an alveolar–arterial gradient greater than 15 mmHg and is caused by intra-pulmonary arteriovenous shunting owing to the development of arteriolar-venous fistulae with dilatation of the peripheral pulmonary arterial vasculature. Patients are dyspnoeic, which is characteristically worse on standing rather than lying because of increased right to left shunting when upright. Rarely, in advanced cases large vessel shunts can occur which result in the patient becoming cyanosed and often requiring home oxygen administration. There is no effective treatment for this apart from liver transplantation, which results in the closing of the shunts and reversal of the hypoxaemia in the majority of patients.

A small number of patients who are hypoxic without evidence of pulmonary vasculature dilatation may have developed pulmonary hypertension, which occurs in about 2% of patients with portal hypertension, whether hepatic or extra-hepatic in origin. This may occur as a complication of the general hyperdynamic circulation seen in cirrhotic patients. Extreme care should be taken with these patients undergoing any type of surgery as they are at risk of intra-operative acute right ventricular failure with an associated high mortality.

Hepato-renal syndrome

This is a reversible condition associated with severe liver disease resulting in progressive renal failure. It is characterised by intense renal vasoconstriction on the background of an otherwise high-output vasodilated state. There is no evidence of primary renal pathology, renal biopsies show essentially normal histology, and the process is a complex functional response to a variety of physiological abnormalities rather than structural damage to the kidneys. The aetiology is complex and likely related to a number of factors including reduced renal blood flow as a result of the hyperdynamic circulation (see above) and bacteraemia because of the increased permeability of the gut mucosa causing vasoconstriction and reduced glomerular blood flow. Patients with apparently normal renal function pre-operatively may develop problems in the post-operative period as a result of relative dehydration during the pre-operative period and are more sensitive to hypotension developing during the procedure because of operative blood loss. Pre-hydration should be considered in all patients with advanced chronic liver disease.

Specific surgical procedures

Hepatic resection

The commonest indication for hepatic resection is for the treatment of colorectal hepatic metastases. Other indications are for primary tumours, both benign and malignant, neuroendocrine metastases and trauma. At present in the UK, there are a few centres that undertake live donor liver resection for transplantation but this is relatively rare.

Resection can be either an anatomical resection (functional segments or entire lobectomy) or non-anatomical wedge resections. The implication of the latter is that liver parenchyma is disrupted as no plane is followed and this type of resection can be associated with greater blood loss. However the advantage is that less liver volume is usually removed, which is important in patients with cirrhosis and impaired function, who need to lose as little functioning tissue as possible.

Following the procedure it is important to make an assessment of liver function, which is dependent upon the volume of liver removed, presence of pre-existing liver disease and biliary tract pathology. Intra-operatively, this will also be influenced by hepatic ischaemic insult and blood loss.

Hepatic ischaemia can be a result of blood loss and hypovolaemia but also because of manipulation of the liver intra-operatively. Blood loss can be significantly reduced during resection by temporary occlusion of the blood supply to the liver. There are a number of manoeuvres described, the commonest being the Pringle which consists of occlusion of the porta hepatis with a soft clamp, preventing both arterial and portal inflow of the portal vein and hepatic artery respectively. However, while reducing the blood flow into the liver, and therefore blood loss, it causes liver ischaemia, a reduction in cardiac output and an increase in left ventricular afterload with potential cardiac compromise. When the occlusion is released, there is the potential for a reperfusion injury, manifested by the reduction in cardiac function, blood pressure and potential arrhythmias. This is because of the release of potassium, inflammatory and oxidative mediators from the ischaemic hepatocytes, which have a profound effect on the myocardium. It is imperative that there is good communication between surgeon and anaesthetist, with the onset and release of every manoeuvre communicated. Management of reperfusion injury is primarily by the use of fluids, vasoactive drugs (e.g. metaraminol and noradrenaline) and calcium. Total time for occlusion should not exceed 15 to 20 minutes without a clamp-free period. It has recently been suggested that it should be avoided in hepatectomies for cancer patients because of its side effects on tumour recurrence and worse prognosis. Many surgeons only use it in situations where there is significant uncontrolled bleeding, preferring to isolate the segment or lobe being resected prior to parenchymal dissection by tying the relevant hepatic artery and portal vein. However this obviously does not apply to non-anatomical resections.

Another method for reducing blood loss is to reduce central venous pressure during the parenchymal dissection to reduce back bleeding from hepatic veins and their branches. This can be achieved by using vaso-dilators such as glyceryl trinitrate and sodium nitroprusside and judicious use of intra-operative fluids. This is not universal practice. Many centres feel the risk of renal dysfunction is too great and that careful surgical technique and the use of argon diathermy and the cavitron ultrasonic aspirator (CUSA) reduces the amount of blood loss.

Cholecystectomy

The commonest approach to cholecystectomy is laparoscopic. This circumvents the need for a painful right sub-costal abdominal or upper mid-line incision and the inherent problems these are associated with. However, the laparoscopic approach is not without issue. Inadvertent insertion of the trocars into a blood vessel or viscera can result in major haemorrhage and potential gas embolism if CO_2 is inadvertently insufflated. As mentioned before, the risk of this occurring is raised in patients with portal hypertension and recanalisation of the umbilical vein. The pneumoperitoneum results in splinting of the diaphragm and an increase in intrapulmonary ventilation pressures is required to achieve and maintain a reasonable tidal volume. The insufflated CO_2 is absorbed by the blood (CO_2 is 20 times more soluble in blood than O_2) and the patient frequently becomes hypercapnic, requiring increased ventilation to prevent the development of a respiratory acidosis. The pneumoperitoneum also reduces venous return, and therefore cardiac output. It is important to have a balance between high intra-abdominal pressures for surgical access and the risk of pulmonary or cardiac complication. This is of particular importance in patients with pre-existing cardiopulmonary co-morbidity.

Post-operatively, the majority of patients (ASA 1–2) can go home within 23 hours. One troublesome complication is shoulder tip pain, because of diaphragmatic irritation. This pain can be reduced by removing as much CO_2 as possible at the end of the procedure.

An open procedure often causes considerable pain on inspiration, which can lead to shallow, inadequate tidal ventilation and subsequent respiratory compromise. Patients require good post-operative analgesia, frequently provided by regional anaesthetic techniques, circumventing the use of opioids, which may worsen the respiratory compromise. As the incision is unilateral and upper abdominal, the techniques used can include intrapleural block/catheter or intercostal blocks. These blocks can produce targeted unilateral dermatomal loss of sensation, with minimal cardiovascular/respiratory sequelae. Severe pain can also be treated with an epidural. Occasionally, a drain is sited for 24 hours post-operatively, which may add to the discomfort.

Whipples resection

A Whipples resection consists of a pancreatico-duodenectomy, followed by anastomosis of the pancreas, liver and stomach to the jejunum using a Roux-En-Y procedure. This is primarily carried out for pancreatic or ampullary carcinoma. The procedure carries a high-risk of post-operative complications, which include anastomotic break down, bile and pancreatic leak and respiratory compromise. Patients with diabetes need good glycaemic control peri-operatively, with vigilance that continues into the post-operative period. Patients who are not diabetic prior to surgery have no increased incidence of diabetes post-operatively.

Intra-operative monitoring consists of arterial and central venous pressure lines. The procedure results in large fluid volume shifts and it is important to ensure that over-zealous fluid administration does not occur. Patients who have received excessive fluid replacement intra-operatively can develop respiratory compromise in the post-operative period. There is still debate regarding the best form of analgesic control. The authors favour epidurals as first-line pain management, but the evidence for improvement in mortality and morbidity remains uncertain.

Patients need to be nursed in a high-dependency unit/area with close monitoring to detect any evidence of complications. In the immediate post-operative period the main complication is significant post-operative bleeding requiring urgent return to theatre. Later complications include chest infections and anastomotic breakdown (most commonly the pancreatico-enteric anastomosis), which classically occurs around day seven to ten after surgery. There is debate regarding the long-term use of drains in these patients; however, the presence of amylase-rich fluid from the abdomen and signs of sepsis (tachycardia, pyrexia, increased respiratory rate, or hypocapnia, and leucocytosis or leucopoenia) must always raise suspicion of anastomotic breakdown. Management is dependent on imaging results and patient condition. Drainage of the collection, antibiotics and continuation of octreotide (which inhibits pancreatic exocrine secretion) may suffice. However, evidence of haemorrhage, uncontrollable fistula and the degree of retroperitoneal damage caused by inflammation will dictate surgical intervention.

Transjugular intrahepatic portal shunt (TIPS)

This is the formation of a portal–systemic connection bypassing the liver to decompress the vascular system and alleviate variceal bleeding and formation of ascites. Although potentially possible under local, this procedure is usually carried out under general anaesthesia because of potential complications, difficulty and duration of procedure. This procedure is undertaken, by definition, in the sickest group of patients, who are awaiting transplantation or for control of severe symptoms. They are at increased risk of encephalopathy post-procedure and need to be nursed in an HDU/ITU environment post-operatively until stable. Complications include pneumothorax, vascular perforation and bleeding, hepatic capsular tear, arrhythmias (intracardiac passage of catheter) and congestive cardiac failure. This last is a result of the blood flow bypassing the liver straight into the systemic circulation and the subsequent increase in venous return. The interventional radiologist usually carries out these cases, within the angiography suite. This raises the challenge of a complex, high-risk case being carried out in a remote setting which may not have all the equipment the anaesthetic team are used to in the theatre environment. It is therefore vital that all involved are aware of the potential complications and the anaesthetic team are familiar with their surroundings.

Surgical porto-systemic shunts

These procedures have largely been replaced by the ability to bypass the liver radiologically (TIPS, see above), but are still occasionally performed when TIPS placement is contraindicated or has failed. The surgical procedure is the formation of a direct connection between the portal and systemic venous systems often using a PTFE graft. Porto-caval and meso-caval shunts are the commonest performed as well as spleno-renal shunts between the splenic and renal veins. Porto-caval shunts can be performed by disconnecting the portal vein completely from the liver and anastomosing it to the side of the IVC rather than using a graft.

Whichever shunt is utilised, the procedure is usually performed as an emergency in the context of current or recent significant variceal haemorrhage as a result of portal hypertension, and therefore the patients are very unstable with a high risk of significant mortality and morbidity. Blood loss can be considerable before the shunt is established and the use of a cell saver should be considered. Such patients are often in established acute renal failure or at significant risk of developing renal failure and it may be necessary to perform haemofiltration continuously during the procedure.

Post-operative management

Patients requiring major hepato-pancreato biliary surgery undergo a massive intra-operative physiological insult, on a background of altered haemodynamics and multiple organ physiological derangement. The vast majority of these patients will require high dependency or intensive care in the first post-operative days.

Specific attention needs to be paid to:

1. Support of already failing organs
2. Identifying and supporting organs that require temporary support in the immediate post-operative period. These are organ systems that are most sensitive to the stress of surgery and include the lungs, heart, brain, kidneys and haematological systems
3. Fluid balance and fluid replacement, avoiding iatrogenic hypo- or hypernatraemia
4. Nutrition – with adequate replacement while avoiding nitrogen overload
5. Glucose control
6. Analgesia

Summary

Liver surgery tests the knowledge and skills of anaesthetists. The patients for most surgical procedures (except elective cholecystectomy) are often presenting in extremes of physiology, and are difficult to manage in the peri-operative period. Excessive blood loss is not uncommon during liver surgery and therefore management of coagulation and careful monitoring of cardio-respiratory parameters are important for best outcomes of the surgical patients. A team-based approach to post-operative care, including analgesia and nutrition, leads to the greatest chance of a smooth recovery.

Chapter 11

Endocrine cases

Pete Hambly and Radu Mihai

Introduction

Endocrine surgery is predominantly focused on the surgery of the thyroid, parathyroid and adrenal glands. The care of patients with the rare endocrine pancreatic tumours and neuroendocrine tumours (carcinoids) is divided between endocrine surgeons, pancreatic surgeons and liver surgeons, based on the local expertise available in individual centres. Pituitary and testicular tumours are outside the remit of this chapter as they are dealt with by neurosurgeons and urologists, respectively.

For all conditions discussed in this chapter, the management of the patient has to follow the sequence described in Figure 11.1. History and clinical examination remain the cornerstone of an accurate diagnosis. For example, observing the subtle signs of Cushing's syndrome will allow the astute clinician to consider this diagnosis in patients previously labelled as obese and depressed. Listening to the description of recurrent 'attacks' might trigger appropriate tests for phaeochromocytoma in patients who were previously treated for anxiety or primary hypertension. The combination of fatigue, depression, insomnia, abdominal discomfort, joint pains and nocturia might be dismissed as normal ageing but should raise the suspicion of hypercalcaemia of primary hyperparathyroidism.

In the context of a suggestive clinical scenario one needs to understand what biochemical tests are necessary for confirming/excluding the diagnosis. Only when the biochemistry is conclusive should one proceed to imaging studies to localise the endocrine tumour. Negative imaging does not exclude the diagnosis of an endocrine disease – for example, at least a third of patients with primary hyperparathyroidism have negative scans and the majority of patients with primary hyperaldosteronism might have no convincing abnormalities on a CT scan of the adrenal glands.

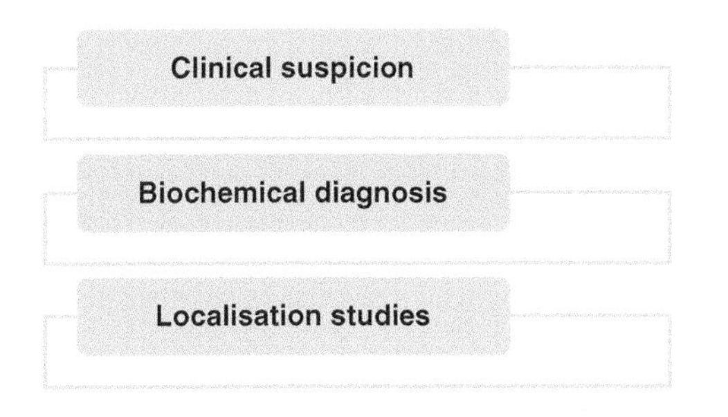

Figure 11.1 Management algorithm for patients with endocrine conditions.

A Surgeon's Guide to Anaesthesia and Peri-operative Care, ed. Jane Sturgess, Justin Davies and Kamen Valchanov. Published by Cambridge University Press.

Thyroid surgery

Thyroid surgery is the most common operation performed by endocrine surgeons. The national audit maintained by the *British Association of Endocrine and Thyroid Surgeons* (BAETS) has published data on thyroidectomies performed by over 140 UK surgeons of whom the majority perform less than 30 operations per year and only a small minority perform in excess of 100 per year. The number of operations undertaken by surgeons not registered with the BAETS might be twice as much.

Depending on the indication for surgery, patients need different operations (Table 11.1). Subtotal thyroidectomy is considered obsolete.

Pre-operative assessment for thyroid surgery

The following parameters need to be assessed in the pre-operative work-up:

1. ***Thyroid function tests (TFTs).*** All patients referred for thyroid surgery need to have TFTs checked (Table 11.2). Routinely these include measurement of TSH and free T4.

Sub-clinical hypothyroidism (i.e. raised TSH in the presence of fT4 in the normal range) is commonly seen in the general population and does not increase the risk of an anaesthetic/operation. Patients with severe hypothyroidism should start thyroxine replacement with the aim of normalising TFTs before proceeding with the planned operation.

Hyperthyroidism needs to be corrected pre-operatively as an operation on a patient with thyrotoxicosis can trigger a thyrotoxic crisis. This is an acute, life-threatening, hypermetabolic state induced by excessive release of thyroid hormone. In patients with uncontrolled hyperthyroidism, it can be precipitated by any form of surgery, as well as trauma or an unrelated acute illness.

Table 11.1 Type of thyroid operations and their indications

Extent of thyroid surgery	Indications
Total thyroidectomy	Graves' disease, multinodular goitre, thyroid cancer
Thyroid lobectomy	Thyroid nodules with biopsy suggestive of follicular neoplasm Asymmetric multinodular goitre Large hot nodules (Plummers' adenoma, > 3 cm)
Isthmusectomy	Small nodules in the isthmus

Table 11.2 Possible results of thyroid function tests and their interpretation. f = free

	Low TSH	Normal TSH	High TSH
Low free T4	Administration of T3 (e.g. in the period before radioactive iodine ablation)		HYPOTHYROIDISM (e.g. Hashimoto thyroiditis)
Normal fT4	Early response to carbimazole (when T4 decreases and TSH is yet to normalise)	EUTHYROID	Sub-clinical hypothyroidism
High fT4	HYPERTHYROIDISM		Pituitary adenoma secreting TSH

2. ***Calcitonin measurement.*** The pre-operative diagnosis of medullary thyroid carcinoma (MTC) relies on cytological features on the needle aspiration biopsy of a thyroid nodule. Because this cytological diagnosis remains challenging, some advocate the routine measurement of calcitonin in all patients with thyroid nodules. Others quote its high false negative rate (i.e. patents with a minimal/moderate rise in calcitonin because of thyroiditis).

In patients with known MTC, calcitonin levels govern the extent of the operation. It is considered that calcitonin <100 pg/ml is associated with disease limited to the thyroid, <200 pg/ml is common when lymph node metastases are limited to central compartment, <500 pg/ml is likely to involve only ipsilateral lateral neck, up to 1000 pg/ml will occur in patients with disease limited to the cervical area and over 2–10,000 pg/ml are associated with widespread metastatic disease. Based on these values a rational decision can be made about the extent of the operation needed for such patients: total thyroidectomy ± ipsilateral or bilateral central compartment dissection ± ipsilateral or bilateral lateral radical neck dissection.

Patients with raised calcitonin levels should have pre-operative 24-hour urine metanephrine measurement to exclude the presence of an associated phaeochromocytoma, as could be the case in familial MEN2 syndrome.

3. ***Anatomical considerations.*** In the presence of obstructive symptoms or if there is clinical suspicion of retrosternal extension of a cervical goitre (patients with positive Pemberton sign) assessment of the extent of the goitre and the severity of tracheal compression is best achieved with CT scan (Figure 11.2). The information required is:

- minimum tracheal diameter (critical if < 5 mm)
- point of maximum tracheal compression (obstruction immediately under the larynx might create additional difficulties for tracheal intubation)
- position of the lower limit of the intra-thoracic goitre in relation to the aortic arch. Generally, goitres above the aortic arch can be removed through a cervical incision, goitres behind the aortic arch may be removed through a cervical incision and goitres distal to the aortic arch will require sternotomy
- the 'shape' of the goitre, i.e. the change in diameter of the goitre at the transition between the neck and the mediastinum, the classical description being that 'carrots' are much easier removed than 'pears'.

4. ***Airway assessment.*** Respiratory function tests (flow loops) are indicated when the respiratory symptoms are excessive, to distinguish between upper airway obstruction (as expected from the goitre) and an associated lung pathology (Figure 11.3).

5. ***Vocal cord function.*** Recent BAETS guidelines encourage routine pre- and post-operative assessment of vocal cord movement through flexible laryngoscopy. Some patients might have asymptomatic unilateral vocal cord palsy (i.e. with no associated voice changes) and being aware of this diagnosis can influence the decision about the extent of the operation. Vocal cord palsy in the presence of a thyroid nodule is suggestive of malignancy.

6. ***Assessment of eye disease.*** Graves ophthalmopathy is caused by an autoimmune process which triggers infiltration of extraocular muscles whose increased volume creates increased intraorbital pressure and leads to protrusion of the eye globes. The presence of periorbital

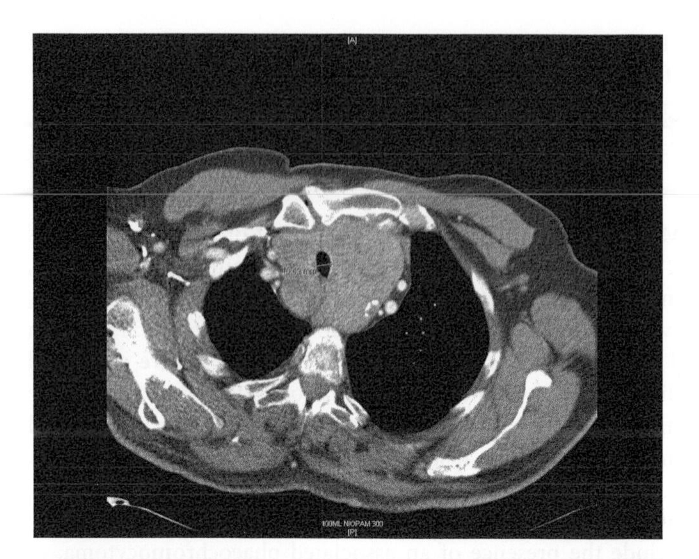

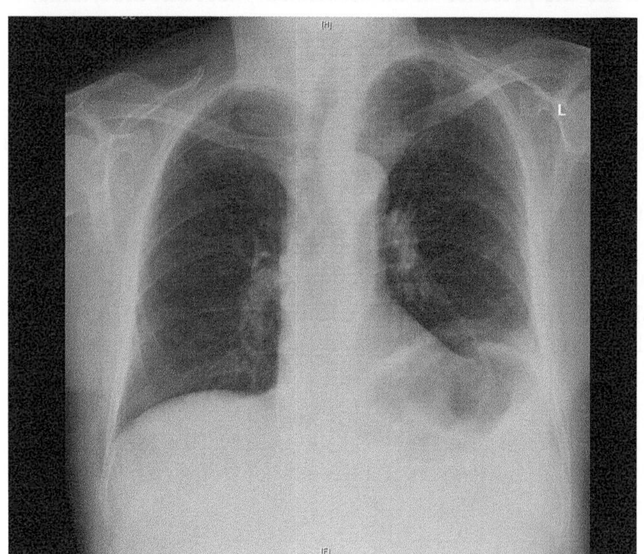

Figure 11.2 (a) CT showing a retrosternal multinodular goitre encircling the trachea and causing tracheal compression. (b) CXR demonstrating an upper mediastinal soft tissue mass displacing the trachea to the right.

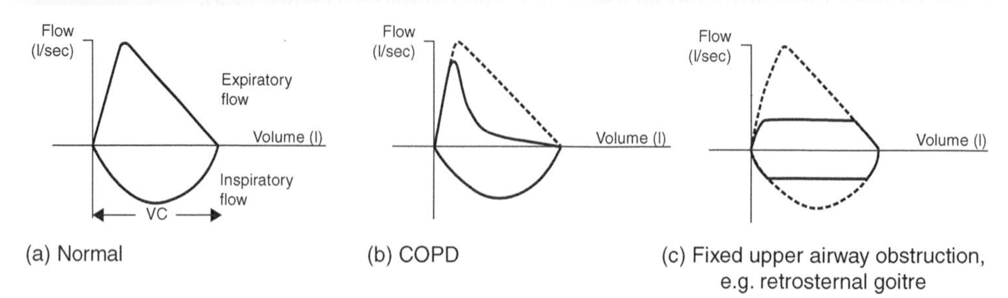

Figure 11.3 Flow volume loops. (a) Normal, (b) COPD, (c) Fixed upper airway obstruction, e.g. retrosternal goitre with tracheal compression.

oedema, chemosis, upper lid retraction, lid lag, difficulties in eye movement and extent of the protrusion of each eye globe should be noted.

7. ***Genetic tests***. RET gene mutation analysis is important in patients with MEN2 syndrome because there is a proven phenotype–genotype correlation, based on which clinicians can advise the age at which a child should undergo prophylactic thyroidectomy with the aim of avoiding the development of medullary thyroid carcinoma.

8. ***Anaesthetic assessment before thyroidectomy***:

a. Airway. Careful airway assessment is essential. Difficult intubation can be anticipated in approximately 6% of thyroid surgery patients. The incidence is much higher in malignant goitre. Presence of stridor or dyspnoea on lying flat should be noted. CT images should be reviewed for tracheal compression (minimum diameter and point of compression).

b. Endocrine status. In all but extreme circumstances, the patient should be euthyroid before surgery. Surgery in the presence of hyperthyroidism is associated with increased gland vascularity and the risk of thyroid storm. Hypothyroidism is associated with depressed myocardial function, hypothermia, sensitivity to anaesthetic agents, respiratory impairment, accelerated coronary artery disease and hyponatraemia. Adequate correction of significant hypothyroidism can take weeks or months, and attempts at rapid correction with intravenous thyroid hormone can precipitate myocardial ischaemia. Where surgery in the presence of hypothyroidism is deemed necessary, treatment with intravenous hydrocortisone has been advocated.

Intra-operative care during thyroidectomy

Anaesthetic technique for thyroidectomy

a. Regional anaesthesia. It is possible to carry out thyroidectomy without general anaesthesia, though this is rarely performed in the UK. Techniques include combined superficial/deep cervical plexus block, or cervical epidural anaesthesia. Both of these carry significant hazards, and close monitoring is essential. It is not our practice to offer 'awake thyroidectomy'.

b. General anaesthesia.

- GA with intravenous induction is the commonest technique. Endotracheal intubation with a reinforced tube is usual. The size of tube should take into account any tracheal compression observed on CT. Tubes are available with built-in electrodes to facilitate intra-operative laryngeal nerve monitoring.
- The laryngeal mask airway (LMA) has been used successfully in thyroidectomy, and has the advantage of allowing vocal cord movement to be observed directly during surgery. The LMA does not provide as secure an airway as an endotracheal tube, however, and this technique requires careful patient selection.
- For patients in whom difficult intubation is anticipated, awake fibre-optic intubation may be preferred. Patients with stridor can be managed by inhalational induction with sevoflurane.

c. Bilateral superficial cervical plexus block provides safe and effective post-operative analgesia.

d. Eye protection with tape, pads and/or lubricant is important, especially in the presence of exophthalmos.
e. Invasive monitoring is not routinely employed, though advisable in high-risk patients or where prolonged or difficult surgery is anticipated.
f. Dexamethasone 8 mg i.v. given intra-operatively reduces laryngeal oedema and post-operative nausea and vomiting.
g. Avoidance of neuromuscular blockade (apart from an initial intubation dose) is often required to allow intra-operative recurrent laryngeal nerve (RLN) monitoring. Remifentanil infusions are rapidly becoming the standard alternative to muscle relaxants, providing excellent operating conditions, reliable suppression of laryngeal reflexes and rapid post-operative recovery.

Thyroidectomy – post-operative care

Most patients can be managed in a standard recovery area, followed by overnight observation on a general ward. Admission to ICU is seldom indicated unless there is concern related to the patency of the airway.

On return from theatre, patients are allowed to drink clear fluids and observed for signs of possible aspiration (suggestive of RLN injury). Normal oral intake is allowed by the evening of the operation. Thyroid hormone replacement is initiated before discharge: thyroxine is prescribed to all patients in a dose dependent on their body weight (100–150 mcg/day), with the exception of patients with thyroid cancer who are started on liothyronine (20 mcg tds).

Transient hypocalcaemia may occur in up to 20% of patients post-operatively, because of inadvertent damage/excision of parathyroid glands. Symptoms of hypocalcaemia include perioral tingling, twitching, tetany, seizures and ventricular dysrhythmias. In some units routine oral calcium replacement is started in all patients while other clinicians use biochemical assessment to identify those at risk of hypocalcaemia (the rate of change of calcium levels post-operatively, the rise in phosphate and/or the concentration of PTH at 4–24 hours post-operatively). In cases of severe hypocalcaemia (serum calcium $<$ 1.8 mmol/l) intravenous calcium gluconate is indicated (10 ml of 10% solution).

Thyroidectomy is associated with a number of post-operative complications, which although rare, may be life-threatening. For this reason, day-case thyroidectomy is declining in popularity and overnight admission is the routine policy in most units.

Post-operative complications

i. ***Haemorrhage.*** This causes tense swelling in the neck and can lead to airway obstruction, because of laryngeal oedema resulting from impaired venous drainage in the presence of a tense haematoma in the central compartment. Management includes release of wound stitches (or staples) and evacuation of the clot, at the bedside if necessary, followed by re-exploration in theatre under GA.
ii. ***Tracheomalacia.*** This is a condition where erosion of tracheal cartilages by a large chronic or malignant goitre leads to flaccidity, and tracheal collapse during inspiration. It is extremely rare in the UK. It presents with airway obstruction and requires immediate reintubation. Tracheostomy is to be avoided in such cases unless the problem

persists after initial conservative management or unless the cause of airway compromise is found to be an unrecognised bilateral injury to the recurrent laryngeal nerves.

iii. ***Recurrent laryngeal nerve (RLN) palsy.*** Acute unilateral RLN palsy presents with hoarseness and difficulties with swallowing/aspiration. It rarely threatens the airway, though a chronic palsy combined with laryngeal oedema can occasionally cause airway compromise. Bilateral RLN palsy can cause stridor and may require reintubation.

iv. ***Pain.*** Pain after thyroidectomy is mild, particularly when bilateral cervical plexus blocks are performed pre-operatively. Sore throat and neck stiffness from positioning are usually more troublesome than the surgical incision. Paracetamol and NSAIDs are usually sufficient.

v. ***Hypocalcaemia.*** Permanent hypoparathyroidism is rare (5% incidence on the national BAETS audit). Long-term vitamin D and oral calcium supplements are indicated. It can take up to 12 months to observe a return of the parathyroid function, hence regular monitoring is necessary.

Parathyroid surgery

Primary hyperparathyroidism (PHPT) remains the commonest indication for parathyroid surgery. It is defined by the presence of hypercalcaemia associated with normal/raised PTH level in patients with normal renal function. It is caused by a single adenoma in the vast majority of patients (90%), while a small minority of patients would be found to have double adenomas and multigland disease. Parathyroid carcinoma is vanishingly rare.

Secondary hyperparathyroidism occurs in response to a biochemical stimulus that triggers multigland hyperplasia. The most common cause is renal insufficiency: raised phosphate levels, decreased levels of vitamin D (because of lack of renal 1α-hydroxylation), and abnormal expression of the calcium-sensing receptor on parathyroid cells all play a role in maintaining diffuse multigland hyperplasia.

Tertiary hyperparathyroidism occurs in a patient with a functioning renal transplant whose renal function has normalised but whose 'physiological' secondary hyperparathyroidism fails to resolve.

Pre-operative assessment for primary hyperparathyroidism

P1. Calcium levels. Hypercalcaemia is present in all patients and can be classified as minimal (<2.8 mmol/l), moderate (<3 mmol/l) or severe (>3.00 mmol/l). Extreme hypercalcaemia (>3.50–4.00 mmol/l) can lead to 'hypercalcaemic crisis', manifested by nausea and vomiting, polyuria, progressive dehydration and hypotonia, leading to hallucinations and coma.

Renal excretion of calcium is assessed in patients suspected of having familial hypocalciuric hypercalcaemia (FHH). In this condition, mutations in the calcium-sensing receptor lead to longstanding mild hypercalcaemia and multigland hyperplasia. The calcium/creatinine clearance ratio on a 24-h urine collection is <1%. Surgical treatment is not indicated for patients with FHH.

P2. PTH levels. PHPT is characterised by inappropriately raised PTH in the presence of a raised serum calcium. In other conditions associated with hypercalcaemia (e.g. metastatic bone disease, myeloma) PTH is inhibited or immeasurable. Current assays measure the concentration of intact molecules of PTH and are not affected by circulating fragments of PTH (whose concentration is raised in patients with renal failure).

P3. Localisation studies. The combination of Tc 99m sestamibi scintigraphy and neck ultrasound is used to localise parathyroid adenomas. When the results are concordant, patients can undergo minimally invasive parathyroidectomy with dissection of the adenoma identified by scans. When scans are negative or conflicting, patients undergo bilateral neck exploration with identification of all four parathyroid glands and resection of the enlarged one. In most centres, the scans are positive only in two-thirds of patients.

Other localisation studies, such as selective venous sampling, MRI or CT, are reserved for patients who have undergone failed surgical exploration.

P4. Anaesthetic assessment. Patients admitted with severe hypercalcaemia and acute symptoms should have calcium levels controlled using vigorous intravenous hydration with saline. Bisphosphonate therapy is indicated only when parathyroidectomy is not feasible. Those who are candidates for parathyroidectomy should have an urgent operation and should not receive bisphosphonates as they increase the risk of post-operative severe hypocalcaemia.

Hypercalcaemia leads to ECG changes (shortening of the QT interval and ST segment elevation), makes the threshold potential in the conducting pathways and contractile cells less negative (increasing cardiac excitability), decreases ventricular conduction velocity and shortens the refractory period. This combination of changes has been postulated to increase the risk of severe/life-threatening ventricular arrhythmias but in clinical practice the incidence of such arrhythmias is rare.

Associated co-morbidity should be sought and assessed. Parathyroid disease commonly co-exists with renal impairment, and may be a presenting feature of multiple endocrine neoplasia (MEN) syndromes especially Type I, which is also associated with tumours of the pituitary and pancreas.

Parathyroidectomy for primary hyperparathyroidism – intra-operative care

Minimally invasive parathyroidectomy for patients with positive concordant scans can be performed with a small incision (2 cm) over the affected gland. Superficial cervical plexus block and/or local infiltration, with or without sedation, are suitable techniques, though many surgeons still prefer general anaesthesia.

Bilateral neck exploration via a collar incision similar to that used for thyroidectomy is necessary for patients with negative scans or when there is no facility for localisation studies. Malignant disease is vanishingly rare and warrants en bloc neck dissection of the parathyroid tumours and ipsilateral thyroid lobectomy.

General anaesthesia is usually required for neck exploration. No one technique carries any particular advantage. Airway maintenance with endotracheal intubation or laryngeal mask airway are acceptable.

- A parathyroid adenoma can be difficult to locate, and operation time can be unpredictable. Warming devices and temperature monitoring are advisable. Maintenance of adequate hydration is essential.
- Methylene blue is sometime used to aid location. An intravenous infusion may be given after induction of anaesthesia. Methylene blue carries a significant incidence of allergic

reaction. It can also confuse a pulse oximeter, causing it to register an erroneously low oxygen saturation. Its use is less popular in recent years after reports of post-operative confusion and neurological deficits in patients treated with antidepressants.

Post-operative care for primary hyperparathyroidism

Measurement of PTH levels at one hour post-operatively is used to demonstrate biochemical cure (levels expected to be unmeasurable at 30–60 minutes after the excision of the overactive adenoma as the half-life of PTH is two to three minutes).

Most patients are discharged within six hours of their operation. Calcium supplements are prescribed to prevent post-operative hypocalcaemia, which is more common in patients with severe pre-operative hypercalcaemia, and in those with severe bone disease where alkaline phosphatase levels are greatly raised.

Calcium levels are rechecked at six weeks and 12 months post-operatively. Repeat bone densitometry (DEXA scan) is postponed for 12–18 months post-operatively because the positive impact on the bone health is slow to occur.

Adrenalectomy for cortical tumours

Functional adenomas derived from the adrenal cortex lead to eponymous syndromes caused by excess production of aldosterone (Conn's syndrome) or cortisol (Cushing's syndrome). Virilising adenomas are very rare.

Non-functional adenomas are frequently diagnosed as incidentalomas on scans performed for other indications.

Adrenocortical cancer is a very rare tumour, with an incidence of 1/million/year and its management raises challenges that are outside the remit of this chapter.

Pre-operative assessment for cortical adrenal tumours

A. ***Conn's syndrome***. The biochemical diagnosis of primary hyperaldosteronism (PHA) is based on the finding of a raised aldosterone/renin ratio in a hypertensive patient. Cross-sectional imaging is used to identify whether PHA is caused by unilateral adenoma. If a small adenoma (<2 cm) is visualised on one side in the presence of a normal contralateral gland many surgeons would proceed to adrenalectomy. Others consider that *selective adrenal venous sampling* should be performed in all patients, not only in those with negative scans. The test consists of measuring the aldosterone/cortisol ratio in blood samples taken from the IVC, left renal vein and right renal vein.

If present, hypokalaemia is corrected by the use of spironolactone and potassium supplements. Hypertension can be resistant to medical management.

B. ***Cushing's syndrome***. The standard biochemical investigation of suspected cortisol excess is the overnight *dexamethasone suppression test*, in which a 1 mg dose of dexamethasone is given at 11 pm, and cortisol levels are measured the following morning. In normal subjects, the cortisol levels are suppressed (below 50 mmol/l), and a failure of this suppression indicates autonomous cortisol production. This test will not distinguish between Cushing's syndrome caused by pituitary adenoma from other causes. A 48-hour high-dose dexamethasone suppression test (8 mg/day for two days) will cause cortisol production to decrease in patients with pituitary tumours but not in those with adrenal tumours or those with ectopic ACTH production from other malignant tumours.

Cross-sectional imaging will confirm the side of the adrenal tumour when biochemical testing demonstrates adrenal disease.

Patients with a unilateral adrenal adenoma are generally operated without the need for pharmacological treatment of the raised cortisol. In the presence of severe clinical signs, the cortisol synthesis inhibitor metyrapone can be used.

Intra-operative care for cortical adrenal tumours

Laparoscopic adrenalectomy is the technique of choice. Most surgeons use a transperitoneal approach though retroperitoneoscopic adrenalectomy is increasing in popularity in recent years.

For Conn's syndrome there are no specific concerns. For patients with Cushing's syndrome hydrocortisone should be administered intra-operatively (*see below*). Patients with Cushing's syndrome are at increased risk of venous thromboembolism and post-operative infections.

Post-operative care for cortical adrenal tumours

Patients with Conn's syndrome will stop the spironolactone and the potassium supplements used pre-operatively. Where multiple antihypertensive drugs have been used, these can be withdrawn gradually while the BP response is monitored closely. The likelihood of long-term cure of hypertension is higher in those with hypertension of $<$ six years duration, those who use no more than two drugs, in women and slim patients (BMI$<$25).

In Cushing's syndrome, an adrenal adenoma causes profound suppression of normal adrenal cortical activity as a result of inhibition of ACTH secretion. This inhibition persists after removal of the tumour, and patients require hydrocortisone replacement for up to 12 months post-operatively. Intravenous hydrocortisone 100 mg qds is used until oral intake is restarted. Oral hydrocortisone is started at high dose (20–20–10 mg) and tapered slowly towards the physiological dose (10–10–5 mg) within the following few months.

Adrenalectomy for phaeochromocytoma

Phaeochromocytoma (PHAEO) (meaning 'dusky-coloured tumour') is a catecholamine-secreting tumour arising from chromaffin cells in the adrenal medulla. Paragangliomas are similar tumours derived from extradrenal paraganglia of the sympathetic nervous system.

Patients present with a variety of symptoms including resistant hypertension, tachycardia, palpitations and anxiety. Some are discovered as an incidental finding on CT. The diagnosis is confirmed by demonstrating biochemical evidence of excessive catecholamine secretion. In recent years 24-hour urinary free metanephrine measurement has become the most reliable test. There appears to be no correlation between the magnitude of biochemical abnormalities and severity of cardiovascular effects. Historically, measurement of vanillyl mandelic acid (VMA) or urine or plasma free catecholamines were used but these assays are affected by the episodic secretion and carry a high false negative rate.

Pre-operative medical management for phaeochromocytomas

Once a diagnosis has been made, pharmacological treatment is started to control symptoms and prevent cardiovascular complications. Classically this is achieved with the alpha-blocker phenoxybenzamine, together with propranolol. Some advocate use of the selective alpha-1 blocker doxazosin as a single drug, as it lacks the side effects associated with the alpha-2 effects of phenoxybenzamine (nasal stuffiness, postural hypotension, somnolence).

Doses of medication that adequately control blood pressure and symptoms without excessive side effects, may provide insufficient protection from cardiovascular changes that occur during surgical manipulation. In the authors' unit, the practice is to admit patients a few days before surgery, to measure lying/standing pulse and blood pressure regularly, and titrate up the dose of medication towards the following end points:

- Controlled systolic BP, preferably ≤ 120 mmHg
- Significant postural drop
- Controlled heart rate, preferably ≤ 80 bpm
- No significant increase in HR on standing

Patients are likely to suffer side effects from the doses required to achieve this, indeed some use their presence as further reassurance that the patient is adequately blocked.

Intra-operative care for PHAEOs

- An anxiolytic premed is advisable and may contribute to cardiovascular stability.
- Invasive monitoring with arterial line and CVP is mandatory. Arterial monitoring should be set up before induction of anaesthesia.
- A range of antihypertensive agents should be available before induction. These vary according to taste but may include labetalol, magnesium, phentolamine, esmolol, metoprolol and sodium nitroprusside. The latter is a powerful vasodilator which has the advantage of not acting via adrenoreceptors.
- A variety of anaesthetic techniques are used and no evidence favours one over any other. The author uses total intravenous anaesthesia with propofol and remifentanil, as both these agents can be used to help control blood pressure surges, while also being relatively short-acting.
- A combination of general with epidural anaesthesia has been advocated, but is usually reserved for open adrenalectomy. A surge in blood pressure may occur on induction of anaesthesia.
- Tracheal intubation is usual, and may also be associated with hypertension.
- Phaeochromocytoma is associated with intravascular fluid depletion, though adequate pharmacological management should prevent this. Fluid requirements during surgery are usually modest.
- Surgical manipulation of the tumour, whether open or laparoscopic, is associated with release of catecholamine and surges of blood pressure. Antihypertensives should be given to treat, and ideally pre-empt, these surges. A pre-eminent concern is to prevent the cardiac and cerebrovascular complications that may result from extremes of blood pressure. It is usually possible to identify the moment the surgeon ligates the main adrenal vein, when blood pressure becomes almost immediately less labile.

Post-operative management for PHAEOs

After successful excision of a phaeochromocytoma, cardiovascular stability is usual. Somewhat surprisingly, the presence of high-dose alpha- and beta-blockade rarely leads to post-operative hypotension. In such cases, a period of post-operative vasopressor support may be required. Post-operative hypertension is rarer still, and may suggest undetected bilateral or extra-adrenal disease. Hypoglycaemia may occasionally occur in diabetics, as a result of the withdrawal of the anti-insulin effects of catecholamines.

An hour or two of invasive blood pressure monitoring in recovery is appropriate, after which patients can be discharged to a general ward. Management in ITU/HDU is rarely required.

Phenoxybenzamine (or doxazosin) can be stopped immediately post-operatively. Propranolol is usually weaned off over a period of days, to prevent rebound tachycardia.

Summary

Endocrine surgery remains a challenging multi-disciplinary medical specialty. It can offer curative surgery and excellent post-operative longevity. Endocrine patients require careful pre-operative investigations and assessment. Team working in the peri-operative settings and careful post-operative monitoring provide the best chance for uncomplicated recovery.

Further reading

http://www.baets.org.uk/guidelines/.

Chapter 12

Vascular cases

Fay Gilder and Paul Hayes

Of all elective surgical sub-specialties, vascular surgery is associated with the highest risk of death (5%). Because of the high incidence of co-morbidities (therefore increasing the baseline risk) among this patient group, patients must be carefully evaluated and informed of the risks and benefits. Although these patients do represent a high-risk group, the consequences of not undertaking an operation must also be considered. These consequences could include limb loss if bypass surgery is deferred, stroke when carotid endarterectomy is delayed and death from aortic rupture when aneurysms are not treated.

Pre-operative evaluation and preparation, intra- and post-operative care all play key roles in minimising risk to the patient. Vascular surgery can be approached through conventional open surgery or via a minimally invasive, endovascular route, and choosing the correct mode of intervention is key to a good result. Successful outcomes after vascular surgery are very much dependent on a multi-disciplinary team approach to care with the anaesthetist, surgeon and interventional radiologist (for endovascular procedures) all playing key roles.

Risk scoring

There are several well-validated guidelines and risk scores used to help inform the requirement for optimisation and to aid discussions with the patient about the risks and benefits of surgery.

The American College of Cardiology and American Heart Association (ACC AHA) guidelines incorporate the risk associated with the surgical procedure with the risk associated with patient co-morbidity (Lee's revised cardiac risk index, see Chapter 22) to guide both work-up and calculation of risk for each individual according to the proposed type of surgery. They are applied as follows:

1. Does the patient need emergency surgery (e.g. ruptured aortic aneurysm)? If 'yes' go to theatre and plan for peri-operative and post-operative risk factor management. If 'no' proceed to step 2.
2. Does the patient have any active cardiac conditions? (unstable coronary syndromes, severe valvular heart disease, decompensated cardiac failure, significant cardiac arrhythmias) – if 'yes' delay surgery for evaluation and treatment. If 'no' proceed to step 3.

A Surgeon's Guide to Anaesthesia and Peri-operative Care, ed. Jane Sturgess, Justin Davies and Kamen Valchanov. Published by Cambridge University Press.

3. Does the patient have a good functional capacity (>4 METs – see below) without symptoms? If yes – proceed to surgery. If no or unknown – proceed to step 4.
4. Does the patient have one or more clinical risk factors (history of – ischaemic heart disease, compensated or prior heart failure, cerebrovascular disease, co-existing diabetes mellitus, renal insufficiency). If yes – consider non-invasive cardiac stress testing and requesting a cardiology opinion to define the patient's cardiac status and peri-operative risk. If no proceed to surgery.

When deciding whether to investigate vascular surgery patients, the potential benefits that may be accrued (or not) through a lengthy series of tests must be weighed up against the cost of delaying treatment. Delaying treatment in a woman lady with an 8 cm abdominal aortic aneurysm (AAA) for six weeks carries around a 5% risk of mortality. Postponing a carotid endarterectomy in a symptomatic patient with a 70% stenosis for two weeks comes with a stroke risk of up to 10%. These risks may well be far greater than any benefit derived from the investigations and subsequent additional treatment required.

The other consideration when investigating patients is the impact of the additional treatment that may be needed. Many vascular patients will exhibit evidence of coronary artery disease if tested. Treatment of this comes with a risk of mortality, which is in addition to that posed by the vascular disorder. Additionally, treatments such as coronary artery stenting will necessitate the patient to continue on dual anti-platelet therapy for three to twelve months depending on the type of stent used, and this may complicate or delay the initial intended surgery further, particularly if an open surgical approach is being considered.

Surgical risk score

Surgery carries an associated risk of death or non-fatal MI. Vascular surgical procedures fall into either high (>5%) or intermediate risk surgery (1–5%). High-risk encompasses major open aortic surgery and complex peripheral vascular surgery in frail patients. Intermediate risk surgery includes endovascular aortic reconstruction (EVAR) and carotid endarterectomy. Surgical scoring systems exist that can calculate the mortality risk for a cohort of vascular surgical patients, but as yet there is no system that will reliably calculate an individual's risk.

The vascular patient

By definition these patients have atherosclerosis affecting all their arteries even if the condition has become overt in only one anatomical region. All organ systems (cardiac, renal, cerebral, splanchnic) should be regarded as having a compromised blood supply. Consequently pre-operative assessment should include careful evaluation of each organ system, where possible, in order to optimise the patient for surgery.

Risk factors for vascular disease include hypertension, hypercholesterolaemia, smoking, family history and diabetes.

Pre-operative evaluation

The most common cause of post-operative morbidity and mortality is pre-existing cardiovascular disease. History taking and physical examination must be targeted towards elucidating symptoms and signs of ischaemic heart disease, pulmonary disease and diabetes.

Systems enquiry must specifically include questioning for the presence of symptoms of heart failure, angina and symptoms of respiratory compromise. An estimate of functional status predicts the need for further investigation and so must be ascertained. A Duke's activity score of 4 metabolic equivalents (METs) or greater tends to predict lower risk. This is equivalent to climbing a flight of stairs without symptoms. Where effort tolerance is limited by claudication, cardiovascular stress testing (myocardial perfusion scanning (MIBI) or dobutamine stress echocardiography (DSE)) may be indicated if high-risk arterial surgery is being considered.

Physical examination of the cardiovascular system must include assessment of blood pressure, heart rate and rhythm, the presence of heart murmurs and auscultatory signs of heart failure. The presence or absence of all peripheral pulses should be documented, not forgetting to palpate the abdomen for an occult AAA. Examination of the respiratory system must include respiratory rate and effort, oxygen saturation and auscultation of the lungs.

Routine laboratory investigations will be guided by the history and examination. However all patients should have a full blood count and urea and electrolytes. HbA1C, arterial blood gases and liver function testing may also be necessary in higher-risk surgery. All patients should have a recent electrocardiogram (ECG).

If the patient has a functional status of less than 4 METs and is undergoing high-risk surgery, the need for further cardiac testing should be discussed with a cardiologist. Testing should only be performed where it will alter the planned management of the patient. For example if the intention is to go ahead with surgery and there is no time to act on the findings of further tests then the tests should not be done at all. However if the results of the test will influence whether or not the procedure should go ahead at all then the testing should occur.

Cardiopulmonary exercise testing is becoming incorporated into many centres' pre-operative assessment pathways. Currently published data do not support this practice. It adds to the cost of the patient's treatment and may well lead to them having a number of unnecessary additional investigations.

Pharmacotherapy

1. *Anti-platelet agents* – Aspirin and clopidogrel both irreversibly inhibit platelet aggregation. When used in secondary prevention, multiple studies have shown significantly improved outcomes in patients with vascular disease or risk factors for vascular disease. There is some evidence that clopidogrel may be more effective than aspirin for patients with peripheral vascular disease, although because of its pharmacogenetics this is not true of all patients. All vascular patients should be taking an anti-platelet agent.

   It is not unusual for some vascular patients to be on dual anti-platelet agents and this obviously increases the patient's potential for peri-operative bleeding. However, there may be a good reason for dual therapy, such as symptomatic carotid disease or recent coronary artery stenting. Carotid surgery is safe to perform with dual anti-platelets onboard, as is EVAR. Unless there are strong reasons for continuing both agents, most surgeons would stop clopidogrel before open aortic surgery. For peripheral arterial surgery a balance exists and it is often best to discuss with the surgical team. Should the patient require neuraxial block, clopidogrel must be stopped 5–7 days before surgery

(use local guidance). Continuing clopidogrel increases the risk of an epidural haematoma if the epidural vein is inadvertently pierced by the spinal/epidural needle. An epidural haematoma can cause spinal cord compression.
2. *Statins* – Statins reduce cholesterol by inhibiting HMG-CoA (3 hydroxy-3-methylglutaryl-coenzyme A) reductase, an enzyme that controls cholesterol production in the liver. By reducing cholesterol levels, statins reduce atherosclerotic plaque size and de novo formation. They are thought to contribute to plaque stabilisation and improve endothelial function. All patients with evidence of vascular disease should be considered for statin therapy.
3. *ACE inhibitors* – angiotensin converting enzyme (ACE) inhibitors are potent vasodilators and are used for the treatment of hypertension and heart failure. The mechanism of action of ACE inhibitors is incompletely understood. What is known is that effects attributable to the use of ACE inhibitors include reduced left ventricular stiffness, improved left ventricular systolic function, improved endothelial function and atherosclerotic plaque stabilisation. Guidelines suggest that this group of drugs should be considered in vascular surgery patients.
4. *Beta-blockers* – the peri-operative use of beta-blockers has been widely investigated and recently re-evaluated in light of the outcomes of the POISE study. Conventional wisdom suggests that beta-blockers should not be discontinued peri-operatively, and that starting beta-blockers should be considered in high-risk patients.

General principles of anaesthesia for patients undergoing vascular surgery

The majority of vascular surgical mortality is due to cardiovascular causes.

Myocardial ischaemia is provoked in circumstances where oxygen demand outstrips supply. All patients undergoing vascular surgery should be treated as if they have coronary artery disease and measures taken to limit provocation of ischaemia. Simply speaking this is achieved by maintaining a normotensive patient with a heart rate of between 55–70 bpm.

Anaesthetic manoeuvres provoking hypertension and tachycardia include intubation, extubation and inadequate anaesthesia at times of surgical stimulus. Post-operatively myocardial ischaemia is provoked by a cold, hypertensive, tachycardic, shivering patient in pain. Oxygen delivery is also affected by haemoglobin concentration, and vascular patients tolerate anaemia less well than other surgical patients. Those with known cardiac disease should be transfused if their Hb falls below 90 g/l.

Myocardial ischaemia and infarction most commonly occur within 72 hours of surgery. One of the contributory factors is the change in sleep pattern induced by anaesthesia – the ratio of rapid eye movement sleep (REM) (associated with hypertension and tachycardia) to non-REM sleep increases. The deleterious effect of change in sleep pattern can be ameliorated to some extent by the administration of low-flow oxygen (2 l/min via nasal cannulae) for three nights post-operatively.

Surgical stress and arterial injury both activate platelets, and so increase the risk of thrombotic events, leading to MI or stroke. For this reason, if it is felt necessary to stop anti-platelet agent peri-operatively, patients should have their platelet inhibition recommenced as soon as possible after surgery.

Surgery-specific considerations

Open aortic aneurysm repair

Open aortic aneurysm repair is major surgery, with an approximate 5% risk of death and myocardial infarction. Pre-operative assessment will optimise any co-existing disease and specifically identify active cardiac conditions that may require intervention prior to surgery.

The anaesthetic plan includes the use of invasive arterial and central venous pressure monitoring and the consideration of an epidural for post-operative pain control.

Intra-operative considerations

Induction: understanding the demands of the surgery is an essential part of the anaesthetist's practice and no more so than for AAA repair. Induction and maintenance necessitates careful attention to heart rate control and preservation of normotension.

Aortic cross-clamping – Overzealous administration of intravenous fluids can have deleterious effects on the heart (secondary to left atrial and/or ventricular distension) and may exaggerate the cardiovascular response to the aortic cross-clamp, when the infra-renal aorta is occluded to allow the AAA sac to be opened. At the time of aortic cross-clamping the patient's systemic vascular resistance increases significantly as the left ventricle contracts against the cross-clamp. It is this point that the patient is most likely to exhibit signs of coronary artery ischaemia because of left ventricular wall distension and consequent coronary artery insufficiency. In most cases this is responsive to the administration of a vasodilator (e.g. GTN, isoflurane) and/or a beta-blocker.

Opening of the aneurysmal sac – once cardiovascular stability has been restored, the surgeon will open the aneurysmal sac and significant bleeding because of the presence of lumbar collateral arteries will occur until the surgeon has managed to ligate them. The bleeding from these 'small' vessels can be surprisingly brisk. Surgeons will usually know from a pre-operative CT if these vessels are larger or more numerous than usual. Prompt fluid replacement and cell salvage is commonly used to reduce the need for homologous blood transfusion.

Release of the aortic cross clamp – reperfusion of the lower limbs is sequential with the surgeon releasing one iliac artery at a time. Hypertension at this point is not usually well tolerated by the surgeon, as aortic anastomoses may not be entirely 'water-tight' until the clotting system has had time to take effect. Cardiac instability (hypotension, myocardial ischaemia or infarction, dysrhythmias) may occur at this point secondary to haemorrhage from vascular anastomoses or to the deleterious effects of ischaemic metabolites on the heart and peripheral vasculature. In the absence of haemorrhage, hypotension responds well to a vasoconstrictor (e.g. metaraminol, ephedrine, epinephrine) but sometimes it is necessary to replace the aortic clamp. Many surgeons will simply constrict the aortic graft to allow a little flow to the lower limbs while maintaining a reasonable perfusion pressure above to the vital organs.

Post-operative care focuses on maintenance of cardiovascular stability, oxygenation and analgesia and is carried out in a high-dependency unit setting.

As EVAR has become more widespread, the complexity of open aortic surgery has increased because many of the straightforward cases are now treated endovascularly. It is common for the remaining patients having open aortic surgery to need the aortic cross-clamp placed above one or both renal arteries. This will lead to a variable period of renal ischaemia, and subsequent renal impairment. These patients need a high level of care post-operatively with a careful fluid balance. Care must be shown in those patients with an epidural in order to avoid hypotension and as such a reduction in renal perfusion pressure, accentuating the renal impairment. It is important to exclude haemorrhagic or cardiac causes of hypotension before attributing hypotension to the epidural block. The use of excess fluid administration as a way of maintaining post-operative blood pressure is not to be encouraged as these patients tip into cardiac failure with relative ease. If the renal ischaemia is prolonged then pre-emptive placement of a haemofiltration line in theatre is useful.

Endovascular aortic reconstruction (EVAR) for abdominal aortic aneurysms

This procedure is classified as intermediate risk. It is less invasive and far less perturbing to the cardiovascular system as the aorta is not cross-clamped or occluded for any significant length of time.

As is the case with all vascular patients, careful pre-operative assessment is required. These procedures can be carried out under local or general anaesthesia. The choice for an elective case is usually dictated by the anticipated length of the procedure, patient preference and local practice.

Anaesthetic plan – ventilation needs to be controlled (breath-holding for angiograms), invasive arterial monitoring is routinely placed and a large bore cannula is required in case of haemorrhage. Post-operative pain is mild because of the relatively superficial nature of the incisions.

Intra-operative considerations – the airway can be managed using a laryngeal mask airway (LMA) in suitable patients or an endotracheal tube (ETT). If an LMA is chosen it must provide a good enough seal to facilitate controlled ventilation. The advantage of an LMA is that it avoids the tachycardic and hypertensive responses associated with tracheal intubation and extubation.

Blood loss is usually less than 500 ml; however, there is a risk of arterial/aortic rupture by the device and should this happen blood loss is brisk and can be extensive. For that reason the placement of a large-bore intravenous cannula is prudent. The patient is most stimulated at the time of groin incision and wound closure. If the procedure is prolonged the reduction of arterial blood flow to the legs may induce ischaemic pain, although this is only a major issue during local anaesthesia. An intra-aortic balloon may be inflated, occluding the aorta temporarily, to seal the stent against the wall of the aorta or to seal the components of the stent. It is rare for this to cause significant adverse cardiovascular effects.

Post-operative care – is undertaken in an HDU setting for the first 12–24 hours. The patient is carefully observed for signs of renal insufficiency and cardiovascular compromise.

The ruptured abdominal aortic aneurysm

There are two surgical approaches to the management of a ruptured abdominal aortic aneurysm – open repair and EVAR. If the patient is stable and the anatomy of the aorta suitable an EVAR is the treatment of choice. The use of an endovascular approach under LA allows the aortic rupture to be sealed off, while the abdominal musculature helps to retain a degree of compression of the rupture site. It is also associated with far less physiological stress, which is an important consideration in these already unstable patients.

In cases where the anatomy is unsuitable, or expertise is not available for EVAR, the aneurysm is repaired as an open procedure. Open repair is associated with an approximate 50% mortality. The patient should be reviewed for fitness to proceed as soon as possible by the anaesthetist and preparations made for an open repair even if an EVAR is anticipated. The prime concern is to get the aortic leak controlled as soon as possible. Prior to commencing surgery the following anaesthetic resources are necessary: two anaesthetic assistants, two anaesthetists – one a vascular anaesthetist if possible, blood components and transfusion on standby, fluid warmer, forced air warmer, rapid infusion equipment, a cell saver and a theatre team who are prepared. The ITU needs to be forewarned.

Anaesthetic considerations – standard anaesthetic monitoring, preparedness for haemorrhage and coagulopathy, patient warming (patients can get very cold in emergency department resuscitation areas and hypothermia impairs coagulation), two large-bore cannulae.

Intra-operative considerations – EVAR – performed under LA. Stent may be a uni-iliac device necessitating a femoro-femoral cross-over (and a GA) or a bi-iliac device which can be performed under LA alone.

Open repair – non-invasive blood pressure measurement is acceptable initially as is permissive hypotension. If the patient is conscious with a systolic blood pressure of 80 there is little need to elevate it until after the aorta is cross-clamped. The higher the blood pressure the greater the potential for further aortic leak or rupture. The procedure should not be delayed by attempts to insert invasive monitoring. Close attention to temperature is essential. Considerable haemorrhage may also occur after the aorta is cross-clamped either from lumbar collateral arteries or iliac artery back-bleeding. Renal impairment is common and the need for haemofiltration post-operatively should be anticipated.

Thoracic EVAR (TEVAR)

TEVAR is undertaken to treat thoracic aortic dissection or thoracic aortic aneurysms. Not all thoracic aortic abnormalities are suitable for EVAR and the anatomy should be studied carefully prior to the procedure. The stent may occlude the left common carotid artery (in which case a carotid to carotid bypass is undertaken prior to stenting) or the left subclavian artery. The stent may also occlude arteries that supply the spinal cord, risking spinal cord ischaemia. In these cases a lumbar drain may be placed to help reduce CSF pressure and improve spinal cord perfusion. These patients are placed on a strict antihypertensive regime at the time of diagnosis to lower the risk of thoracic aortic rupture or extension of the dissection.

Anaesthetic plan – these cases are undertaken in either an endovascular theatre or an interventional radiology suite remote to theatres. In the latter case the anaesthetist must ensure they have all the necessary equipment with them. Intra-arterial blood pressure monitoring is routine. The need for a lumbar drain should be discussed, and placed prior to the procedure if used. Post-operative pain is mild to moderate.

Intra-operative considerations – induction of anaesthesia includes careful attention to attenuating the hypertensive response to endotracheal intubation. The arterial line should be placed in the right radial or brachial artery if the left subclavian artery is to be occluded. Cardiovascular disturbance is commonly induced by:

1. The proximal ends of catheters used by the interventional radiologist, because they are placed just distal to the aortic valve, easily stimulating ventricular arrhythmias.

2. The anaesthetist – because of the strength of the aortic impulse at the level of the aortic arch the systolic pressure must be lowered to 70 mmHg prior to deployment of the stent in order to ensure the stent comes to rest in the correct place. Suitable pharmacological agents include propofol boluses, increasing volatile agent concentration, short-acting beta-blockade (esmolol) or GTN.

Patients require intra-operative anticoagulation. Heparin dosing varies between centres.

Patients should be placed in an HDU where cardiovascular and neurological status can be closely monitored.

Hybrid procedures – combined open and endovascular cases

In very extensive aortic aneurysms, the origins of the two renal arteries, the superior mesenteric artery and coeliac artery, may all arise from within the AAA. Through an open surgical approach, it is possible to move the blood inflow site to these vessels from the abdominal aorta to the common or even external iliac arteries. This then allows an endovascular stent to be placed from the thoracic aorta all the way down to the aortic bifurcation. Understandably, these major cases carry a very high peri-operative risk. Cases are managed as for open aortic procedures although a lumbar drain may also be required. Renal impairment is an expected complication. All patients require intensive care post-operatively.

Carotid endarterectomy

Carotid endarterectomy is considered to be intermediate-risk surgery. It is a prophylactic operation and should only be performed when the benefit of surgery outweighs the risks. Large-scale trials have determined this to be symptomatic patients presenting with a carotid artery stenosis of >50%. The risk of a stroke following a transient ischaemic attack (TIA) is around 10–15% in the first two weeks after the event. Associated ischaemic heart disease is common. Peri-operative risk of stroke is determined by the extent of carotid disease in both arteries. Bilateral carotid stenosis of >85% is considered to be high risk – these patients are at risk of intra-operative ischaemic stroke because of reduction of cerebrovascular blood flow at the time of the endarterectomy even if a shunt is used, and post-operative haemorrhagic stroke because of the resultant relative cerebral hyperperfusion. The anaesthetic technique and post-operative care can significantly reduce the impact of both on the patient.

Anaesthetic plan – careful evaluation of the anatomy of carotid disease with attention paid to both carotid arteries is essential. The procedure can be performed under local (LA) or general anaesthetic. The recent GALA trial established no advantage of one technique over another. The LA can be performed by the surgeon, the anaesthetist or both. Local infiltration and cervical plexus blocks are the most common techniques applied. The perceived advantage of an LA technique is that an awake patient is the gold standard for cerebral monitoring. Patients need to understand what will be required of them if they opt for LA and nervous patients are not best placed for this technique. If surgery is performed under GA, ventilation needs to be controlled. The airway can be managed with an LMA or endotracheal tube. Invasive arterial monitoring is routinely placed.

Intra-operative considerations – consideration must be given to the fact that two hours is the most any patient can remain motionless – a GA technique is chosen under such circumstances. In those undergoing general anaesthesia, the advantage of an LMA, in addition to those mentioned before, is that it is very unusual for the patient to cough or strain on an LMA, thereby lowering the risk of post-operative haematoma formation. A potential disadvantage is that LMAs can displace on manipulation of the head or trachea intra-operatively. Intra-arterial blood pressure monitoring is usual and necessitated by the direct relationship between arterial blood pressure and cerebral blood flow. Some form of cerebral monitoring is required for carotid endarterectomy. Techniques include the awake patient, stump pressure monitoring, EEG monitoring, near infra-red spectroscopy and transcranial Doppler (TCD). The TCD is the most common device used. It measures blood flow across the middle cerebral artery (MCAv) which, if decreased significantly on carotid cross-clamping, is used as an indication to insert a shunt from the common carotid to the internal carotid artery. The TCD has the additional benefit of detecting particulate micro-emboli – the frequency of which alerts staff to the risk of embolic stroke.

In addition to standard anaesthetic care, careful management of the patient's blood pressure can assist in the prevention of cerebral ischaemia and preserve cerebral blood flow. Prior to carotid endarterectomy cerebral blood flow is impaired. It is further reduced by carotid artery cross-clamping and in patients with a compromised circle of Willis, cerebral ischaemia will occur. A reduction in MCAv as detected by TCD or deterioration in the awake patient is indicative of cerebral ischaemia. A shunt can be placed to augment cerebral blood flow but carries the risk of air or plaque embolisation, intimal tears and carotid dissection. Decision to place a shunt varies between centre and surgeon. Supplemental oxygenation and raising blood pressure to 20% greater than the pre-operative level are effective measures. Once the endarterectomy is complete the cross-clamp will be removed. Gaseous and particulate emboli are commonly heard if a TCD is used but are usually neurologically inconsequential. Cerebral blood flow will increase, carrying with it an increased risk of haemorrhagic stroke. Systolic blood pressure should be less than 160 mmHg (140 mmHg in high-risk patients, such as those with a large recent infarct) at the time of cerebral reperfusion.

Heparin is given prior to carotid cross-clamping. Bleeding from stitch holes can occur and usually resolves quickly. Protamine to reverse the effects of heparin should not be used as there is evidence of an increase in post-operative ischaemic events with it. Rarely platelet function is significantly inhibited by the effects of clopidogrel and a platelet transfusion is required.

Post-operative concerns include cardiovascular status (both hypo- and hypertension are common), neurological status and observation for neck haematoma. Hypertension must be controlled as it places the patient at risk of cerebral hyperperfusion and haemorrhagic stroke. Hypotension can compromise both coronary artery blood flow and cerebral blood flow. Pain is usually mild.

Surgery for peripheral vascular disease (including both limb salvage surgery and amputation)

These procedures are classified as high-risk surgery. This is because of the fact that when peripheral arteries are atheromatous, so are coronary arteries. Pre-operative assessment is key as is the need for a cardiovascularly stable anaesthetic, good post-operative analgesia and oxygenation in the post-operative period.

Anaesthetic considerations – where possible and appropriate, co-morbidities require definition and optimisation and the patient informed of the risks of surgery. Except for particularly lengthy surgery, either regional or GA can be used. Invasive monitoring is not required unless the patient's condition dictates it. An LMA or ETT may be used although an LMA is preferable for reasons mentioned above. Arterial bypass surgery is not stimulating except at incision and formation of the tunnel through which the bypass graft is passed. Post-operatively the patient should be pain-free, free of nausea and vomiting, normothermic and well oxygenated to avoid the hazards associated with tachycardia and hypertension. Analgesic options for below- and above-knee amputation should include a regional block and regional nerve catheter where possible. These techniques are morphine-sparing thus reducing the potential for respiratory depression and confusion in the post-operative period.

Summary

Vascular surgery carries a high-risk of mortality and cardiovascular morbidity. Meticulous pre-operative assessment is essential to establish which patients will benefit from it. This is not possible in patients who require emergency vascular surgery and would die without immediate intervention. The advent of endovascular and hybrid procedures has improved the peri-operative morbidity for many patients and is likely in the future to offer additional health benefits. Careful patient selection for these procedures offers maximum patient benefit.

Further reading

Devereaux PJ, Yang H, Guyatt GH, *et al.* Rationale, design, and organization of the Peri-operative Ischemic Evaluation (POISE) trial: a randomized controlled trial of metoprolol versus placebo in patients undergoing noncardiac surgery. *Am Heart J* 2006; **152**: 223–30.

GALA Trial Collaborative Group. General anaesthesia versus local anaesthesia for carotid surgery (GALA): a multicentre, randomised controlled trial. *The Lancet* 2008; **372**: 2132–42.

2011ASA/ACCF/AHA/AANN/AANS/ACR/ASNR/CNS/SAIP/SCAI/SIR/SNIS/SVM/SVS. Guideline on the management of patients with extracranial carotid and vertebral artery disease. *Circulation* 2011; **124**: e54–e130.

Chapter 13

Organ transplant cases

Nicola Jones and Christopher J.E. Watson

Transplantation

Allogeneic transplantation is one of the biggest medical breakthroughs of the 20th century. It has saved many patients' lives and dramatically improved more. Rapidly developing progress in this area will undoubtedly improve safety and long-term results. Along with its success, transplantation offers more questions than answers in the area of medical ethics.

Kidney transplantation

Donor considerations

Kidneys for transplantation may come from live or deceased donors, and in the UK a third of kidneys come from live donors. Each type of kidney has different peri-operative considerations.

Live donor kidneys

Live donor kidney transplants may be conducted in parallel, with the donor in an adjacent theatre, or in tandem with the recipient procedure following the donor procedure. When in parallel there is often a period of time when the recipient is anaesthetised and ready to receive the donor kidney, and the donor kidney has yet to become available. In this case it is important to maintain muscle relaxation and anaesthesia, since the surgeons may have left the operative field while preparing the donor kidney.

ABO incompatible live donor kidneys

While it is usual to transplant blood group compatible kidneys, it is possible to pre-treat the recipient with plasmapheresis or antibody absorption columns to remove anti-blood group antibodies. This has two consequences. First, any blood products (e.g. fresh frozen plasma) need to be of donor type, and not recipient type. Second, plasmapheresis often removes clotting factors and it is common for patients to be depleted of fibrinogen. It is important to check fibrinogen and clotting before surgery since deficiency is readily treated by cryoprecipitate.

HLA incompatible live donor kidney transplant

The presence of high levels of antibodies to the donor's human leucocyte antigens (HLA) is a contra-indication to surgery. However, as with ABO incompatible transplantation, it is

A Surgeon's Guide to Anaesthesia and Peri-operative Care, ed. Jane Sturgess, Justin Davies and Kamen Valchanov. Published by Cambridge University Press.

possible to remove the donor-specific HLA antibodies if they are of relative low levels. This is done by plasmapheresis and has the same consequences of depletion of clotting factors as described above.

Deceased donor kidneys

Unlike live donor kidneys, where immediate function may be anticipated in over 95% of cases, kidneys from deceased donors often do not start to work immediately. In particular, the incidence of delayed function is over 50% with kidneys donated after circulatory death. The recipient is therefore more likely to need to continue dialysis after surgery, and will not clear potassium or fluid unlike a kidney in which diuresis occurs immediately.

The recipient anaesthetic should not begin until the donor kidney has been examined and is known to be transplantable. It is not uncommon for arterial injuries, tears or parenchymal tumours that may preclude transplantation to become obvious during bench work preparation. It is important to avoid an unnecessary anaesthetic for the disappointed potential recipient.

Pre-op preparation

Recipient assessment

The potential recipient should be assessed in a waiting list clinic before listing for transplantation. A history should screen for cardiac symptoms and vascular insufficiency in the legs. Examination should assess whether there is sufficient space in the abdomen for transplantation where renal failure is because of polycystic kidney disease, and look for evidence of central vein occlusion where these have previously been used for access. Follow-up investigations looking for occult cardiac or vascular disease may also be indicated.

Recipient preparation

Before surgery it is important to check the serum potassium, which may be raised, particularly if the patient is on haemodialysis. It is generally considered unsafe to start a transplant if the potassium is over 5 mmol/l. If this is the case the patient should undergo a short period of haemodialysis to lower the potassium before anaesthesia begins. This is because anaesthetic drugs, and blood if required, may raise potassium intra-operatively.

Following induction of anaesthesia it is usual to place a central line. This must be done using ultrasound guidance, and may be particularly difficult if the patient has previously had internal jugular lines placed. It is important not to use a subclavian vein approach for central access since this is associated with stenosis, which will compromise subsequent arterio-venous dialysis fistulae on the affected side.

Peripheral venous access is also important, and it is important to avoid cannulating the cephalic vein in the forearm since this vein may be used for later dialysis access. It is important to realise that for most patients one transplant will not last them forever, and it is likely that they will need to return to dialysis before a subsequent transplant is possible. Never place a cannula on the same side as an arterio-venous dialysis fistula.

Where arterial monitoring is required, use of the distal radial artery is preferred.

The patient is placed supine on the operating table with one arm out. Ideally that should be the arm with the A-V fistula, but if this is placed by the patient's side it needs to be padded to protect it. The authors prefer not to place both arms out in the crucifix position because of the risk of brachial plexus injury. A urinary catheter is placed to distend the bladder while performing the ureteric anastomosis and to monitor the function of the new transplant.

Operative considerations

Surgical approach

In the adult, kidneys are placed through an incision in one iliac fossa. The external iliac vessels are approached extra-peritoneally. The renal vein is placed end-to-side on the external iliac vein. The recipient vein does not usually require much mobilisation although if the donor vein is short, as may happen with a live donor kidney, some internal iliac vein tributaries may need to be ligated. There is a risk in doing this that the short internal iliac vein stump is not adequately secured and bleeding starts, which can be difficult to control. Live donor kidneys, or deceased donor kidneys with a diseased aortic patch, are often placed on the recipient's internal iliac artery; otherwise the external iliac artery is controlled and clamped for the duration of the anastomosis. In older patients, those with diabetes or those who have been on dialysis for a long time, the recipient iliac artery may be diseased or the intima calcified, with the risk that clamping may result in a distal arterial dissection.

Paediatric patients

In small children the kidney is often placed on the aorta and inferior vena cava through a mid-line incision, either with a retro-peritoneal or trans-peritoneal approach. An adult kidney requires a significant volume of blood to perfuse it, and in a small child half the circulating volume may be required to perfuse it. The anaesthetist needs to be aware of the significant haemodynamic changes that may ensue.

Reperfusion

Reperfusion of the kidney may be accompanied by haemorrhage as well as release of potassium from the donor kidney and ipsilateral leg as the clamps are removed. In addition, blood replacement at this stage may further exacerbate hyperkalaemia.

Following reperfusion the ureteric anastomosis is usually a relatively straightforward procedure, unless it is done to an ileal conduit, in which case the peritoneal cavity is opened.

Closure

With the completion of the anastomoses it is important that the patient remains paralysed until the wound is closed. Failure to do this may result in the kidney being ejected forcibly from the wound when the retractors are removed, avulsing the artery and vein with catastrophic haemorrhage.

A transversus abdominis plane (TAP) local anaesthetic block provides excellent post-operative analgesia, and enables avoidance of large doses of opiates. This is particularly desirable where renal function is slow to return, since opiates are not metabolised normally in patients with renal failure and tend to accumulate, potentially causing respiratory depression and arrest. If a PCA is prescribed, fentanyl is preferable to morphine. The dose and dosing interval will need to be adjusted according to the patient.

Post-operative management

Following surgery there are two main considerations. The first is to recheck the serum potassium and arrange haemodialysis if it is high. Haemodialysis should also be performed if the potassium has been high intra-operatively since, although measures such as insulin and dextrose may reduce the potassium in the short term, it will rebound early after surgery. The second consideration is volume replacement. Following transplantation some kidneys, particularly live donor kidneys, may undergo a profound diuresis with 500 ml/h or more urine output. Typical regimens are to give half-strength normal saline at a rate equivalent to the previous hour's urine output plus 25 ml/h.

Pancreas transplantation

Donor considerations

The donor pancreas requires considerable pre-operative preparation before it can be transplanted. In particular the donor iliac vessels are used to unite the donor superior mesenteric artery and splenic artery, and the mesenteric and splenic vessels must be ligated distal to the pancreas. This may take two hours or more, and the recipient anaesthetic should be timed to begin once the pancreas is deemed transplantable but before the benchwork is complete to avoid unnecessary prolongation of the ischaemic time. Long ischaemic times are associated with significantly poorer outcomes for the pancreas.

Pre-op preparation

Recipient assessment

Most patients undergoing a pancreas transplant are in renal failure secondary to their diabetes and are receiving the donor's kidney at the same time. A small proportion will have previously received a kidney, commonly from a live donor, while a minority will be receiving the pancreas as a treatment for life-threatening hypoglycaemia.

Recipient assessment is primarily aimed at identifying the co-morbidities of the recipient, in particular detecting occult cardiac ischaemia. In addition, older patients, those with a long history of dialysis, and those with peripheral vascular disease should have computed tomography of the iliac arteries to ensure the vessels are suitable to receive both kidney and pancreas.

Recipient preparation

Patients undergoing pancreas transplantation require large volume venous access to enable management of brisk haemorrhage that sometimes accompanies reperfusion. In addition epidural analgesia is desirable for post-operative pain relief.

Most patients coming to pancreas transplantation have significant autonomic neuropathy, and should be assumed to have gastroparesis. Careful airway protection is essential during intubation.

Operative considerations

The pancreas may be implanted by revascularising it either from the common or external iliac arteries, with venous drainage to the external or common iliac veins, IVC, or a superior mesenteric venous tributary for portal venous drainage. Local practice is to use systemic venous drainage to the IVC, controlling this with a side-clamp, and with the pancreas orientated head up. Exocrine drainage is either to a loop of intestine (we use a Roux-en-Y loop of jejunum) or to the dome of the bladder.

Reperfusion

The most critical part of the operation is reperfusion of the pancreas. Many arterial branches and venous tributaries pass though the pancreas bloc and, in spite of meticulous bench preparation, these may bleed briskly on reperfusion. It is not unheard of to lose one or two litres of blood in a matter of minutes, and occasionally immediate pancreatectomy is necessary to control such bleeding. Awareness of this potential, and clear communication between the surgeon and anaesthetist is essential to manage this period successfully.

Most diabetic recipients will be on an insulin infusion at the time of surgery. This should be stopped just before reperfusion, and the glucose checked then and shortly after reperfusion. Occasionally a poorly preserved graft may release large amounts of insulin into the circulation when revascularised, resulting in profound hypoglycaemia.

Following revascularisation the exocrine drainage is fashioned, and then the kidney transplanted. This may be extra-peritoneal or intra-peritoneal. From the renal viewpoint the same concerns exist with respect to hyperkalaemia and opiates.

Consideration may be given to placing a feeding jejunostomy in those patients with marked gastroparesis. This will enable enteral feeding and drug administration post-operatively, and may be continued at home until gastric emptying returns. In addition it avoids parenteral nutrition, which inevitably stresses the new pancreas because of its high glucose loads.

Closure

The addition of pancreas and kidney can result in abdominal compartment syndrome on closure. Previous pregnancy or peritoneal dialysis tend to make the abdominal wall more flaccid so this complication is less likely. If the abdomen appears tight at closure it is best to reopen and place a 'gusset' of hernia mesh between the two sides of the linea alba, or alternatively simply close the skin leaving the muscle open.

Post-operative management

The principle cause of graft loss in the first month after pancreas transplantation is graft thrombosis so patients tend to be anticoagulated to a greater or lesser degree. This, together with the number of vessels passing across the gland, mean that post-operative haemorrhage requiring re-exploration is common in the early post-operative period. The timing of anticoagulation should be checked to ascertain the best time to manipulate or remove the epidural catheter.

Liver transplantation

Liver transplantation is one of the largest operative insults. The principal concerns relate to pre-existing co-morbidity, risk of haemorrhage, cardiovascular instability during the anhepatic phase, and the risk of cardiac arrest following reperfusion. Unlike kidney transplantation where patients are stable on dialysis, patients with liver failure may range from the relatively fit patient with a metabolic liver disease, to a patient in coma with fulminant liver failure. Current allocation schemes allocate livers to the sickest patient rather than the one waiting longest.

Donor considerations

The donor liver may be from a live donor (right lobe for an adult, left lobe for a child) or from a deceased donor. The best deceased donor livers tend to be split ex vivo such that the right lobe goes to an adult and left lobe to a child. In the UK the adult receiving the right lobe also receives the IVC, right portal vein and common hepatic artery and common bile duct. Where the right lobe is from a live donor there is no IVC, and extensive bench surgery is required to ensure venous drainage of all segments.

Increasingly livers from donors after circulatory death are being used. Such livers are less likely to work well immediately after transplantation, with a greater proportion never working such that the recipient requires an immediate retransplant to avoid death. This higher risk is justified by the considerable mortality on the waiting list (10 to 15% at one year in the UK).

Pre-op preparation

Recipient assessment

Patients listed for liver transplantation undergo an extensive inpatient assessment for suitability.

Recipient preparation

Patients are anaesthetised and prepared for surgery. This includes arterial line, central line for manometry, volume lines in the central veins in the neck and peripheral cannulae. Before lines are placed, coagulopathies are corrected using factor concentrates or fresh frozen plasma, together with platelets where indicated. Clotting is monitored throughout the procedure using thromboelastography as well as inspection of the surgical field and corrected as indicated.

Operative considerations

There are three phases of surgery: hepatectomy, anhepatic and reperfusion.

Hepatectomy

During the hepatectomy phase the liver is freed from its peritoneal attachments and the portal vein, hepatic artery and bile duct are isolated and divided. The liver may be removed from the IVC, or with retrohepatic IVC. The ease of hepatectomy depends on whether the recipient has undergone previous upper abdominal surgery, the extent of any portal hypertension and the presence of portal vein thrombosis. All are associated with significant risk of bleeding.

Anhepatic

During the anhepatic phase the donor liver is implanted. The IVC will be side-clamped, and thus partially occluded, if the liver has been removed without the native retro-hepatic IVC. Implantation is then by a 'piggy-back' or a 'cavo-cavostomy technique, where the donor

IVC is anastomosed either end-to-end onto the confluence of the recipient hepatic veins or side-to-side to the recipient IVC. Venous return is usually adequate to maintain cardiac perfusion, and renal function is relatively preserved, although oliguria is common during hepatectomy.

Where the retro-hepatic IVC has been removed en bloc with the liver, a clamp is placed above the confluence of the renal veins and a second above the confluence of the hepatic veins just caudal to the diaphragm. If the cardiac output is suboptimal when these clamps are applied it may be necessary to use veno-veno bypass to shunt blood from the IVC below the clamps to the superior vena cava. This is achieved by placing a large bypass cannula (e.g. 24Fr) into the right femoral vein at the sapheno-femoral junction, and two smaller (10Fr) cannulae in the right internal jugular vein. These latter cannulae are usually placed at induction, or smaller cannulae placed which can then be rail-roaded by the larger cannulae. Such a circuit is usually not heparinised, relying instead on the coagulopathy present in the recipient to avoid clot formation. The major risks of bypass are that it tends to cool the recipient thus exacerbating any bleeding, the bypass circuit may thrombose, particularly if the flow rate is low, or the circuit may be disrupted allowing air to enter causing an air embolism. It is important for the surgeon and anaesthetist to communicate clearly with the perfusionist for the duration of bypass with minimal ambient noise.

Reperfusion

Once the IVC and portal vein and/or hepatic artery anastomoses have been fashioned, the clamps are removed allowing the new liver to be perfused with recipient blood. The effluent from the liver is cold, high in potassium (in part from the preservation fluid, in part because of cell necrosis) and acidotic. As it passes to the heart it causes instability and may lead to cardiac arrest. This risk can be minimised by flushing the liver with saline, colloid or recipient portal blood before completing the portal and caval anastomoses. In addition the anaesthetist can minimise the risk by keeping the serum potassium under control before reperfusion and giving calcium at reperfusion. If cardiac arrest does occur it is usually biochemical, rather than because of coronary artery disease, and responds to sustained cardiac massage. Massage is best delivered externally, since attempts to open the pericardium by splitting the diaphragm may result in inadvertent opening of the distended right atrium or ventricle.

Bleeding from suture lines is also common on reperfusion, but it is seldom as brisk as during the hepatectomy phase. Once the portal vein flow is restored, the hepatic artery is reconstructed and hepatic arterial flow restored (unless this was done with the portal vein). Occasionally where the hepatic artery is too small, or thrombosed, a conduit of donor artery is used. This is anastomosed to the donor hepatic artery and recipient aorta, usually infra-renal but occasionally supra-coeliac. The aorta may be cross-clamped or side-clamped during this anastomosis. Once fully perfused with portal venous and hepatic arterial blood the liver should assume a normal colour, and the serum lactate start to fall and acidosis correct. Attention is then turned to achieving haemostasis before the bile duct anastomosis is completed.

Post-operative management

The main peri-operative complications are primary non-function, hepatic arterial thrombosis, bleeding and biliary leak. The patient is returned to an intensive care unit where close monitoring for these potential complications is carried out. Lactate and blood gases are checked regularly, hepatic arterial patency is confirmed the day following surgery by duplex ultrasonography, and the drains are monitored for bile and blood.

Heart transplantation

Heart transplantation is an established treatment option for patients with end-stage heart disease. Since the first human heart transplant by Barnard in 1967 more than 100,000 cardiac transplants have been performed worldwide. Advances in patient management have led to improved outcomes and five-year survival is now in excess of 70%.

Donor considerations

Acceptance of a potential heart donor requires diagnosis of brain death and confirmation of cardiac viability. As the primary factor limiting heart transplantation is the shortage of donors, criteria for donation have been relaxed, with increased acceptance of older donors and those with evidence of coronary or valvular heart disease. However, the presence of intractable ventricular arrhythmias, discrete wall motion abnormalities or left ventricular ejection fraction <40%, despite optimisation of haemodynamics with inotropic support, remain contra-indications to transplantation.

Brain death is associated with significant cardiovascular aberrations, including arrhythmia, hyper/hypotension and myocardial depression, which may jeopardise post-transplant cardiac function. Invasive monitoring is necessary to optimise haemodynamics by guiding administration of fluids and vasoactive drugs. Where possible, the use of high-dose inotropes and vasopressors, which increase myocardial oxygen demand and deplete myocardial high-energy phosphates, should be avoided. Non-depolarizing muscle relaxants are commonly used during organ recovery to prevent spinal reflex-mediated muscle movement.

Pre-operative considerations

Heart transplantation occurs on an emergency basis and there is usually limited time for anaesthetic pre-operative assessment. However, the recipient will have been under the care of a team experienced in the management of end-stage cardiac failure, and the patient's medical therapy will have been optimised. Timing is critical to successful transplantation and requires close communication between the retrieval team and the transplant centre. Induction of anaesthesia should not occur until the heart has been definitively accepted; however, it needs to proceed expeditiously in order to minimise cold ischaemia time (ideally to less than four hours). The aim is for the recipient to be on cardiopulmonary bypass (CPB), with the native heart explanted as the donor heart arrives. More time should be allowed when difficulties are expected (for example in patients who have had multiple line insertions or previous cardiac surgery).

Recipient assessment

Assessment should include when the person last ate and drank, whether they, or a family member, have had any reactions to anaesthesia and an evaluation of the airway. The current level of cardiovascular support should be determined, including recent deteriorations and the need for intravenous inotropes or mechanical circulatory support. The presence of pulmonary hypertension (PH) should be noted as this is a predictor of post-operative right ventricular (RV) failure and mortality. Methods used to quantify the severity of PH include calculation of pulmonary vascular resistance and the transpulmonary gradient (mean pulmonary artery (PA) pressure – pulmonary capillary wedge pressure (PCWP)). Patients with an implantable device should be identified as these will need re-programming to a non-sensing mode and, if present, the defibrillator function disabled and external defibrillator pads applied. Recent laboratory and chest radiograph results should be sought to assess renal, hepatic, haematological and pulmonary function, which may be deteriorating secondary to low cardiac output or be affected by concurrent medication (e.g. warfarin or angiotensin-converting-enzyme inhibitors). For patients who have undergone prior cardiac surgery, previous exposure to the antifibrinolytic aprotinin should be noted, as re-exposure is associated with an increased risk of anaphylaxis. Appropriately cross-matched blood should be available.

Recipient preparation

Pre-medication is avoided on the ward as even small doses may increase pulmonary vascular resistance (PVR) (through hypoxia and hypercapnia) and reduce circulating catecholamines resulting in haemodynamic collapse. On arrival in the anaesthetic room peripheral venous access is established and at this stage sedation may be administered judiciously together with supplemental oxygen. Next an arterial catheter is inserted; placement can be difficult in patients with an axial flow ventricular assist device (VAD) as no arterial pulse can be palpated and in these instances ultrasound may be helpful. The drugs used for induction are less important than the way in which they are administered and utmost appreciation must be given to the delayed response associated with the slow circulation time of end-stage heart failure. Inotropic support is initiated or increased before inducing anaesthesia and any disturbances in heart rate or blood pressure should be treated promptly. It is important to keep in mind that there is significant down-regulation of the β receptors in the recipient heart, which decreases the responsiveness to β agonists. Following induction of anaesthesia, multi-lumen central venous and pulmonary artery catheters are inserted along with adequate large-bore intravenous access (typically more than one in patients undergoing re-sternotomy or VAD explant). Careful attention must be paid to aseptic technique with consideration given to use of impregnated venous catheters and antimicrobial dressings. Access is often difficult because of multiple previous line insertions and ultrasound is useful. Unless contra-indicated a transoesophageal echocardiography (TOE) probe is inserted to guide haemodynamic management. All patients receive antibiotic prophylaxis, and immunosuppression must be given as ordered by the transplant team.

Operative considerations

Surgical approach

The vast majority of heart transplants are orthotopic. The recipient is placed on standard CPB, the diseased heart explanted and the donor allograft inserted anatomically in its place. Implantation may be via the biatrial or bicaval technique. There is some evidence to suggest that the bicaval technique may result in fewer post-operative rhythm problems, less tricuspid regurgitation, lowered thromboembolic risk and improved right heart function. Heterotopic transplantation is a rarely performed procedure in which the recipient's heart remains in place, and the donor heart is attached to its right side so that the flow in each is in parallel. This procedure is primarily reserved for patients with pulmonary hypertension as a strategy to avoid acute right heart failure in the unconditioned donor heart.

Anaesthetic management

Prior to CPB the aim of anaesthesia is to maintain haemodynamic stability and adequate end-organ perfusion. An antifibrinolytic, such as tranexamic acid, is commenced to attenuate the haemostatic activation associated with CPB and reduce peri-operative blood loss. Heparin is administered once the heart is exposed and the pulmonary artery catheter is withdrawn from the heart into the sterile sheath before the superior vena cava is cannulated.

Once on CPB, ventilation is ceased. Filtration may be necessary on bypass as patients with end-stage heart failure are commonly volume overloaded and have a degree of renal impairment. Prior to aortic cross-clamp removal the heart is de-aired and adequacy assessed by TOE. At this stage high-dose steroid (e.g. methylprednisolone) is often administered to reduce the likelihood of acute rejection.

Prior to weaning from CPB the patient must be re-warmed and any electrolyte or acid–base disturbances corrected. Ventilation is re-commenced with small tidal volumes and a low positive end expiratory pressure in order to prevent mechanical compression of the pulmonary capillary bed and an increase in PVR. In patients with PH, consideration should be given to pre-emptive ventilation with inhaled nitric oxide (NO) or aerosolised prostaglandin. A direct-acting chronotrope (e.g. isoprenaline) and/or epicardial pacing are used to achieve a heart rate of 90–110 beats per minute. Donor heart function is supported with an inotrope(s) (e.g. dopamine, epinephrine). The choice of agent varies between centres and depends upon the clinical situation but will be particularly necessary after a long ischaemic time or when the donor heart was marginal. If the mean arterial blood pressure has been low on CPB then a vasopressor (e.g. vasopressin, norepinephrine) may be commenced to maintain vascular tone.

On weaning from CPB the heart is slowly filled while carefully monitoring the arterial and central venous pressures and watching the right ventricle directly in the surgical field and the left ventricle with TOE. Once the majority of the venous return is passing from the right atrium through the right ventricle, it is usually possible to advance the pulmonary artery catheter into the pulmonary artery and thereby perform cardiac output studies to guide haemodynamic management. If pharmacological support is ineffective in achieving an adequate cardiac output then early consideration should be given to mechanical support with an intra-aortic balloon pump, and if this fails implantation of a temporary right or left VAD or extracorporeal membrane oxygenation (ECMO).

After satisfactory haemodynamics are achieved, protamine is given to reverse the effects of heparin. This must administered with caution as it is associated with systemic hypotension. If bleeding persists in the absence of a surgical cause then functional tests of coagulation (e.g. thromboelastography) may be helpful in identifying the cause of coagulopathy. Transfusion of large volumes of blood products should be avoided as the right ventricle is particularly sensitive to over distension; consideration should be given to the use of factor concentrates (e.g. prothrombin complex concentrate). Chest closure must be done cautiously as it can result in compression of the often swollen heart by the lungs and result in a tamponade-like effect. If previously stable haemodynamics remain unsatisfactory in this situation, re-opening and leaving the chest open is an option, though not without risk in the immunosuppressed patient.

Post-operative considerations

Once the patient has achieved stable hemodynamics and there is no significant bleeding, consideration can be given to decreasing sedation and weaning ventilatory support. It must be remembered that the donor heart is denervated so reflex-mediated heart rate responses will be absent and drugs acting indirectly on the heart through the autonomic nervous system (e.g. atropine) will be ineffective. Instead the heart only responds to direct acting agents (e.g. catecholamines). Careful attention should be paid for signs of rejection and infection.

Lung transplantation

Following the first lung transplant in 1963 over 40,000 lung transplants have been performed worldwide for carefully selected patients with end-stage lung disease, such as chronic obstructive pulmonary disease (COPD), cystic fibrosis (CF), idiopathic pulmonary fibrosis (IPF) and idiopathic pulmonary arterial hypertension (PAH).

Donor considerations

Lungs are traditionally retrieved from individuals who have died after brain death. However, in order to meet the growing demand for transplantation, lungs are increasingly used from donors after circulatory death. To maximise the potential for the lungs to be transplanted, excessive fluid loading should be avoided. Furthermore the inspired oxygen concentration should be kept as low as possible to minimise the risks of oxygen toxicity and protective ventilation used to avoid ventilator-induced lung injury. Physiotherapy should be undertaken regularly and strict asepsis should be observed during suction.

Pre-operative considerations

Lung transplantation is complex treatment with a significant risk of peri-operative morbidity and mortality and patients must undergo rigorous assessment prior to listing. At the time a patient is placed on the active waiting list, the transplant team must identify the specific procedure for which the patient is listed. For most candidates, the choice is between single and bilateral lung transplant; however, in certain circumstances heart–lung transplantation may be required (e.g. pulmonary vascular disease). The decision between single and bilateral transplantation is chiefly dictated by the underlying disease. Patients with cystic fibrosis and other forms of suppurative lung disease require bilateral transplant as leaving behind an infected native lung would run the risk of infecting the allograft, whereas single lung transplantation can be considered in those with obstructive and restrictive disease.

Recipient assessment

The patient should be asked whether they have deteriorated since they underwent pre-operative investigations and about symptoms of recent respiratory infections. The anaesthetist should establish when the patient last ate and drank, and whether they or a family member have had any reactions to anaesthesia. Particular attention should be given to evaluation of the airway so as to identify those in whom intubation may be difficult. The patient's height should be determined in order to select an appropriate-sized double-lumen tube (DLT). It is important to determine whether the patient has suppurative, obstructive or restrictive end-stage lung disease, as each is associated with different ventilation strategies. The current level of respiratory support should be noted (e.g. home oxygen, overnight ventilation) and arterial blood gases, pulmonary function tests and the lung perfusion scan reviewed so as to determine how well the patient will tolerate one-lung ventilation (OLV). Left and particularly right ventricular function should be determined and whether there is pulmonary hypertension as these are associated with increased operative risk. Microbiology should be reviewed to identify patients who are colonised with resistant organisms. Medications, including use of long-term steroids should be noted. Peri-operative analgesia should be discussed with the patient. Thoracic epidural analgesia provides superior analgesia compared with systemic opioids but pre-operative insertion is associated with increased risk and delayed diagnosis of epidural haematoma, because of potential heparinisation for CPB, development of coagulopathy and post-operative sedation. Alternative strategies include inserting an epidural, if needed, post-operatively or using a paravertebral block/catheter in the case of single-sided surgery.

Recipient preparation

Because of the lack of respiratory reserve, sedation is not recommended on the ward and should be given with extreme caution in the anaesthetic room, as it can precipitate cardio-respiratory arrest because of hypoxaemia, hypercapnia, increased PVR and acute right ventricular failure. Peripheral venous access is established and an arterial catheter inserted; placement can be difficult, as patients will likely have had multiple admissions to hospital and repeated arterial blood gases. If a pre-operative epidural is to be inserted this usually occurs before induction of anaesthesia; attention must be paid to positioning and care taken to avoid a bloody tap. Induction of anaesthesia can be very challenging and the surgeon and perfusionist must be present and prepared to perform urgent sternotomy and initiation of CPB in the event of cardiovascular collapse. Goals of induction are to avoid factors that increase PVR (hypoxia, hypercapnia and high intra-thoracic positive pressure) and to preserve systemic vascular resistance and myocardial contractility. Inotropes and vasopressors need to be started pre-induction in patients at high risk of right ventricular failure. Following induction of anaesthesia the patient is intubated. A substantial number of lung transplants are performed through a sternotomy, and a normal tracheal intubation is adequate. However, if lung isolation is required a DLT (usually left-sided) is used to facilitate OLV and the position checked with a fibre optic bronchoscope (FOB). The DLT is trickier to insert than single lumen endotracheal tubes and in case of difficulty a bronchial blocker can be used with an endotracheal tube to provide lung isolation. However performance is inferior to that of a DLT. The endobronchial tube should be suctioned thoroughly before commencing ventilation and consideration given to bronchial lavage, particularly in patients with suppurative lung disease. Ventilation will invariably be difficult and an ICU-level ventilator may be required. Ventilator settings should take into account the underlying pathophysiology, in patients with obstructive lung disease long expiratory times are used and external PEEP avoided, while in those with restrictive disease a long inspiratory time will be necessary and higher peak inspiratory pressures will be expected. If not inserted pre-induction, multi-lumen central venous and pulmonary artery catheters are then inserted along with adequate large-bore intravenous access. Careful attention must be paid to aseptic technique with consideration given to use of impregnated venous catheters and antimicrobial dressings. Access is often difficult because of multiple previous line insertions and ultrasound is advised as patients will not tolerate a pneumothorax. Unless contra-indicated a TOE probe is inserted to guide haemodynamic management. Broad spectrum antibiotics are given for prophylaxis; for patients with suppurative lung disease or a current chest infection, the choice of antibiotics will be determined by the actual or suspected microbiological burden. Immunosuppression is administered as directed by the transplant team. The patient is then positioned supine (bilateral lung) or in right/left lateral decubitus (single lung) position dependent on the procedure planned with particular attention to pressure areas.

Operative considerations

Surgical approach

Single-lung transplantation is performed using a standard posterolateral thoracotomy through the bed of the excised fifth rib, while double lung transplantation is performed via median sternotomy, clamshell incision or bilateral anterior thoracotomies via the fourth or fifth intercostal space. Surgery can be done with or without CPB; indications for bypass include patients with severe PH or those who do not tolerate OLV or PA clamping. The CPB provides haemodynamic stability but is associated with activation of pro-inflammatory cascades that increase the risk of lung injury and greater need for transfusion of blood and blood products because of haemodilution, coagulopathy and platelet dysfunction.

Anaesthetic management

Anaesthesia can be maintained with inhalational or intravenous agents; the latter may be preferable as difficulties/interruptions to ventilation can result in inadequate depth of anaesthesia and awareness. Lungs should be ventilated to their baseline arterial carbon dioxide tension ($PaCO_2$). A large alveolar dead space makes the end tidal carbon dioxide underestimate the $PaCO_2$ by an unpredictable amount and frequent correlation to arterial blood gases is required. The initial dissection may be prolonged especially if pleural adhesions are present and the anaesthetist must be vigilant as significant blood loss may occur. Many centres set up a rapid infuser system to provide rapid resuscitation with blood products.

The OLV is testing and associated with hypoxaemia and hypercapnia, particularly when the patient is in the supine position. If a perfusion asymmetry exists, the lung with the lower perfusion is transplanted first. Strategies to manage hypoxaemia include suction, recruitment and application of PEEP to the ventilated lung. Hypercapnia may be controlled by increasing minute ventilation. Despite these measures profound hypoxia and respiratory acidosis can result, leading to increased PVR and right ventricular dysfunction, which will be exacerbated on clamping the PA. The TOE can be very helpful in guiding management and the right heart may be supported with judicious fluid loading, inotropes/inodilators, adequate systemic arterial perfusion pressure and reduction in PVR. If unsuccessful, CPB will be necessary. Good communication between surgeon and anaesthetist is essential.

Once the bronchial anastomosis is completed the anaesthetist should perform a FOB to inspect the anastomosis and toilet the airways. Before completing the atrial anastomosis, the lung should be inflated to a sustained pressure of 15–20 cmH_2O in order to de-air the graft. De-airing and reperfusion can be associated with severe hypotension, which requires volume loading and intravenous boluses of calcium or epinephrine. To reduce lung injury, initial ventilation should be with a low inspired oxygen concentration, peak inspiratory pressure and PEEP. In bilateral lung transplantation settings are then adjusted to provide adequate oxygenation and ventilation ahead of the implantation of the next lung. Reperfusion of the donor lung can be associated with acute hyperaemia, which manifests as pulmonary oedema with persistent hypoxaemia, elevated pulmonary artery pressures, and potentially decreased cardiac output. Inappropriate fluid loading should be avoided, PEEP increased and consideration given to diuretics, inotropes and pulmonary vasodilators. If medical management is unsuccessful ECMO should be considered early.

Post-operative considerations

The DLT is changed to a single lumen tube at the end of surgery. Differential synchronous ventilation may be needed if the lungs vary significantly in compliance as may be encountered after single-lung transplantation. The aim is to extubate the patient as soon as possible in order to avoid complications such as ventilator-acquired pneumonia. Adequate analgesia is essential to the success of extubation and spontaneous breathing. Care must be taken to avoid unnecessary fluid administration.

Heart–lung transplantation

The number of heart–lung transplants undertaken is decreasing with less than ten performed annually in the UK over recent years. Indications include congenital heart disease, idiopathic PH and respiratory disease with secondary PH. Surgery is performed via median sternotomy on CPB thus anaesthetic preparation is similar to that for heart transplantation. Patients tend to be high risk and have poor outcomes compared to patients requiring only heart or lung transplantation.

Summary

Anaesthesia for transplant surgery is a challenging area. Smooth team working and communication in the peri-operative period are essential for optimal patient care. Most of the transplant operations are time consuming. Care with positioning, antibiotic prophylaxis and immunosuppression is required from both teams. Anaesthesia for heart and lung transplantation is particularly challenging, as these patients would normally be declared unfit for any other surgery as the risk of mortality is overwhelming. Thus these are carefully conducted cases and require amicable interaction by all peri-operative practitioners. Once the new organs are implanted sound knowledge of transplant physiology is required to avoid damaging the new organs and maintain other organ functions.

Further reading

Clavien PA. Petrowski H. Deoliviera ML, et al. Strategies for safer liver surgery and partial liver transplantation *NEJM* 2007; **356**: 1545–59.

Organ donation and transplantation activity data: www.organdonation.nhs.uk/statistics/down loads/united-kingdom-dec13.pdf.

Chapter 14

Otorhinology, head and neck cases

Helen Smith and Neil Donnelly

Surgery on the head and neck requires excellent communication between surgeon and anaesthetist for a successful and safe outcome. The shared and often complex airway means that the anaesthetist and surgeon are integral in facilitating the work of each other and require a clear understanding of the needs of the other. Airway difficulties can mean that speed is of the essence and both parties need to work quickly together to obtain a safe airway.

Pre-operative assessment

The age range covered in routine otolaryngology and maxillofacial surgery spans from cradle to grave and covers a wide variety of pathology. Those patients who are generally fit and well with no significant cardiovascular or respiratory pathology require no more than standard pre-operative assessment appropriate for the age of the patient and nature of the surgery. Many cases are suitable for treatment as a day case. There are some notable exceptions where a more detailed pre-assessment is required.

Head and neck malignancy

A significant number of upper aerodigestive tract malignancies are associated with a prolonged history of smoking. The cardiovascular and pulmonary effects of this exposure need to be ascertained to establish any potential pre-operative optimisation or contraindications to surgery.

Airway obstruction

Airway obstruction secondary to chronic disease or malignancy can pose a challenge to maintaining an airway during induction of anaesthesia, intubation, intra-operative ventilation and post-operative management. The most challenging cases require an impressive amount of co-operation between surgeon and anaesthetist, with the surgeon scrubbed and prepared to perform a surgical airway or rigid bronchoscopy as induction starts. In these cases time is of the essence and it is essential to anticipate the potential difficulties that might arise in advance.

Chronic sleep apnoea may result in raised pulmonary pressures and right ventricular hypertrophy. This can result in pulmonary oedema once the obstructive cause has been

A Surgeon's Guide to Anaesthesia and Peri-operative Care, ed. Jane Sturgess, Justin Davies and Kamen Valchanov. Published by Cambridge University Press.

surgically removed. These patients are exquisitely sensitive to the respiratory depressant effects of anaesthetic agents and particularly opiates. Such cases require a pre-operative echocardiogram and the availability of high-dependence observation post-operatively.

Airway obstruction at the level of the pharynx, supraglottis and glottis can usually be adequately assessed pre-operatively with a flexible nasal endoscope. In conditions where there is concern regarding sub-glottic or tracheal narrowing (e.g. retrosternal goitre) the airway may require more detailed assessment with CT or MR imaging.

Surgery on secreting tumours and lesions

There are a small number of head and neck tumours and conditions that result in the secretion of vasoactive substances that could have an adverse effect on the patient during surgery. Such tumours include paragangliomas (5% secreting) and toxic thyroid nodules. Graves' disease is another condition where the pre-operative endocrinology requires specialist work-up with the involvement of an endocrinologist in the pre-operative period (see Chapter 11 Endocrine cases).

Day case surgery

More and more cases are being performed as day of surgery admission. This means that pre-assessment and pre-operative work-up needs to be completed and reviewed prior to surgery. In addition, the number of day case procedures is increasing. Good pre-operative work up must be combined with good communication with the patient and their general practitioner. Information should be provided regarding the procedure, potential complications, post-operative recovery and necessary pain relief. A detailed discharge summary along with written information regarding post-operative care should also be provided to ensure that patients and their carers understand any problems that may arise and how to access the care they need should problems occur.

The emergency airway

Difficulties with the airway may arise before surgery, during induction, post-induction, during intubation or post-operatively.

Some of the most challenging cases for surgeon and anaesthetist are those airways that present as an emergency and are difficult to maintain prior to reaching theatre. These are usually critical, life-threatening airways that need immediate attention. The priority is for the team to bring the patient to a controlled environment such as theatre. Senior help from both anaesthetic and surgical side should be requested. The surgical team should be prepared to perform a surgical airway or needle cricothyroidotomy with jet ventilation, if required. Essential equipment must be available and full monitoring placed on the patient before attempting any procedure, including induction of anaesthesia. It is vital that a plan is made before the start and that back-up plans have also been worked through should the first plan fail. Once the patient is no longer self-ventilating there is very little time to find a solution.

There may be several different options available to deal with the difficult airway, dependent on the patient and the skills of the team. These include an awake fibre-optic intubation, inhalational induction, intravenous induction, awake tracheostomy, or awake needle cricothyroidotomy.

Intubation

The choice of tracheal tube type and route of intubation route is one that the anaesthetist and surgeon must discuss prior to each case. The decisions made are usually dictated by the nature of the surgery but where there are options, personal preference is exercised if both parties are in agreement. The principal choice is between endotracheal tube and laryngeal mask. It is best to avoid having to switch from one to the other intra-operatively.

Factors that support the choice of an endotracheal tube include:

- Risk of aspiration
- Longer length of surgery
- Greater anticipated bleeding within the shared airway
- The use of the laser within the shared airway
- Requirement for laryngeal nerve monitoring
- Repeated positioning of the head

The absolute indication for intubation is:

- Protection of the airway

A majority of cases will require a standard oral intubation. There are times when limited mouth opening, challenging anatomy or site of surgical interest will require nasal intubation. Nasal intubation may be required for oral surgery. Whichever tube type is selected and intubation route used, it should be adequately secured with tape and/or ties.

Awake fibre-optic intubation can be performed as an oral or nasal procedure and is particularly useful in cases that have a patent glottis and normal subglottic airway but have difficult direct laryngoscopy views – for example, poor mouth opening, craniofacial abnormalities and neck deformities (ankylosing spondylitis, rheumatoid arthritis, unstable neck). This requires pre-treatment with an antisialogogue in preparation to allow effective administration of local anaesthetic to render the airway insensitive.

In certain situations, such as a large glottic tumour, difficulties may be anticipated or arise when intubation is attempted. In this situation, the surgeon must be comfortable with and prepared to perform a tracheostomy. In certain cases, performing a tracheostomy under local anaesthetic as a first-line approach should be considered.

For major head and neck surgery, feeding post-operatively may be a challenge and the insertion of a nasogastric tube (NG tube) is an essential part of patient care. Under these circumstances the NG tube can be placed in advance of the surgery at induction and secured preferably by suture to prevent displacement in the peri-operative period.

Throat pack

There are many procedures in ENT and maxillofacial surgery where it is beneficial to have a throat pack inserted in the posterior oropharynx in order to prevent aspiration of blood. It is essential to record the presence of the throat pack in an obvious location on the patient as well as on the white theatre board. The entire theatre team should note removal before the patient leaves theatre.

Positioning

The standard positioning for ENT and maxillofacial surgery is with the patient supine on a head ring, shoulder roll, or both. Complex otological cases require the patient to be strapped to the table to facilitate rolling of the table for surgical access. This requires careful padding of the patient to prevent pressure-point injury and the displacement of access lines. It is often helpful to have the patient head up to limit venous congestion in the head.

For cases that take longer than six hours consideration of the use of a urinary catheter is appropriate for patient comfort and safety and also to measure urine output.

Unlike most surgical specialties, the surgeon is at the 'head end' of the patient, with the anaesthetist situated towards the toes. The surgically draped patient does not provide rapid access to the airway and it is essential that the utmost care is taken to prevent accidental extubation.

Maintenance of anaesthesia

Muscle relaxation

Many otolaryngological procedures, in particular ear surgery (facial nerve), parotid surgery (facial nerve) and thyroid cases (recurrent laryngeal nerve) require a non-paralysed patient to enable the use of active nerve monitoring. It is important for anaesthetist and surgeon to discuss whether nerve monitoring is required prior to intubation to ensure that the patient has no muscle relaxation when nerve monitoring is required.

Local anaesthesia and vasoconstrictors

It is common to use a combination of local anaesthesia and vasoconstrictor at the beginning of surgery to improve the surgical field. This must be discussed prior to surgery to ensure that there are no anaesthetic contraindications.

The most common injected preparation is lignocaine and adrenaline. The maximal dose of lignocaine is 3 mg/kg alone and 7 mg/kg with adrenaline. The total dose of adrenaline should not exceed 500 mcg.

Cocaine preparations are commonly used in nasal procedures because of the rapid penetration of mucous membranes, resulting in excellent vasoconstriction. The maximum dose of cocaine is 1.5 mg/kg up to a maximum dose of 100 mg. Cocaine has sympathomimetic effects which when used in conjunction with adrenaline can cause significant arrhythmias and possible cardiac ischaemia, even within the maximum dose in the elderly patient with susceptible pathology; care should be taken with these patients.

Hypotensive anaesthesia

When performing surgery in small anatomical spaces such as the ear, nose or larynx, a small amount of bleeding can significantly impede progress. Having a hypotensive anaesthetic within the bounds of what can be tolerated by the patient is advantageous when combined with other techniques such as head-up positioning and vasoconstrictors. Again, caution is required in those patients with poor functional reserve, particularly the elderly, those with ischaemic heart disease and hypertension. In such cases the use of this technique may result in a stroke or a myocardial infarction.

Ventilation

Typically, intermittent positive pressure ventilation is the most common method of maintaining ventilation throughout the operation. For some procedures such as microlaryngoscopy other forms of ventilation may be utilised such as jet ventilation or spontaneous respiration. This requires anaesthetic to be given intravenously (i.v.) and access to the i.v. line becomes very important.

Special considerations

Microlaryngobronchoscopy (MLB)

The requirements for an MLB need to be discussed in advance of the procedure. It is necessary to establish whether spontaneous ventilation is required throughout or if intermittent positive pressure ventilation is also needed. Alternatively jet ventilation may be used instead. Factors determining means of ventilation include which method will provide the optimal surgical conditions and whether the necessary specialist equipment is available. Patients at either end of the age spectrum can be particularly difficult to manage as their respiratory reserve is reduced.

The procedure requires good analgesia at the level of the vocal cords to prevent stimulation during surgery. This is best achieved by spraying local anaesthetic directly on to the cords. In order for this to work effectively the patient needs an antisialogogue such as glycopyrrolate or atropine to be given in advance. With complete analgesia of the vocal cords, the patient should remain nil by mouth until they are capable of protecting their own airway.

Removal of bronchial foreign body

Maintaining spontaneous ventilation throughout the procedure is important to prevent pushing the foreign body even further down the airway but this may be difficult when the operation takes a long time as atelectasis may occur and oxygen saturations difficult to keep within normal limits. Breaks in the procedure may need to take place to ensure good ventilation of the patient.

Laser surgery

The primary concern during laser surgery is damage caused by the laser such as unintended burns and fires, particularly airway fires. Draping adjacent areas with saline soaked swabs, the use of special laser endotracheal tubes, filling the endotracheal tube cuff with saline and keeping oxygen and nitrous oxide out of the area to be lasered help to prevent this occurring.

Thyroid surgery

An enlarged thyroid gland can result in pressure on or distortion of the trachea, which in turn may lead to difficulty in intubation after induction of anaesthesia. The retrosternal goitre is more likely to compress and distort the trachea and can lead to some degree of tracheomalacia. Surgery for the large retrosternal goitre can provide a major challenge with the potential requirement to open the chest and the complications associated with this, including major haemorrhage.

Attention to haemostasis intra-operatively is important as bleeding can quickly cause airway obstruction, posing a difficult airway post-extubation that may be challenging to re-intubate. Smooth extubation is the ideal way to reduce the risk of haemorrhage triggered by coughing post-operatively. In the event of a post-operative haematoma, the swift removal of sutures or staples will release the pressure and allow airway control. Any vocal cord palsy caused during surgery may impact on airway management post-operatively.

Neck dissection

Potential complications during neck dissection include vagal stimulation leading to severe bradycardia and associated hypotension. Injury to the jugular vein may lead to air embolism. Injury to the carotid artery can also occur during dissection. The risk of blood loss may be high and the operation may be difficult and prolonged, in which case invasive monitoring with arterial line +/- central venous access may be required to take regular blood samples and monitor fluid requirements.

Head and neck major reconstructive surgery

For reconstructive surgery the use of free flaps means that certain limbs will be used by the surgical team and not available to the anaesthetist for line insertion – this needs to be planned and discussed in advance. These operations are complex and often lengthy; considerations for positioning, padding of the patient and deep vein thrombosis prophylaxis are particularly important.

Tracheostomy

Tracheostomy can be relatively straightforward when the anatomy is easily identifiable and the airway easily managed. However, there are some very challenging patients who require tracheostomy. These can be divided into two: those that require a tracheostomy as emergency airway technique as discussed above and those that are intubated on the intensive care unit who have multiple pathologies with poor respiratory and cardiovascular function.

This second group can be a challenge to transfer from one area to another and, in addition, the transfer from bed to operating table can cause major problems. A team approach again is vital. Consideration may be given to performing the procedure on the bed. Many patients will manage very little apnoeic time even with prolonged preoxygenation. The transition from endotracheal tube to tracheal tube needs to be smooth and quick. The tube must be adequately secured with sutures and/or ties. The potential complications of false passage, bleeding and tube displacement can lead to very poor outcomes.

Post-operatively tracheostomies can provide a nursing challenge. Humidification is important to overcome drying of the mucosal surfaces. Frequent suction may be required with occasional problems of obstruction and potential desaturation. Critically ill patients should be managed within the intensive care setting; however, many patients with a tracheostomy are managed safely on wards with appropriately highly skilled nursing staff.

Ear surgery

In complex ear surgery it is often preferable to have the patient intubated with an endotracheal tube. The reason for this is having the head rotated away from the surgeon, which runs the risk of displacing a laryngeal mask or putting too much pressure on the side of the pharynx leading to post-operative pain.

The majority of otological cases require active monitoring of the facial nerve and as such need a non-paralysed patient within the first half-hour of surgery. The microscopic size of the surgical field means that it is essential to limit bleeding into the field. For this reason the peri-auricular region is injected with adrenaline, usually combined with local anaesthetic. In addition a hypotensive anaesthetic with a systolic blood pressure of less than 100 mmHg is beneficial.

In cases such as stapedectomy or cochlear implantation, where the inner ear is opened, it is important to have a slow and smooth extubation to prevent coughing and raised intracranial pressure that may result in a loss of perilymph and hearing loss. Patients are often dizzy and nauseated following ear surgery and require adequate provision of anti-emetics.

Extubation

Once surgery has concluded within the shared airway, prior to extubation, it is essential to check that haemostasis has been adequately established. This is particularly important as the vocal folds may have been anaesthetised prior to intubation. It is vital to ensure that potential reservoirs of coagulated blood have been checked and cleared. An example of this is checking the postnasal space after tonsillectomy, an area in the past that has been overlooked to the extent that any blood in this area is referred to as the 'coroner's clot'. Any throat pack placed needs to be removed prior to extubation and a record made of this.

Patients who have had airway compromise may benefit from ventilation post-operatively in the intensive care unit to allow time for airway swelling to subside. Alternatively tracheostomy may be performed if appropriate.

Immediate post-operative care

All the problems associated with the difficult airway pre-operatively can potentially be worse post-operatively. Smooth extubation of all patients following removal of all blood and clots with excellent post-operative monitoring is required for most ENT and maxillofacial surgical procedures. Patients may require major input from both the anaesthetist and the surgeon in this period to ensure that the airway is well maintained.

In any procedure where obstruction of the airway has been a concern, the use of opioids may increase the risks of complete obstruction in the post-operative period. If opioids are required for pain relief in such cases, then post-operative care will need to be within a high-dependency area.

Summary

In the ENT and head and neck surgical cases the main challenge is that both the anaesthetic and surgical team work on the same area of the body. While none has sole ownership, it is important to have a detailed pre-operative discussion of the steps each team takes, aiming to ensure a smooth surgical procedure, and minimise the risk of post-operative complications.

Paediatric cases

Simon Whyte and Sonia Butterworth

Peri-operative care of paediatric patients presents unique challenges and opportunities for surgeons and anaesthetists to work synergistically. No subpopulation of patients is more heterogeneous with respect to physiology or spectrum of pathology.

Pre-operative

Having decided that the child before them requires an operation, surgeons must consider a number of areas peculiar to paediatric patients.

Need for general anaesthesia

Many procedures that would be done in adults under local anaesthesia, or with conscious sedation, cannot be achieved without general anaesthesia in children. Examples include MR imaging studies, GI endoscopies and most minor body surface surgery.

Assessment and optimisation

Most elective procedures in children are performed on a day case basis. Prudent selection and referral of patients who require pre-operative anaesthetic assessment for optimisation is critical, to avoid both unnecessary additional hospital visits and day of surgery cancellations.

Planned pre-operative admission

This is an indication for a detailed pre-operative anaesthesia assessment. The admission is likely a function of some combination of the magnitude of surgery, existing co-morbidity and the need for advanced post-op pain management modalities. Adequate time needs to be provided for optimisation of co-morbidities, and for the risks and benefits of anaesthesia and post-op pain management strategies to be presented and digested by the patient and family.

Consent and assent issues

Consent needs to include consent for surgery and for blood transfusion. The laws on when and which children are able or allowed to consent, or refuse consent, to undergo surgical procedures vary between jurisdictions. The following principles, however, are generic:

A Surgeon's Guide to Anaesthesia and Peri-operative Care, ed. Jane Sturgess, Justin Davies and Kamen Valchanov. Published by Cambridge University Press.

I. All physicians must act in the best interests of the child. This allows for emergency surgery, which should not be delayed or withheld in the absence of informed consent from the patient or legal guardian.
II. Informed consent for a surgical procedure should always be sought from the legal guardian and/or the competent patient if possible.
III. Children should be involved in decisions made about them as far as is possible. *Assent* from a child for any intervention should be sought; explanation of and agreement to the procedure has a positive effect on outcome. The importance of obtaining assent increases with the maturity and understanding of the child.
IV. A legally competent child is legally entitled to withhold consent. However, in some circumstances, this can be over-ridden by their parents/guardians. If the treating physician believes the child's decision to be detrimental to their wellbeing, the clinician can seek legal opinion. A court may need to rule on whether the child can be treated against their expressed wishes. If legal guardians agree with the competent child's refusal to consent, but the treating doctor believes this not to be in the child's best interest, legal advice will be needed.
V. An incompetent child can neither consent to, nor refuse treatment. The legal guardians must provide consent on the child's behalf. If the guardians refuse consent for a procedure that the treating physician believes is in the child's best interests, court intervention must be sought. This is classically the scenario when consent for blood transfusion is refused by Jehovah's Witness parents.
VI. A consent process must outline the procedure, its rationale, risks and alternatives to the competent patient and legal guardians. A clear discussion with the patient and family about the diagnosis, planned intervention and expected outcome, with and without intervention, is critical. The known common complications must be outlined, with their respective frequencies. In addition, rare but severe complications (organ or life threatening) require discussion. It is often very helpful for families to have the surgeon illustrate the anatomy and the procedure on the back of the consent form. When discussing interventions with a family, both surgeon and anaesthetist must ensure that there are no language barriers. Most institutions have interpreters available.
A registered translator is considered more likely to provide the most accurate translation. Family members are very useful but may not convey the entire/accurate message.

Peri-operative

Operations planned on children require particular attention to age, physiological needs and development. The younger the child, the less they are able to tolerate fasting without developing hypoglycaemia. In addition, children with diabetes or specific types of metabolic disorders may become hypoglycaemic with fasting and may require a glucose infusion to be started at initiation of fasting. Ordering of the operating list should account for:

- physiological and psychological tolerance of fasting
- co-morbidities
- likely bed availability

Thus neonates and infants, children with diabetes, and autistic children are all legitimate candidates for the first slot of the list.

The prospect of undergoing an operation can be overwhelming for some children and the engagement of their caregivers in the process decreases anxiety. For children over a year of age, having a parent present in the anaesthetic room until they are anaesthetised, and present in recovery once they are aware, decreases anxiety for the patient and the family.

Any existing fluid volume deficit must be corrected before taking a child to theatre. Hypovolaemic children maintain their cardiac output by a combination of vasoconstriction and increasing their heart rate. During general anaesthesia, heart rate and vascular tone fall, and hypotension may result if a volume deficit persists. Normal saline or Ringer's lactate is typically used for volume correction. Particular attention must also be paid to ongoing evaporative fluid loss during open body cavity surgery, as additional fluid loss can be significant (10–20 ml/kg/h in neonates).

Antibiotic prophylaxis for the paediatric population follows the same principles as for adult surgical cases. Clean procedures without insertion of a prosthetic material do not require antibiotics.

Thermoregulation

The ability to thermoregulate is extensively compromised by general anaesthesia, for multiple reasons:

- Cold operating room environment
- Inhibition of shivering by anaesthesia
- Administration of 'cold' (room temperature) i.v. fluids and drugs
- Use of non-humidified inspired gases

Neonates, infants and small children rapidly become hypothermic (core temperature $<36^\circ$C) following induction of anaesthesia, owing to their large surface area/body mass ratio. Core temperature monitoring is thus standard in paediatric anaesthesia practice, and multiple strategies are employed to avoid intra-operative hypothermia. These may include:

- Increasing ambient room temperature
- Forced air warming
- Intravenous fluid warming (especially blood products)
- Warmed blankets to cover exposed areas outside the operative field, especially the head

Surgeons can contribute to maintaining patient normothermia by:

- Limiting post-induction examination
- Minimising time interval between anaesthesia and start of surgery
- Warming surgical and irrigation fluids

Technical adjustments – according to size and age of patient:

Diathermy

- 10–15 in infants

Sutures

- 2–0 for fascia and 5–0 for skin in infants
    - Disposable wherever possible to avoid the need for removal

Laparoscopy

- Intra-peritoneal pressure <10 mmHg in infants
  - Intra-peritoneal pressure <12 mmHg for children
  - Pressures limited to avoid compromise in haemodynamic parameters, ventilation and cerebral perfusion

Intra-operative fluoroscopy

- Settings adjusted for patient weight and exposure of limited duration Children are particularly susceptible to radiation-induced malignancies

When **draping** the patient, it is critical to be attentive to all the lines and tubes. The operating field is small. Lack of space should prompt the surgeon to communicate clearly with the anaesthetist. Awareness by the operating team of the position of all tubes and lines during the procedure is important to prevent inadvertent occlusion or disconnection. Care, attention and communication at completion of the operation when removing the drapes will minimise complications such as accidental extubation, or line removal.

Regional anaesthesia

Clear communication between anaesthetist and surgeon regarding who is giving which local anaesthetic agent and in what quantity is particularly important in paediatric patients. Maximum recommended doses of the commonly used local anaesthetics are given in Table 15.1.

Bupivacaine with epinephrine is the most widely used intra-operative local anaesthetic. It is supplied in concentrations of 0.25% and 0.5%. These solutions contain, respectively, 2.5 mg/ml and 5 mg/ml of bupivacaine. As the maximum dose of bupivacaine with epinephrine is 2.5 mg/ml, the maximum permissible volume of bupivacaine 0.25% is easily remembered as the child's weight, in kg.

Caudal epidural analgesia is the most commonly employed regional technique, being used for many infra-umbilical surgeries. The epidural space is accessed by cannulating the sacral hiatus. This typically ossifies towards the end of the first decade, making access more difficult. With maximal dosing, a block to T10 can be achieved.

Table 15.1 Maximum recommended local anaesthetic doses in children

Local anaesthetic	Maximum dose
Lidocaine (lignocaine) – plain	3 mg/kg
Lidocaine (lignocaine) – with epinephrine	7 mg/kg
Bupivacaine – plain	2 mg/kg
Bupivacaine – with epinephrine	2.5 mg/kg
Ropivacaine	3–4 mg/kg

Post-operative

Pain management

The basic principles apply equally well to children as to adults:

- All children, of all ages, including premature neonates born at the limit of viability, are capable of experiencing pain

- Amelioration or elimination of pain is a critical duty of, and the shared responsibility of, the peri-operative care team
- Analgesic modalities should be tailored to the expected magnitude of discomfort, and adjusted according to regular clinical assessment
- Heterogeneity in developmental pharmacokinetics, and pharmacogenetics, generates greater variability in responses to 'standard' dosing in the youngest paediatric patients. Prescribing should be weight-based and paediatric formularies consulted
- Simple analgesics are highly effective, act synergistically and suffice for many minor surgical procedures. They should be given regularly, at the correct dose and interval. Decreases in dose size and frequency are necessary for neonates and some infants. Simple agents are opioid sparing and should be used in combination with more advanced techniques, as part of a multimodal analgesia plan, if required

A dedicated acute pain service team should oversee all opioid infusions in infants, patient-controlled analgesia (PCA), nurse-controlled analgesia (NCA), and continuous regional anaesthetic infusion techniques.

Fluid management

Wherever possible, return to oral intake is preferred.

When i.v. fluids are required, maintenance requirements and ongoing losses must be considered before writing the prescription. It is also important to consider the type, volume and tonicity of fluid required for maintenance and to replace ongoing losses.

Maintenance fluids should be isosmolar, and contain glucose only if the child is fasting. Certain patient groups require special consideration – TPN dependent children, the premature neonate and those with metabolic syndromes predisposing to hypoglycaemia.

Controversy exists over the most appropriate choice of maintenance fluid for replacement of insensible and urinary loss, but the weight of opinion among experts leans in favour of isotonic fluids.

Maintenance fluid calculations: 4/2/1 rule

4 ml/kg/h for the first 10 kg of bodyweight
2 ml/kg/h for the second 10 kg
1 ml/kg/h for each kg thereafter

e.g.: 17 kg child requires $(10\times4) + (7\times2) = 54$ ml/h.
33 kg child requires $40 + 20 + 13 = 73$ ml/h.

Ongoing loss:

Replace like with like. Non-haemorrhagic loss typically resembles extracellular fluid, and is usually replaced with normal saline.

Volume resuscitation:

Isotonic fluid should be given for non-haemorrhagic shock as a bolus of 20 ml/kg. Albumin can be considered. This can be repeated a further two times before resorting to blood products. **Haemorrhage** should be replaced with appropriate blood products.

Children who are unwell and/or are recovering from surgery have multiple stimuli for non-osmotic arginine vasopressin secretion, and are at increased risk of hyponatraemia. This is compounded by injudicious choices in fluid management. Children are more susceptible to cerebral oedema caused by acute hyponatraemia because of relative differences in brain and skull volumes. They become symptomatic at less marked levels of hyponatraemia than adults. Symptomatic hyponatraemia is a medical emergency that may require intensive care management.

All children receiving intravenous fluid therapy should have baseline electrolytes checked and then every 24 hours.

Nutrition

Children have increased nutritional requirements and decreased reserves compared to adults. If enteral nutrition is not possible, parenteral nutrition will be required in infants (1–3 days), children (4–5 days) and adolescents (7–10 days). The composition of parenteral nutrition is tailored to the patient, the younger the child, the greater the nutritional needs (Table 15.2).

Table 15.2 Total parenteral nutrition requirements in children

Age (yrs)	#Fluid (ml/kg/d)	Energy (kcal/kg/d)	Protein (g/kg/d)	Fat (g/kg/d)	*Carbohydrate (g/kg/d)[mg/kg/min]
<1	100	85–100	2–3	2–3	14.4–17.3 [10–12]
1–7	100 (first 10 kg) + 50 (next 10 kg)	75–90	1–3	2–3	11.5–14.4 [8–10]
7–12	100 (first 10 kg) + 50 (next 10 kg) + 20 (>20 kg)	50–75	1–3	2–3	11.5–14.4 [8–10]
>12	As for 7–12 yrs	30–50	0.8–1.5	1–2.5	7.2–8.6 [5–6]

Daily maintenance fluid requirements
* Glucose requirements are usually presented as mg/kg/min

Deep venous thrombosis (DVT)

Complications relating to DVT are rare, occurring with a frequency of <1% of hospitalised children. Risk factors to develop a DVT include post-pubertal age, high injury severity score, vascular injury, ICU stay > three days and central venous catheter (especially femoral).

The paediatric peri-operative history and examination

The ease with which a full history can be gained is dependent on the age, maturity, ability and willingness of the child to provide it. It may be best to obtain information from multiple sources.

From the anaesthetist's perspective, the following are important:

1. Presenting complaint: highlighting any disturbance of airway anatomy, cardiorespiratory reserve, hepatic and renal function, CNS status, risk of gastro-oesophageal reflux

2. Past medical history: co-existing disease (e.g. diabetes, epilepsy, asthma), syndromes, previous surgeries and hospital/ICU admissions. For infants, include gestational age at birth and current corrected gestational age
3. Previous problems with general anaesthesia
4. Family history of severe reactions to anaesthesia (malignant hyperpyrexia or suxamethonium apnoea)
5. Current medications – including recent use or discontinuation of steroids; allergies, including to latex or foods that may cross-react with latex
6. Focused systematic enquiry:

   Snoring/obstructed breathing at night/apnoea
   Loose teeth
   Recent upper respiratory tract infection
   Exercise tolerance
7. Fasting status. Current recommendations:

   6 h for solid food and formula milk
   4 h for breast milk
   2 h for clear fluids

Examination:

- Airway inspection – often external only +/- mouth opening to examine loose teeth +/- tonsils. Assess dysmorphic/syndromic features relevant to airway anatomy, e.g. micrognathia
- RS assessment
  - observation of rate and work of breathing
  - baseline SaO_2 in air
  - auscultation of lung fields
- CVS assessment
  - volume/hydration status. Check capillary refill, baseline heart rate and hydration of the mucous membranes.
  - precordial auscultation for murmurs
- Potential for i.v. access
- 'End-of-bed' impression of child and parent ability to cope with impending induction.

Paediatric issues of anaesthetic importance

Respiratory and cardiovascular reserve

As a general rule, and with certain exceptions, young children have excellent cardiac function and good reserve. In neonates, cardiac output is mostly heart rate dependent. However, their respiratory reserve is distinctly limited, for a variety of anatomical and physiological reasons:

- narrow upper airways
- high oxygen consumption (VO_2) and increased metabolism
- reduced functional residual capacity (FRC)

Post-operative apnoea

There is a risk of post-operative apnoeas in infants whose corrected gestational age is less than 60 weeks. Apnoeas typically occur in the first 12 hours and may persist up to 72 hours post-operatively. The risk is independently increased by ex-prematurity. The risk of post-operative apnoea in an infant whose post-conceptional age is 48 weeks is significantly higher if that infant was born at 28 weeks' gestation (post-natal age now five months) versus term (post-natal age now two months). There is debate around whether a low haematocrit (Hct) is an independent risk factor for post-operative apnoea. It is common practice to delay surgery if Hct <30%.

Recent upper respiratory tract infection (URTI)

Children with, or recovering from, an URTI are at up to ten-fold increased risk of peri-operative adverse respiratory events (PRAE), a composite outcome comprising laryngospasm, bronchospasm, desaturation (<95%), and severe coughing. The practical decision that the anaesthetist needs to make, in conjunction with the surgeon, is whether the risk of proceeding with anaesthesia outweighs the benefit of surgery at that moment in time. Clearly this is an individualised decision for each child. As a rough rule of thumb, children who have purulent sputum or nasal secretions, children who are systemically unwell, and children who have a cough as part of their URTI symptomatology should be postponed for two to three weeks unless the surgery is imperative. Children who are fully recovered from an URTI more than two weeks ago have returned to baseline risk of airway complications. The vast majority fall into a grey area that encompasses resolved – or resolving – URTI within the preceding two weeks. Decision-making in this large group is partly art, partly science, and depends upon anaesthetist comfort level, parental attitude to risk and the planned procedure. For example, the same child in whom it might be reasonable to proceed with an MRI scan (requiring no airway manipulation) might be postponed for a tonsillectomy (requiring intubation and hence a much higher risk of PRAE).

Neurotoxicity

Experimental work in multiple animal species, including primates, has demonstrated accelerated neuroapoptosis after exposure to many anaesthetic drugs. Exposure at times of critical synaptogenesis has subsequently been associated with neurobehavioural deficits. Whether these findings translate to humans is a controversial research area.

Syndromes

Many syndromes have anaesthetic implications. For common syndromes, these are usually well understood. As an example, in trisomy 21, the commonest syndrome encountered in paediatric anaesthesia, there are multiple considerations: potential difficult airway, risk of hypothyroidism, obstructive sleep apnoea, corrected or uncorrected congenital heart disease, difficult i.v. access, variable degrees of co-operation, to name a few. For rare ones, there may be little or no literature on experience of anaesthesia. Adequate time for research, and thorough pre-operative evaluation are the key guiding principles when planning anaesthesia for such children.

Emergence delirium (ED)

ED is a post-anaesthetic acute confusional state, characterised by agitation and disorientation, which typically lasts 20–90 minutes. It is extremely distressing for parents and healthcare workers to witness, and may disrupt the surgical wound. It is associated with rapid emergence facilitated by short-acting volatile anaesthetics, especially sevoflurane. It typically occurs in the two- to five-year age group and can be mistaken for uncontrolled pain, with which it may co-exist. It can be very challenging to distinguish between the two in young children, who cannot verbalise or articulate the cause of their distress. Emergence delirium is not especially responsive to opioid analgesia; the mainstay of treatment until recently has been i.v. ketamine, which blunts the severity of the delirium. As the nature and frequency of ED have become more widely recognised, its prevention and treatment have become areas of active research. Avoiding volatile exposure, by using propofol-based total intravenous anaesthesia, significantly reduces the incidence of ED, while treatment of established ED with i.v. dexmedetomidine, an alpha-2 adrenoceptor agonist, has shown promise.

Paediatric issues of surgical importance

Vascular access

In infants and children, vascular access can be challenging. However several routes are available. In the acute phase, intravenous access is typically gained via the percutaneous route. When emergency vascular access is required, if there have been three unsuccessful attempts and/or more than two minutes has passed since attempted percutaneous access, it is recommended an intraosseous needle is placed. Intraosseous needles are temporary lines and should be removed as soon as additional access is achieved. It is not recommended to leave intraosseous needles in for greater than 45 minutes because of risks such as dislodgement, compartment syndrome and osteomyelitis. Percutaneous central venous lines are typically placed in the internal jugular, subclavian or femoral locations. Femoral lines have a significantly increased risk of thrombosis in the younger patients.

For infants and children requiring long-term venous access, percutaneous or surgical central lines are employed. Percutaneously inserted central catheters (PICCs) may be inserted by a radiologist, anaesthetist or intensivist. Line position is radiologically confirmed. Surgical lines have subcutaneous tunnels and are placed by either venous cut down or via the percutaneous route. Complications of long-term central lines include infection, thrombosis, malposition and compromise of line integrity.

Correctable congenital abnormalities

The most common congenital abnormalities of the gastrointestinal tract are related to atresias. In infants with oesophageal atresia with or without fistula, patients have excessive secretions and may present with desaturations because of aspiration. Infants must be placed with the head of the bed 30 degrees upright, have a replogle (double-lumen) tube inserted to decompress the oesophagus and be placed on intravenous antibiotics. Patients need to be assessed for associated malformations (vertebral, anorectal malformation, cardiac, trachea-oesophageal, renal and limb (VACTERL)). Operative correction is open or thoracoscopic via the right hemithorax. A chest tube is typically placed and the patient kept on antibiotics and nil by mouth until a post-operative contrast study confirms patency of the oesophageal anastomosis without leak.

Intestinal atresias can occur anywhere, but are typically found in the small bowel. With duodenal atresia, an increased incidence of cardiac malformations occurs. Principles of management for intestinal atresia include nasogastric decompression, intravenous antibiotics and operative correction. Primary repair is often possible, although for some patients stomas are required because of patient or intestinal factors. Post-operatively, gastric decompression is needed until bowel function begins.

The most common abdominal wall defects are gastroschisis and omphalocoele. At the time of birth, infants with gastroschisis require nasogastric decompression, intravenous antibiotics, fluid resuscitation and protective covering of the intestinal contents to prevent evaporative heat loss and damage. Some infants with gastroschisis have relatively supple bowel and a plan is made for urgent primary closure. This may be performed at the bedside or in the operating room. Sutures may or may not be used. For those infants whose bowel has signs of significant matting, the surgeon may choose to place a silo and achieve reduction of the contents over several days. Closure of the defect is typically planned prior to five days (the risk of infection increases after five days). During either primary or delayed closure, attention is paid to the ventilation pressures; peak pressure measurements are critical to determine if it is safe to close the defect. Ventilation pressure in excess of 30 cmH_2O necessitates abandoning the closure and placement of the silo. Post-operatively, infants require nasogastric decompression and parenteral nutrition as patients with gastroschisis take on average three weeks before feeds can be initiated.

Infants born with omphalocoele have associated abnormalities 50% of the time. The most common associations are congenital heart disease, chromosomal and renal abnormalities as well as pulmonary hypoplasia. Giant omphalocoeles ($>$10 cm in diameter) are more likely to be associated with pulmonary hypoplasia. Timing of closure of the abdominal wall defect is dependent on the severity of the associated conditions. The more severe the pulmonary hypoplasia, the less likely patients will tolerate closure of the abdomen, therefore those with large omphalocoeles and pulmonary hypoplasia may be managed with topical dressings and the defect closed in a delayed fashion.

Congenital diaphragmatic hernia typically presents immediately after birth with severe respiratory distress. Intubation and a nasogastric tube are required. Patients often have significant pulmonary hypoplasia as well as pulmonary hypertension; support with high-frequency oscillating ventilation, jet ventilation, inotropes, paralysis, pulmonary vasodilators, and ECMO (extracorporeal membrane oxygenation) may be employed. Strategies are aimed at achieving adequate oxygenation with minimal barotrauma. Timing of surgical repair is dependent on the clinical status of the infant. Most commonly, once the patient is off inotropic support and pulmonary vascular reactivity has stabilised, repair of the defect is performed. This is done either open, through a left upper quadrant transverse incision or, in selected patients, thoracoscopically. The decision about when to operate requires discussion with the anaesthetist as well as the neonatal intensivist.

Congenital heart defects

Surgical intervention for children with congenital heart disease (CHD) is classified as palliative, partially corrective or completely corrective. Palliative procedures decrease negative effects of the given disorder without correcting the underlying cause. Surgery for congenital cardiac disease is typically performed via a median sternotomy and may be done on or off bypass. Closure of the sternotomy, which may be delayed, is accomplished with trans-sternal wire fixation.

Children with CHD may, of course, present for elective or emergent non-cardiac surgery, with attendant challenges for the anaesthetist. While the considerations for specific CHD lesions are beyond the scope of this text, the anaesthetist will want to ascertain the following information, wherever possible:

- Original CHD lesion(s)
- Surgical interventions for the lesion(s)
- Current anatomy of the heart and great vessels
- Functional cardiac status
- Findings of last cardiology review/ECHO/cath lab investigation

Neural tube defects

Children with neural tube defects may have associated anomalies, including cutaneous, orthopaedic, spinal, anorectal, urological abnormalities and congenital cardiac disease. Details of cardiac and renal abnormalities will concern the anaesthetist pre-operatively. For children with a myelomeningocoele, the defect is typically closed within 72 hours of birth, to decrease the chances of infection. Patients are placed prone and closure is achieved by approximating the lateral edges of the open neural plate. Patients are carefully monitored for hydrocephalus, which occurs in up to 60%. For patients with a tethered cord, a prone position is also used, a laminectomy performed and the filum terminale sectioned. Pre-operative antibiotics are given for operative correction of neural tube defects. Prone positioning mandates endotracheal intubation.

Urological abnormalities

Hypospadias results from displacement of the urethral opening and is associated with an abnormal penile curvature (chordee). Repair is one- or two-staged and the first operation is performed typically at approximately six months of age. If a second stage is required, the operation often occurs at 12 months. There are a wide variety of techniques employed to achieve correction. Caudal anaesthesia is widely used to supplement general anaesthesia and is highly effective for immediate post-op analgesia.

Paediatric orthopaedic surgery

As in adults, the array of procedures is vast, and only the most generic principles are outlined.

- Many of these children have underlying neurological co-morbidity that both accounts for their orthopaedic condition and complicates peri-operative management. Cerebral palsy, neurodegenerative disease and myopathies are all over-represented in this population. Thorough pre-op assessment and optimisation is essential, as is pre-planning of multimodal analgesia and post-op disposition.
- Major lower limb orthopaedic surgery is always associated with risk of clinically significant blood loss. Invasive haemodynamic monitoring and cell salvage techniques may be warranted.

- Lower limb surgery is highly amenable to continuous neuraxial or regional nerve block techniques that supplement general anaesthesia and provide optimum post-operative analgesia. The benefits of such techniques typically outweigh the risks of compartment or cast compression syndromes, but careful post-op monitoring protocols are essential.

Anaesthetic and peri-operative considerations for common paediatric surgical procedures

In this section we illustrate how the principles outlined above are applied in commonly encountered conditions that present to paediatric surgeons.

Pyloric stenosis

Results from hypertrophy of the pyloric muscular layers and occurs typically in infants aged two to six weeks. Patients develop dehydration and a hypokalaemic hypochloraemic metabolic alkalosis as a result of loss of gastric contents. Later, metabolic acidosis supervenes if dehydration becomes severe. Upon presentation, infants require repletion of the volume deficit with normal saline, and ongoing fluid maintenance with 5% dextrose saline +20 mmol potassium chloride/l. Re-evaluation of the infant's hydration status, electrolyte deficits and acid–base status is critical. Once the volume deficit is corrected, the chloride is greater than 100 mmol/l and the bicarbonate is less than 30 mmol/l, pyloromyotomy can be planned. Pyloromyotomy is performed either laparoscopically or open. The open approach is either through a periumbilical incision or a transverse right upper quadrant approach. If the umbilical approach is taken, peri-operative antibiotics are required. All infants with pyloric stenosis are considered to have a full stomach at induction. Paracetamol is usually sufficient for post-operative pain control.

Intussusception

Caused by telescoping of a proximal segment of bowel into the distal intestine. It is most common in children six to 24 months of age and presents with cramping abdominal pain, emesis and bloody bowel movements. Image-guided hydrostatic or pneumatic reduction is successful in the majority of cases. For children in whom radiological reduction fails, immediate operative intervention is required. Patients need fluid resuscitation and antibiotics. At operation, a transverse lower quadrant incision is most often used and attempts made to manually reduce the bowel; failing this, resection may be required. The laparoscopic approach also has been utilised. Post-operatively, ongoing fluid replacement, bowel rest and morphine are typically required.

Inguinal hernia/hydrocoele

Repairs of these conditions are among the most common surgeries performed in children. In children $<$ six months of age, the risks of incarceration increase; therefore, operative intervention is recommended at the time of diagnosis. The approaches include open and laparoscopic for hernia repair and inguinal or scrotal for hydrocoele repair. Caudal block, ilioinguinal nerve block and/or local anaesthetic infiltration are options for analgesia. Post-operatively, paracetamol is usually adequate for pain control.

Testicular torsion

Usually occurs in the prepubertal boy and presents with acute testicular pain. Emergency surgery is required to maximise the chance for testicular salvage. The incision is either bilateral transverse hemiscrotal or mid-line scrotal. The testicle is detorsed and viability assessed. If it is not viable, orchidectomy is performed. Contralateral orchidopexy is often performed at the same operation. Regional analgesia is supplemented with intra-operative local infiltration and post-operatively intravenous morphine may be required. This is emergency surgery that cannot be delayed. If the patient is not fasted a rapid-sequence induction is required.

How to estimate patient weight

APLS formula

Weight (kg) = 3 (age) + 7

(For APLS course manual see: www.alsg.org/uk/APLS)

Resuscitation Council formula, 2011

(used for the ease with which it can be remembered)

Weight (kg) = (age + 4) 2

Or:

Infants < 12 months

Weight (kg) = (age in months + 9)/2

Children aged 1–5

Weight (kg) = 2 × (age in years + 5)

Children aged 5–14

Weight (kg) = 4 × age in years

(Dieckman RA. The dilemma of paediatric drug dosing and equipment sizing in the ear of patient safety. *Emerg Med Australas* 2007; **19**(6): 528–34.)

Or:

The Broselow Paediatric Emergency Tape – a colour-coded tape measure that relates the child's height to weight. It is useful up to 12 years.

There is currently no consensus about the calculation of drug doses for the obese child.

Definitions (from European Resuscitation Council)

Neonate: child aged between birth and 28 days of life

Infant: a child under 1 year

Child: from first birthday to puberty

Chapter 16

Plastic, reconstructive and cosmetic cases

Andrew Bailey and Charles Malata

General considerations

Plastic surgery may be the last remaining true general surgical specialty. All areas of the body remain within the remit of the plastic surgeon, from hand and limb surgery, body surface surgery, breast and head and neck oncology and reconstruction, to body cavity surgery, harvesting jejunum or intra-abdominal omentum as part of a reconstructive procedure, or using body wall tissue to obliterate intrathoracic cavities. This makes the life of the plastic surgery anaesthetist varied and testing.

Plastic surgery anaesthesia similarly encompasses the full range of anaesthetic challenges, including the extremes of age, significant patient co-morbidities and the obstructed, difficult and shared airway. In addition the anaesthetist may be required to manipulate the cardiovascular parameters to minimise bleeding or ensure adequate blood flow to a flap reconstruction. Both general and regional anaesthesia skills are essential, along with a finesse to ensure smooth emergence from anaesthesia and minimal post-operative pain, nausea and vomiting.

In addition to procedure-specific anaesthetic concerns, plastic surgical procedures present some general challenges.

Multiple-team involvement

Many plastic surgical procedures are performed in conjunction with other surgical teams. Breast, maxillofacial, ear nose and throat or other surgical teams may resect a tumour, for which the plastic surgeon is required to provide a reconstructive solution, while the orthopaedic surgeon may require plastic surgical involvement while reconstructing a severely damaged limb. This requires meticulous pre-operative planning, which must include the anaesthetist. It is essential that the anaesthetist is aware of what procedures are to be performed, what position the patient is required to be in, whether any position changes are required intra-operatively and what sides and sites can or cannot be used for vascular access and invasive monitoring. Particularly with regards to resection of head and neck tumours, a plan of airway management both intra- and post-operatively is required including whether a tracheostomy is planned. Such planning needs to be made well in advance and should be re-confirmed at the surgical (WHO) team brief in theatre.

A Surgeon's Guide to Anaesthesia and Peri-operative Care, ed. Jane Sturgess, Justin Davies and Kamen Valchanov. Published by Cambridge University Press.

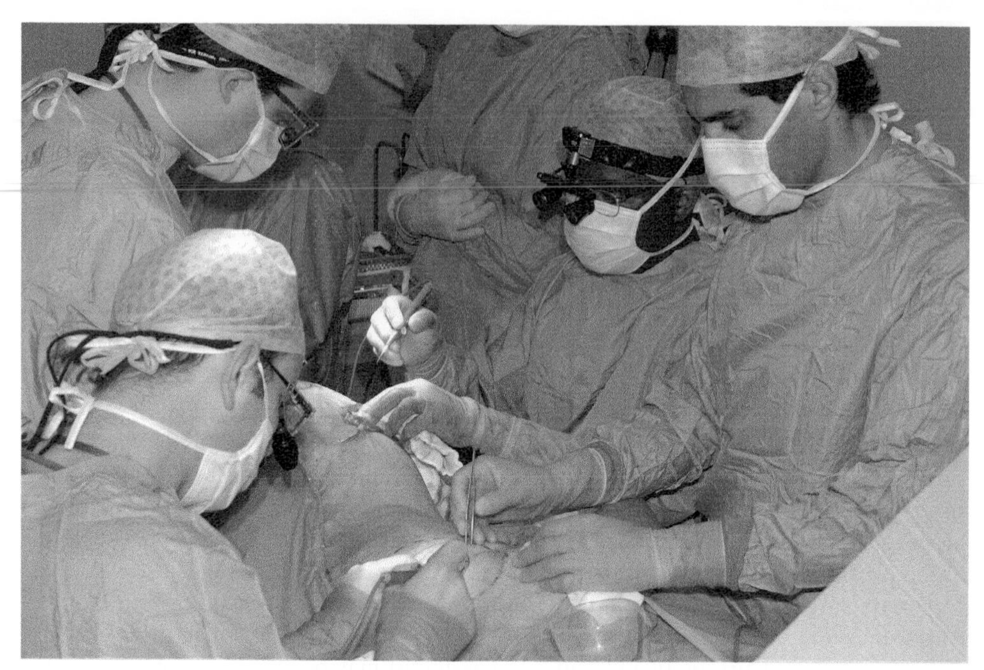

Figure 16.1 Multiple surgeons operating simultaneously during microvascular free flap breast reconstruction. Access to the patient for the anaesthetist is difficult and exposure of the patient to the cold during a prolonged procedure must be guarded against. Gluteal free flap harvest at the same time as internal mammary recipient vessel preparation following mastectomy on a patient in the left lateral decubitus position.

Intra-operative patient access

Multiple-team involvement also raises the issue of intra-operative access to the patient in theatre. In the case of a mastectomy and immediate breast reconstruction with a free abdominal flap and contralateral balancing breast surgery, it is quite common for three surgical teams to be operating at once (Figure 16.1), reducing access to the airway, intravenous lines, monitoring etc. Consequently the anaesthetist must be meticulous in the positioning and securing of all vascular catheters and ensure that there are distant injection ports to administer drugs. In addition, the anaesthetist needs to keep an eye on inadvertent leaning on the patient by surgical assistants, movement of limbs to unacceptable positions and accumulated blood loss from multiple sites.

Prolonged surgery

Major plastic surgery, particularly when combined with tumour resection, can be a lengthy affair, lasting many hours. Blood loss may be insidious, requiring constant monitoring and preparation for transfusion. Fluid balance must be monitored, with a urinary catheter inserted and regular checking of acid–base status, serum haemoglobin/haematocrit and electrolyte and glucose levels. Appropriate pressure care of patients is essential, ensuring that all pressure points are well padded and that pressure is not applied to peripheral nerves. Similarly, padding of the eyes is essential to avoid corneal damage or inadvertent pressure damage. Thromboprophylaxis should also be considered, although many plastic surgeons do not administer thromboprophylaxis prior to surgery, because of concerns of bleeding. Elasticated compression stockings and intermittent pneumatic calf compression devices should be used intra-operatively. Post-operative thromboprophylaxis with low molecular weight heparin is then required.

As with any prolonged surgery, temperature control is important. Hypothermia is associated with coagulopathy, acidosis, cardiac arrhythmias and increased post-operative oxygen requirements. In addition, in the case of free tissue transfer, it is particularly undesirable (see later). Adequate room ambient temperature, warmed intravenous fluids and warm air blankets are required.

Control of bleeding

Although control of bleeding is ostensibly a surgical consideration, the very history of the development of anaesthesia for plastic and reconstructive surgery highlights the role of the anaesthetist in reducing surgical bleeding, making procedures safer by reducing blood loss and transfusion requirement, and by making procedures easier by reducing bleeding into the surgical field, creating a relative 'bloodless field'.

The major means by which a 'bloodless field' can be achieved are:

1. Position: Elevation of the surgical site above the level of the heart, e.g. use of the reverse-Trendelenburg position for head and neck surgery.
2. Local vasoconstrictors: Infiltration of the tissues with a solution containing a vasoconstrictor, e.g. epinephrine, usually combined with a local anaesthetic, or direct topical application to mucous membranes, e.g. cocaine to the nasal mucosa.
3. Ventilation: The use of positive pressure ventilation, particularly when combined with the reverse-Trendelenburg position and the application of PEEP, and vasodilator drugs (including volatile anaesthetic agents) can markedly reduce pre-load, and reduce bleeding in head and neck surgery.
4. Control of arterial carbon dioxide levels: Hypercarbia leads to peripheral vasodilatation, while hypocarbia causes vasoconstriction.
5. Induced or deliberate hypotension (see Table 16.1 and 16.2): This technique was popularised for plastic surgery in the late 1940s and involves the use of drugs to reduce blood pressure during anaesthesia by more than 30% of resting values or to a systolic of around 80 mmHg (mean arterial pressure 50–60 mmHg).

Historically, the blood pressure was slowly returned to normal in the belief that this was less likely to dislodge haemostatic clots. With pharmacological advances and the development of rapidly acting drugs, many surgeons like to see normalisation of the blood pressure before surgical closure, and ensure complete haemostasis. After head and neck surgery, some surgeons also request the anaesthetist to perform a Valsalva manoeuvre or a steep head down position on the patient to increase venous pressure to further assist in identifying bleeding points.

Emergence from anaesthesia and post-operative nausea and vomiting

Coughing, straining and retching can all raise arterial and venous pressure, and contribute to increasing the risk of post-operative haematoma formation. Meticulous attention to the choice of anaesthetic technique is required and its management, along with the

Table 16.1 Contraindications for induced or deliberate hypotension

Cardiovascular pathology	Ischaemic and valvular heart disease Hypertension Cerebrovascular disease Hypovolaemia Anaemia
Other organ pathology	Severe respiratory disease Hepatic disease Renal disease Diabetes Pregnancy

Table 16.2 Drugs commonly used to induce hypotension

Pharmacological agent	Example
Anaesthetic	Intravenous or volatile Epidural or spinal regional technique
Acting on autonomic nervous system	Beta blockade, e.g. atenolol Alpha adrenergic blockade, e.g. phentolamine Combined alpha and beta blockade, e.g. labetalol
Vasodilator drugs	Sodium nitroprusside, glycerine trinitrate, hydralazine

administration of suitable analgesia, to ensure that the patient emerges smoothly from anaesthesia. The use of propofol both for induction and maintenance along with the laryngeal mask airway, avoiding the need for tracheal intubation, has proved a very useful technique for many plastic surgical procedures.

Post-operative nausea and vomiting (PONV) is a common and distressing side effect. Certain risk factors have been identified including:

- Female sex
- Non-smoker
- History of previous PONV or motion sickness
- Post-operative opioids

Patients with risk factors should receive prophylactic anti-emetics. Where no risk factors are identified, there is little value in administering prophylactic anti-emetics except where the procedure is associated with a high incidence of PONV or where the symptoms may compromise the success of the procedure. Many plastic surgical procedures may fit into this final category. For an adult, dexamethasone 4 mg i.v., administered at the start of the surgical procedure, and cyclizine (50 mg i.m. or i.v.) or ondansetron (4 mg i.v.) administered towards the end of surgery is common practice.

Cosmetic surgery

While no different in requirements to any other plastic surgical patient, cosmetic surgery brings its own challenges, both in terms of the expectations of the patients, the

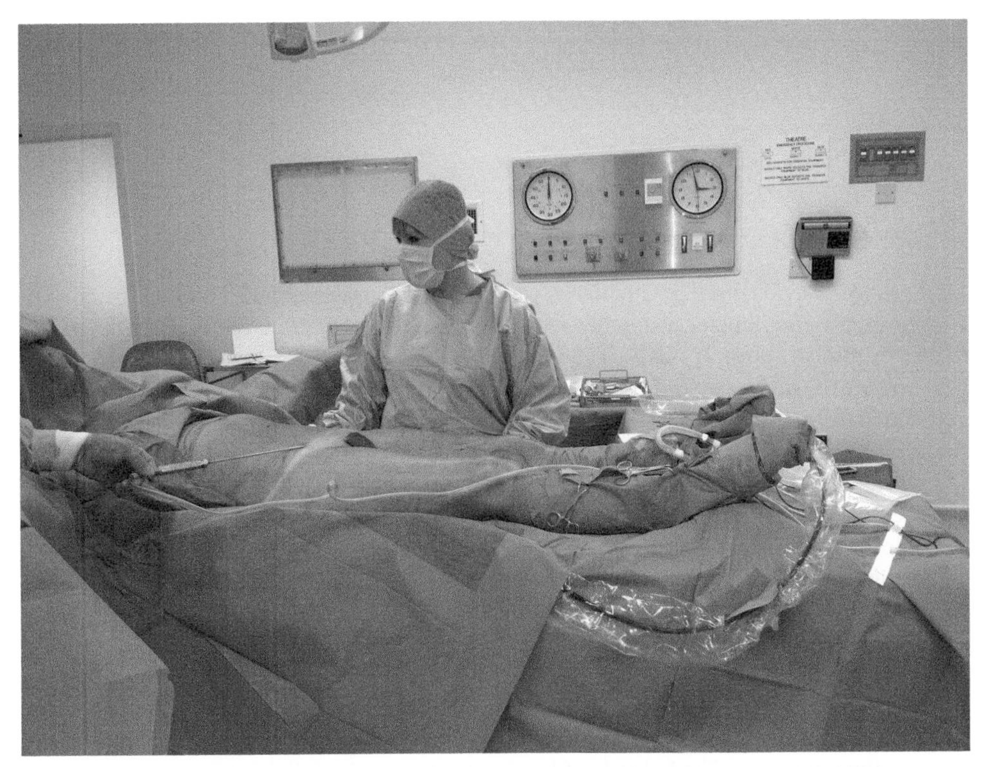

Figure 16.2 Combined cosmetic surgery presents a particular anaesthetic challenge. A 55-year-old lady undergoing simultaneous thigh lifts, arm lifts and abdominal liposuction. Venous access is difficult as is monitoring. After the arm lifts no BP cuffs could be placed on either arm, hence a BP cuff was put on the right calf and its tubes covered in a sterile laparoscopy 'camera bag'. Such exposure of large areas of the body to the environment can quickly lead to reduced core body temperature, especially if cold liposuction fluids are administered. Following the arm lifts the upper third of the body has been covered with sterile drapes and a Bair Hugger® applied. A bladder catheter enabled accurate urine output monitoring and facilitated fluid administration.

consequences of post-operative haematoma formation and the requirement for multiple refining procedures. Combination cosmetic surgery presents a particular anaesthetic challenge because of various problems it poses including exposure with difficulty in keeping the patient warm (see Figure 16.2), monitoring the patient, difficult venous access, multiple changes of position and several potential sites for blood loss to mention but a few.

Safe local anaesthesia for plastic surgery

Although many plastic surgical procedures are performed under general anaesthesia, many others can be performed under local anaesthesia, either in the operating theatre (with or without an anaesthetist), or by the surgeon alone, in an outpatient setting. Local anaesthetic techniques used can include:

- Local infiltration
- Peripheral nerve block
- Plexus block, performed by the surgeon or anaesthetist (e.g. brachial plexus)
- Central neuraxial block (spinal or epidural)

Table 16.3 Recommended safe doses of local anaesthetic

Drug	Safe dose – no adrenaline	Safe dose – with adrenaline
Bupivacaine	2 mg/kg	2 mg/kg
Lidocaine	3 mg/kg	7 mg/kg

Limb surgery lends itself particularly well to local anaesthetic techniques, usually in conscious patients, but occasionally with sedation or general anaesthesia. Local anaesthetic administration is also widely used within plastic surgery to supplement post-operative analgesia and is often administered with adrenaline to provide local vasoconstriction to minimise surgical bleeding and reduce the systemic absorption of the local anaesthetic, allowing greater doses to be used and prolonging the duration of the block.

The use of local anaesthetic agents requires the operator to have knowledge of the safe use of local anaesthetic (including knowledge of how much they are administering), as well as the signs and symptoms of local anaesthetic toxicity and its immediate management. Allergy with the local anaesthetics commonly used in the UK, which all belong to the amide group of local anaesthetics (lidocaine, bupivacaine, levobupivacaine, ropivacaine, prilocaine), is exceptionally rare.

The concept of a safe dose of local anaesthetic is perhaps something of a myth, as in truth it is high, toxic blood concentrations of local anaesthetic that lead to systemic toxicity and not the dose alone. Toxic levels of local anaesthetic arise following:

- The administration of excessive amounts of the drug
- Rapid absorption from the site of administration, which is dependent upon the site of administration (e.g. absorption from an intercostal injection is greater than epidural injection, which in turn is greater than peripheral or subcutaneous injection), tissue blood flow and solubility of the local anaesthetic
- Impaired metabolism can contribute to systemic toxicity
- Accidental intravascular injection. When injecting in a large surgical field, a continuously moving injection cannula reduces the risk of significant intravascular injection.

Despite all of this, it is considered good practice to restrict local anaesthetic doses to their maximum recommended doses.

Systemic local anaesthetic toxicity

1. Manifests as cardiovascular and central nervous system effects.
2. Slow injection allows time to identify the initial symptoms, allowing the injection to be stopped before significant dangerous toxicity arises.
3. Initial symptoms of toxicity include perioral tingling, a metallic taste and tinnitus, progressing to visual and speech disturbance.
4. Significant toxicity may manifest as alteration in mental status, severe agitation, and loss of consciousness, convulsions, cardiac arrhythmias and respiratory or cardiac arrest.

Table 16.4 The use of intravenous 20% lipid emulsion in the management of cardiac arrest caused by systemic local anaesthetic toxicity

Time	Action	Dose of lipid emulsion
Immediately	20% lipid emulsion bolus dose	1.5 ml/kg over 1 minute (100 ml for a 70 kg patient)
	Start infusion of 20% lipid emulsion	15 ml/kg/h
After 5 minutes	Give a maximum of two repeat bolus doses at 5-minute intervals	1.5 ml/kg
	Double the infusion rate if cardiovascular instability continues or further deteriorates	30 ml/kg/h

NB. It is important to know the location of the lipid emulsion before using local anaesthetics

Treatment of systemic toxicity

1. Stop injection and call for help, including anaesthetic support.
2. Maintain the airway and administer 100% oxygen.
3. Treat seizures with incremental midazolam, or propofol or thiopentone.
4. Supportive treatment is required for hypotension or cardiac arrhythmias, including intravenous fluids, vasopressors and antiarrhythmic agents.
5. Treat cardiac arrest with standard BLS/ALS algorithms.
6. Expect prolonged resuscitation (especially with bupivacaine).
7. In cardiac arrest, give intravenous 20% lipid emulsion (Table 16.4).

Terminology of local anaesthetics solutions

Understanding the terminology of the strength of local anaesthetics is essential to ensure the administrator knows what he/she is administering and consequently how much can be given. Most local anaesthetic preparations are labelled as either '%' or mg ml^{-1}

- 0.25% solution means 0.25 g in 100 ml, which equates to 2.5 mg ml^{-1}.
- 0.5% solution means 0.5 g in 100 ml, which equates to 5 mg ml^{-1}.
- 1% solution means 1 g in 100 ml, which equates to 10 mg ml^{-1}.

i.e. multiply the % by 10 to get the mg ml^{-1}.

Terminology of epinephrine (adrenaline) solutions

Epinephrine is often added to local anaesthetic solutions to reduce systemic absorption of local anaesthetics and prolong action or to reduce bleeding. If not ready-mixed with the local anaesthetic, it is supplied as either 1 ml ampoules, containing 1 mg epinephrine (1:1000), or 10 ml ampoules, containing 1 mg epinephrine (1:10,000).

- 1:1,000 means 1 g in 1,000 ml or 1,000 mg in 1,000 ml or 1 mg ml^{-1}
- 1:10,000 means 1 g in 10,000 ml or 1,000 mg in 10,000 ml or 1 mg in 10 ml or 100 mcg ml^{-1}

It is common practice for surgeons to add epinephrine to 20 ml of local anaesthetic to make a 1 in 200,000 solution. This requires the addition of 100 mcg epinephrine (0.1 ml of 1:1,000 epinephrine).

If a plastic surgeon adds 1 ml of 1:1,000 epinephrine to a 1 litre bag for infiltration a 1:1,000,000 solution is created.

Specific procedures

Rhinoplasty

Pre-operative

Patients are generally young and fit and undergo surgery for obvious or perceived abnormalities of appearance. The latter group may bring additional difficulties of unrealistic expectations and may undergo several repeat procedures.

Intra-operative

The main intra-operative requirement is to have a relatively bloodless field. In addition to head up positioning and possible use of a deliberate hypotensive technique, local administration of vasoconstrictors (often cocaine and/or epinephrine) is usual practice.

A throat pack is inserted to soak up any blood in the pharynx, which must be visible throughout the procedure, and removed at the end.

Cocaine is an ester local anaesthetic (the only vasoconstricting local anaesthetic), but it also inhibits the re-uptake of norepinephrine in pre-synaptic sympathetic nerve terminals, leading to peripheral vasoconstriction, as well as hypertension and tachycardia. It is readily absorbed from the nasal mucosa. In addition to the cardiovascular effects, an overdose of cocaine leads to excitement, restlessness and confusion, with further toxicity leading to hyperpyrexia, convulsions, coma and death. Epinephrine is occasionally used in addition to cocaine to provide further vasoconstriction, while theoretically reducing the absorption of the cocaine. This latter effect is inconsistent. The combined use of epinephrine and cocaine has the potential effect of increasing the risk of unwanted sympathetic overactivity, and should be used with extreme caution in patients with cardiovascular pathology.

Cocaine is supplied as a solution or a paste in various strengths (4–10%) and the administered dose should not exceed 1.5 mg kg^{-1}.

Post-operative

Pain following rhinoplasty can usually be treated with simple oral analgesia (paracetamol, non-steroidal anti-inflammatory drugs). The most distressing side effect is often the blocked nose, particularly if a nasal pack is inserted. Swallowing of postnasal bleeding can also lead to nausea and vomiting.

Facelift (rhytidectomy)

Pre-operative

Patients requesting facelifts tend to be older and may have co-morbidities. Again expectations may be high or unrealistic. The procedure may be combined with other aesthetic procedures, including brow or eyelid surgery.

Intra-operative

In the UK this procedure is usually performed under general anaesthesia, while in the USA it is commonly performed under local anaesthesia with sedation or sedo-analgesia (ketamine and benzodiazepines, being a popular combination). Some advocates claim a reduced incidence of post-operative haematoma, as intra-operative hypotension is avoided and post-operative nausea and vomiting is less likely.

When general anaesthesia is employed the choice of airway needs to be discussed with the surgeon and is determined by the areas to be operated on (south facing oral tube or north facing nasal tube). Similarly the method of fixation of the airway needs to be discussed. Some surgeons accept taping of the tube, while others suture or wire the tube to teeth. It is the authors' preference not to fix the tube at all, assuming that no difficulty was encountered in its insertion, allowing the surgeon complete freedom in moving the tube to get to all areas of surgery. Of course this relies upon an understanding with and a confidence in the surgeon that the endotracheal tube will not be dislodged from the trachea. Constant vigilance is essential.

The surgery is performed with head up tilt; blood pressure manipulation may be used, along with local anaesthetic and vasoconstrictor infiltration, to improve surgical conditions. It is essential that haemostasis be confirmed before surgical closure.

Post-operative

Emergence from anaesthesia should be as smooth as possible, avoiding coughing and post-operative vomiting to reduce the risk of bleeding and haematoma formation. Tight or bulky dressings can make airway management difficult should a problem arise in the immediate post-operative period. Post-operative bleeding requires a speedy return to theatre.

Analgesic requirements are generally minimal, particularly if local infiltration or facial nerve blocks have been used, although a single dose of morphine prior to completion of surgery adds a welcome degree of sedation in the post-operative period.

Most patients are discharged from hospital the day after surgery.

Liposuction

Liposuction may be used to reduce the volume of body areas such as breast tissue, or abnormalities following other procedures (dog ears, post abdominoplasty, or post-reconstructive surgery). Alternatively it is used to change body shape for aesthetic reasons (liposculpture). Although volumes are usually restricted to 3 litres, much larger volumes have been aspirated (10–12 litres).

Pre-operative

Pre-operative investigations are dictated by the co-morbidity of the patient, and the expected volume of liposuction to be performed. Patients undergoing large volume liposuction should have a full blood count and serum electrolytes measured, along with a group and save.

Intra-operative

Minor liposuction can be performed under local anaesthesia, supplemented with sedation, but large volume or prolonged procedures are usually performed under general anaesthesia,

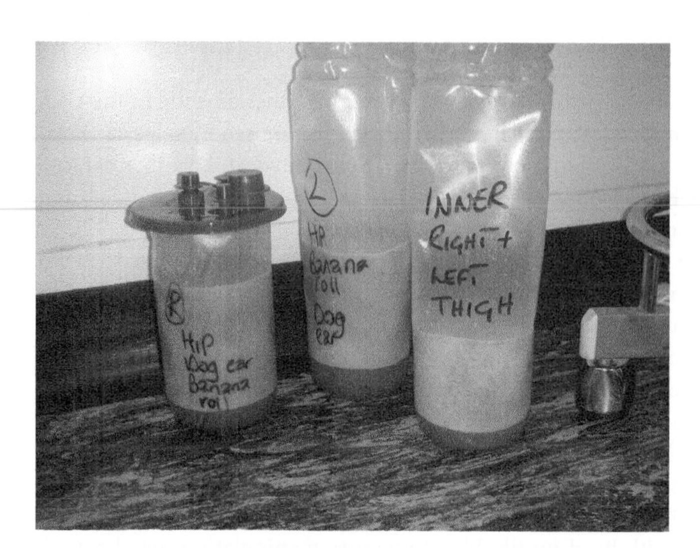

Figure 16.3 Canisters of aspirate obtained during ultrasonic liposuction. The emulsified fat is located above the aqueous (fluid) component. The aspirated volume should be accurately monitored and fluids replaced adequately but judiciously to avoid fluid overload. The blood content varies according to the colour of the aspirate.

particularly in the UK. Position of the patient depends upon which areas are to be aspirated and several intra-operative changes in position may be required. Temperature maintenance may be difficult because of the area of the body that needs to be exposed and forced warm air blankets and warm intravenous fluids should be used.

Assessment of blood loss during the procedure is difficult and depends upon the area being aspirated, the quality of the aspirate and what infiltration has been performed prior to aspiration. Estimates range from 1–40% of the volume aspirated (see Figure 16.3).

The terminology around liposuction techniques reflects the volume of infiltration fluid that is injected into the area prior to aspiration, to assist in the breakdown of the fat and aid aspiration. Terms such as 'dry', 'wet', 'super wet' and 'tumescent' techniques are used, reflecting the volume of injectate and the proportion of the aspirate that is blood. The super wet technique involves the infiltration of 1 ml of infiltrate per ml of aspirate, while the tumescent technique infiltrates two to three times as much fluid. Blood loss with these two techniques is approximately 1–4% and less than 1% of aspirate respectively. A common infiltration regime combines 50 ml 1% lidocaine with 1 ml 1:1,000 adrenaline per litre of Hartmann's solution. As a result, the patient can be exposed to large fluid volumes, with absorption of infiltrate, and high lidocaine and epinephrine doses. Maximum doses of lidocaine of 35–55 $mg.kg^{-1}$ have been advocated using the tumescent technique, well above the standard recommended maximum dose of 7 $mg.kg^{-1}$ lidocaine with epinephrine. Such doses are thought to be tolerated because of the epinephrine, causing vasoconstriction and slowing absorption, fat being relatively avascular and some of the infiltrate being removed with the aspirate. Peak lidocaine concentrations may not be reached for up to 12–24 hours. Nevertheless deaths have occurred following liposuction from infection, haemorrhage, viscus perforation, thromboembolism and fluid overload, but lidocaine toxicity has also been implicated.

Post-operative

Large-volume liposuction resembles a burn injury, with fluid loss that requires intravenous replacement and monitoring of urine output. A post-operative full blood count should also be performed, although the need for transfusion is rare. Analgesic requirements depend upon the site and extent of the procedure. Again oral analgesia is usually sufficient. Where extensive or prolonged surgery has been performed, consideration must be given to thromboprophylaxis.

Anaesthesia for breast plastic surgery

Plastic surgery of the breast ranges from aesthetic surgery, correction of congenital anomalies to reconstructive oncoplastic surgery of the breast.

Breast augmentation surgery

Pre-operative

Patients undergoing this type of surgery are usually young, fit and thin. In a young female population a full blood count and a pregnancy test are usually performed. Blood loss is minimal, so group and save or cross-match is not normally required.

Intra-operative

General anaesthesia for this procedure usually involves airway maintenance with a laryngeal mask or endotracheal tube and spontaneous or positive pressure ventilation. Laryngeal mask airways enable a smoother emergence from anaesthesia in many cases, possibly minimising the risk of coughing.

The patient is positioned with her arms abducted on well-padded arm boards or with the arms by the side, the elbows slightly flexed, padded and resting on 'D' boards, with the hands secured under the buttocks. Care must be taken to ensure that the fingers are flat, to avoid injury. The patient is positioned on the operating table in such a way that they can be sat up, flexing at the hips for inspection of size and symmetry.

Post-operative

Intra-operative intravenous opioids and local anaesthesia provide early post-operative analgesia. Thereafter, paracetamol, oral opioid and non-steroidal analgesia is sufficient in most cases. The surgery is usually performed as a day case or 23 hours stay procedure.

Pneumothorax is a well recognised but rare complication of breast augmentation surgery, arising during preparation of the breast pocket or during injection of local anaesthetic.

Symptoms of dyspnoea and chest pain with hypoxia should trigger investigation and treatment of pneumothorax. Tension pneumothorax requires immediate decompression with a wide-bore intravenous cannula in the second intercostal space, prior to formal insertion of a chest tube.

Reduction mammoplasty and mastopexy (breast lift)

Pre-operative

Historically, this procedure was associated with significant blood loss but advances in electrocautery, with cutting and coagulating diathermy, have revolutionised the procedure, along with the infiltration of the breast with adrenaline containing local anaesthetic solutions, e.g. 300 mg lidocaine plus 1 mg epinephrine in 1,000 ml saline. Nevertheless a group and save sample is usually advised, along with a pre-operative full blood count.

Intra-operative

General anaesthesia is conducted with the use of a laryngeal mask airway or endotracheal tube, usually with positive pressure ventilation. Patients are positioned with the arms abducted on well-padded boards, avoiding abduction further than 90 degrees to avoid brachial plexus injury. Positioning on the table should allow flexion at the hips, when sitting up to inspect symmetry and size.

Post-operative

Intravenous opioid analgesia, paracetamol and non-steroidal anti-inflammatory drugs are used for analgesia and patient-controlled intravenous analgesia can be considered post-operatively. Patients may require intravenous fluids until eating and drinking. Thromboprophylaxis should be prescribed, e.g. low molecular weight heparin and elasticated compression stockings.

With any breast surgery, regular inspection by the nursing and surgical teams is required to detect post-operative haematomas, requiring surgical evacuation. Consideration should be given to the urgency of need of evacuation and balancing it against the risk of aspiration if the patient is not starved.

Breast onco-plastic surgery

All patients requiring mastectomy should have the opportunity to discuss reconstruction, which may be immediate (at the time of mastectomy) or delayed. The options are outside of the scope of this book. Two common reconstructive procedures are detailed below.

Latissimus dorsi pedicled flap

Pre-operative

Pre-operative investigations are dictated by patient age, co-morbidity and cancer treatment. Previous chemotherapy is common and a full blood count is essential. The chemotherapy drugs paclitaxel and epirubicin can cause direct cardiotoxicity, acute coronary syndromes and impaired cardiac conduction leading to arrhythmias. A pre-operative electrocardiogram and an echocardiogram should be considered. Trastuzumab (Herceptin®) has also been associated with cardiac toxicity and these patients have regular echocardiograms to assess left ventricular function, the results of which must be available to the anaesthetist.

Blood loss is gradual over the first few post-operative days and transfusion may be required; a group and save is advised.

Intra-operative

Mastectomy and raising of a latissimus dorsi pedicled flap (LD flap) are often performed simultaneously, with the patient positioned in the lateral position, operative side upper most. Access to the axilla for axillary lymph node clearance requires the arm to be abducted to almost 90 degrees with the elbow flexed, with the forearm and elbow secured to a well-padded L-bar. Once the mastectomy and lymph node dissection have been completed and the flap raised, the donor site is closed and the patient turned supine, again with arms abducted on well-padded boards, ready for insetting of the flap into the mastectomy site with or without insertion of an expander or implant.

Anaesthesia is performed using a laryngeal mask airway or endotracheal tube and positive pressure ventilation. A urinary catheter is useful because of surgical duration, peri-operative fluid losses and limited patient mobility in the day or so after surgery.

Post-operative

Analgesia is provided by intra-operative opiates, paracetamol and non-steroidal anti-inflammatory drugs, followed by post-operative patient-controlled opiate analgesia. Paravertebral block(s) can also be used.

Post-operative thromboprophylaxis with elasticated compression stockings and subcutaneous low molecular weight heparin should be prescribed.

Free flap surgery (8–12 hours)

Free flap reconstruction can be used to provide tissue coverage of defects caused by trauma, burns or surgical excision, where local simpler alternatives are not feasible or where the bulk of a flap containing skin, subcutaneous tissue or muscle will provide a more aesthetically satisfactory result or facilitate function. Free flap or free tissue transfer involves disconnecting a piece of tissue from its arterial and venous circulation, transferring the tissue to a distant site and then using microvascular surgical techniques to re-anastomose the blood vessels to arteries and veins at the new site.

Free flap reconstruction of the breast can be achieved using abdominal tissue, e.g. transverse rectus abdominus myocutaneous flap (TRAM) or deep inferior epigastric perforator flap (DIEP) or buttock tissue, e.g. superior or inferior gluteal artery perforator flap (SGAP or IGAP). During breast reconstruction using a free flap, the following stages occur:

- Mastectomy (if immediate)
- Harvesting of the free flap, including dissection of the artery and vein
- Dissection of the recipient blood vessels
- Disconnection of the free flap from its blood supply
- Anastomosis of the free flap to the recipient blood vessels
- Reperfusion of the flap
- Insetting of the breast and closure
- Closure of the donor site

Several of the stages may occur simultaneously. Consequently these procedures require detailed pre-operative planning so that the whole team are aware of what will happen and the anaesthetist is aware of what access they will have to the patient, the airway and vascular access.

Pre-operative

Pre-operative assessment requires a full and detailed history from the patient to identify significant co-morbidities, drug treatments and oncologic treatment history, with subsequent investigations guided by the findings.

Adequate pre-operative preparation of the patient includes a full explanation by the surgeon of the procedure and its magnitude and discussion of the risk of flap failure.

Obesity is associated with a higher incidence of flap failure and necrosis. The anaesthetist needs to explain any invasive monitoring that is planned and what post-operative analgesia will be used and where the patient will be cared for post-operatively.

Disruption of vascular anastomoses to intrathoracic or axillary blood vessels, although uncommon, can lead to sudden brisk haemorrhage so patients undergoing this type of surgery should be cross matched (usually 2–4 units).

Intra-operative

During the period of disconnection, the tissue is not perfused and is therefore ischaemic (primary ischaemia) and metabolism consequently becomes anaerobic. The tissue becomes acidotic, with the accumulation of lactate, calcium and inflammatory mediators. To prevent irreversible damage, this period must be kept as short as possible (less than 2–4 hours depending on the tissue involved, flaps containing muscle being more at risk of primary ischaemia). Following reperfusion, the flap remains at risk of further ischaemic insults (secondary ischaemia) because of vasoconstriction, vessel spasm or kinking, thrombosis, venous obstruction or haematoma. Inadequate blood flow may also arise as a result of interstitial oedema because of excessive crystalloids, trauma or ischaemia, exacerbated by the absence of lymphatic drainage.

The main principle in the peri-operative management of free flap surgery is to maximise blood flow by ensuring a good cardiac output and a vasodilated circulation. Although perhaps a huge assumption, if blood flow to the free flap is assumed to be laminar, it can be described in terms of the Hagen Poiseuille equation:

$$\text{Laminar flow} = \frac{\Delta P \, \pi r^4}{8 \eta l}$$

Where:

ΔP is the pressure difference
r is the radius of the blood vessel
η is the viscosity of the blood
l is the length of the blood vessel

Consequently the aims of anaesthesia are to ensure:

1. Vasodilatation (and avoid vasoconstriction)
2. A good perfusion pressure
3. A low viscosity

1. The anaesthetist can aid vasodilatation by:

- Avoiding hypovolaemia and ensuring that the patient is well hydrated
- Avoiding hypothermia
- Providing adequate anaesthesia and analgesia
- Avoiding vasoconstrictors whenever possible

Although the free flap tissue is denervated, its blood vessels still respond to physical, humeral and chemical stimuli, including temperature, circulating catecholamines and drugs, while the artery and vein to which it is anastomosed still retain an intact nerve supply responding to sympathetic neuronal activity too.

Topical vasodilators are applied to blood vessels intra-operatively by the surgeon, e.g. papaverine or verapamil. Further vasodilatation may be provided by sympathetic blockade caused by regional anaesthesia (see later).

2. An adequate perfusion pressure is essential, but efforts to raise blood pressure at the expense of vasodilatation should be avoided since changes in radius of blood vessels have a much greater effect on blood flow (fourth power). Hypotension should initially be treated with intravenous fluids rather than vasoactive medications. Although traditional teaching and logic is to avoid vasopressors (e.g. phenylephrine, metaraminol) and to use drugs such as dobutamine to increase blood pressure if required, there is very little evidence to suggest that judicious use of vasopressors to maintain an adequate blood pressure is actually detrimental, if hypovolaemia is avoided.

3. Blood viscosity depends largely on haematocrit, increasing exponentially as haematocrit rises. Consequently, haemodilution increases blood flow but reductions in haematocrit are associated with a reduction in blood oxygen content and therefore delivery to the tissues. A haematocrit of 30% is aimed for to achieve the best balance.

A balanced anaesthetic technique is used, with agents that favour a rapid but smooth extubation at the end of the procedure. Maintenance of anaesthesia with desflurane or a propofol infusion is common practice, supplemented with the ultra-short acting opioid remifentanil by infusion, providing a vasodilated circulation. The airway is usually secured with an endotracheal tube, although some units have reported using the Pro-Seal® laryngeal mask airway, with an oesophageal Doppler probe placed down the drain tube, guiding fluid management.

A more traditional approach to monitoring and guiding fluid therapy is to insert arterial and central venous catheters and a urinary catheter and aim to maintain blood pressure, central venous pressure and a good urine output. Measurement of the difference between the core and peripheral temperatures is a useful indicator of fluid status, with the difference increasing with peripheral vasoconstriction in response to hypovolaemia. A difference of less than 2°C, suggests the patient is warm and well filled. Fluid management should include judicious use of crystalloids, to provide maintenance fluids and replace pre-operative deficits and insensible losses and synthetic colloids and blood to replace blood loss. Excessive use of crystalloids can lead to interstitial oedema of the flap. Intravenous dextrans have also been used because of their effect on improving blood flow and reducing platelet aggregation. The evidence for any benefit in flap outcome is not strong and they are associated with undesirable side effects, including impaired coagulation, renal failure and anaphylaxis.

As stated, hypothermia is a potent cause of vasoconstriction, as well as increased blood viscosity. The core temperature should be monitored during surgery with a nasopharyngeal probe and the patient actively warmed with warm air blankets, operating table warmers, warmed intravenous fluids and ensuring the temperature of the operating theatre is adequate (24–25°C). Circle breathing systems also help to minimise heat loss.

Free tissue transfer procedures can be lengthy. During the peri-operative period, care should be taken in the positioning of the patient, to avoid nerve compression, e.g. ulnar nerve in abducted arms on arm boards and to avoid pressure sores. Similarly awareness of the degree of abduction of the arms is required to avoid hyperabduction and risk of brachial plexus injury, especially as the arms may be moved during the surgery to provide access for the surgical team.

Positional discomfort following the surgery is a real problem, with the patient being in one position for many hours. Some advocate intermittent passive movement of limbs during the case.

Fatigue and boredom may affect the medical team and regular breaks for staff should be encouraged and alarms for vital sign parameters should be set.

Post-operative

Although a lengthy operation, in most units, extubation at the end of surgery is the norm and return to a post-operative plastic surgery ward, rather than a critical care area.

Post-operative analgesia is usually provided by intravenous opioids often in the form of a PCAS (patient-controlled analgesia system), supplemented by regular paracetamol. Non-steroidal anti-inflammatory drugs are often avoided because of a concern about bleeding and haematoma formation. Thoracic epidural analgesia has been used for post-operative analgesia, with the theoretical benefits of good analgesia, a reduction in the stress response to surgery, reduced incidence of venous thromboembolism and more rapid recovery. The vasodilatation produced should be beneficial to the flap. However it has been suggested that vasodilatation of other areas may lead to diversion of blood flow away from the free flap ('Steal' phenomenon) and vasodilatation in the presence of hypovolaemia may markedly reduce blood flow to the free flap.

The principles of free-flap management must not be forgotten post-operatively:

- Normothermia, nursed in a warm environment
- Adequately filled, with a high cardiac output and a vasodilated circulation
- A good urine output (>0.5 ml/kg)
- Haematocrit of 30%
- Good analgesia
- Regular observation of the flap, including colour, capillary refill time and Doppler signal

If the flap becomes pale and cold, arterial thrombosis should be suspected, whereas a congested flap with a brisk capillary return suggests venous obstruction. A prompt return to theatre for surgical re-exploration is indicated in order to salvage the free flap. Where vessel thrombosis is suspected, direct infusion of streptokinase or urokinase into flap vessels may be required, avoiding flushing the solutions into the systemic circulation.

Further reading

Quinlan J, Lodi O. (2009). Anaesthesia for reconstructive surgery. *Anaesthesia and Intensive Care Medicine* 2009; **10(1)**: 26–31.

Simpson P. (1992). Peri-operative blood loss and its reduction: The role of the anaesthetist. *Brit J Anaesthes* 1992; **69**: 498–507.

Chapter 17

Neurosurgery cases

Jane Sturgess and Ramez Kirollos

Anaesthesia is one of the major determinants of a successful outcome after neurosurgical procedures. Pre-operative assessment, induction of anaesthesia, maintenance of anaesthesia, the process of extubation, and immediate post-operative care are interlinked and enable surgery to proceed smoothly. Good neuroanaesthesia produces a relaxed brain and optimal operating conditions. Additional manipulation of the patient's physiology may be necessary according to the procedure. The care of the patient and the maintenance of a favourable intracranial/intraspinal environment remain with the anaesthetist into the recovery room and, at times, the intensive care unit.

Pre-operative assessment

The anaesthetist faces a number of challenges when assessing the neurosurgical patient.

1. Many patients will be transferred as an emergency directly to theatre from other hospitals. Communication regarding the patient's intracranial pathology, the proposed position for surgery and the expected time of arrival can speed the time to incision, and allow the anaesthetist to prepare for the case. Excellent communication between the transferring and receiving team is essential. It must include the patient's medical history as far as is known, mechanism of injury, neurology at scene, treatments received so far, and other injuries identified. Limited information will be available from blood investigations.
2. Patients with intracranial pathology may have receptive or expressive dysphasia, a low GCS, neuropsychiatric disorders or capacity issues.
3. Patients with low GCS, or neurological weakness of whatever cause do not exert themselves physically and assessing cardio-respiratory reserve is a challenge.
4. Patients with sudden acute elevation of intracranial pressure can have a 'sympathetic surge' and subsequent myocardial events – myocardial infarction, Takatsubo (stress-induced) cardiomyopathy, arrhythmias.
5. Patients frequently require surgery without delay to avoid devastating complications – paralysis, blindness and death. Conditions that can be readily optimised should be; conditions that require lengthy investigation or treatment will often be postponed until after surgery, if it is safe to do so.

However, pre-operative assessment and preparation will focus on issues related to maintaining normal homeostasis of the intra-cranial or spinal environment, taking steps to avoid aggravating deranged physiology and improving pathophysiology.

Patients with neurosurgical pathology have certain unique differences to the majority of other surgical patients.

Those with raised intracranial pressure from tumour with surrounding oedema will be on steroids, and often have impaired glycaemic balance. This is not a reason to cancel the patient.

Anticoagulants and antiplatelets must be stopped well in advance of surgery (and may necessitate a cancellation if not stopped). The consequences of bleeding complications like intracranial or spinal haematoma are devastating.

In appropriate patients evidence of neuroendocrine disturbance should be sought, and abnormalities corrected where possible. Neuroendocrine problems can be the indication for surgery (e.g. acromegaly, pituitary apoplexy), or may be predicted to occur during surgery (e.g. diabetes insipidus). These complications should be anticipated.

Seizure disorder is more common in this cohort of patients. Steps must be taken to control seizures, especially at the times of induction and emergence from anaesthesia.

Intra-operative management

Induction of general anaesthesia and endotracheal intubation

It is important to appreciate that careful induction of anaesthesia for neurosurgery can take more time than for other operations, and speed is not essential. A smooth induction and intubation is particularly important in patients with increased intracranial pressure (ICP) or an unsecured ruptured intracranial aneurysm. Any further rise in ICP should be prevented by avoiding cough or straining at intubation, and avoiding periods of hypoventilation resulting in a rise of $PaCO_2$. Adequate pre-oxygenation is applied to avoid even brief periods of hypoxia to the already compromised brain.

In cases of spinal instability fibre-optic intubation is recommended to avoid hyperextension or excessive manipulation of the neck. In some cases this is performed with the patient awake to assess for neurological damage associated with intubation.

The positioning of the head and neck in the supine, prone and lateral (park bench) positions may include neck rotation and hence avoidance of kinking of the tube is necessary. An armoured tube is most often used, although these are not without potential disadvantages. A throat pack is sometimes added to avoid passage of blood, particularly in cases of skull base trauma, trans-sphenoidal or extended endonasal endoscopic anterior skull base surgery.

There are periods of stimulation, that may produce spikes of high blood pressure (and thereby ICP), following induction of anaesthesia. These should be anticipated and obtunded to ensure smooth haemodynamics throughout the operative period. The times of stimulation are intubation, insertion of head pins, skin incision and dural incision.

Maintenance of anaesthesia

Brain relaxation

Many pathologies requiring surgery result in brain swelling. There are a number of anaesthetic practical or therapeutic manoeuvres that can be instituted to avoid aggravation of brain swelling and to counteract the rise in ICP.

1. An excessively rotated or flexed neck may compress the jugular vein and reduce venous drainage of the ipsilateral hemisphere. Similarly care should be taken to ensure that tapes or fixing devices for the endotracheal tube do not compromise venous drainage. In patients with severely raised intracranial pressure jugular venous lines may not be desirable.
2. Simple head elevation improves venous drainage.
3. Avoidance of high PEEP.
4. Avoidance of ventilatory compromise and rises in $PaCO_2$ or falls in PaO_2.
5. Adequate muscle relaxation ensures good ventilation and avoids straining. Both reduce intrathoracic pressure and improve venous drainage.
6. The choice of anaesthetic is aimed at avoiding agents which significantly elevate the ICP. A total intravenous anaesthetic technique with balanced continuous infusions of propofol +/- an opioid (most commonly remifentanil) is often chosen. Propofol causes a fall in cerebral metabolism, and maintains homeostatic flow/metabolism ratios. Remifentanil suppresses the cough reflex. Inhaled anaesthetic agents alter the flow/metabolism ratio, some to a greater degree than others. Even though metabolism is decreased, flow is increased and intracranial blood volume increases along with the ICP. Sevoflurane appears to maintain the best intracranial environment and is the inhalational agent of choice. It has a number of other properties that are favourable for neurosurgical cases – smooth gas induction, fast onset, fast offset and minimal residual after effects.
7. Knowing the underlying reason for brain swelling aids in choosing the appropriate therapeutic options. Swelling may be because of oedema or vasomotor reasons from impairment of auto-regulation. Tumour oedema responds to steroids and intra-operative doses of dexamethasone achieve relatively rapid control of swelling during tumour surgery.
8. Brief periods of hyperventilation may be necessary during the initial steps of surgery following opening of the dura to allow access to the lesion to be resected. Precautions should be taken to avoid prolonged hyperventilation, which may result in ischaemic complications.
9. Mannitol 20% not only decreases ICP by acting as an osmotic agent but also by improving the blood rheology and capillary circulation. Together these improve perfusion to relatively ischaemic brain regions resulting in improved autoregulation. This in turn corrects the vasomotor relaxation, which resulted in brain swelling and explains the rapid onset of action of intravenous mannitol 20%.

These manoeuvres for lowering the ICP are particularly important at the start of surgery until other added measures such as surgical CSF drainage from the ventricles or basal cisterns, drainage of cystic lesions or resection of mass lesions are completed.

It has to be noted that the changes from all these manipulations matters most in those cases that are on the steep part of the intracranial volume–pressure curve (see Section 1 Chapter 2 'System-specific physiology') where a relatively small reduction of the intracranial volume (such as reducing brain swelling) would have a greater impact on lowering the ICP.

Maintenance of cerebral perfusion pressure (CPP)

Hypovolaemia and hypotension result in a significant drop in cerebral blood flow (CBF) and CPP in patients with raised ICP. The maintenance of cerebral perfusion depends on

Table 17.1 Summary of the options available to maintain maximal brain relaxation

Avoiding aggravating brain swelling	Non-surgical therapeutic manoeuvres
Head position	Steroids for tumour oedema
Adequate ventilation	Brief hyperventilation
Choice of anaesthetic agent and neuromuscular blockade	Mannitol 20% or hypertonic saline
Correct hyponatraemia	

optimum mean blood pressure and control of elevated ICP. Many studies have shown poor neurological outcomes of traumatic brain injury patients with even the briefest of periods of hypotension.

Cerebral perfusion pressure = Mean arterial pressure – intracranial pressure

Cerebral autoregulation does not remain uniformly intact throughout the injured brain. In some instances, the intracranial pressure response to manipulations of mean arterial pressure are less predictable, and there are zones of brain tissue that respond in completely different ways to one another. On the whole elevating the MAP will reduce the ICP, but there is a small cohort of patients in whom the opposite will occur.

Current advice remains to maintain a MAP of 90 mmHg in brain-injured patients with raised ICP

Homeostasis

Electrolyte disturbances, with deranged serum sodium levels in particular, are encountered in a variety of intracranial pathological conditions.

Hyponatraemia may induce seizures and exacerbate brain swelling. The compromised brain is particularly vulnerable to even relatively minor degrees of hyponatraemia. Correction of hyponatraemia in cases of SAH not only relies on saline administration hypertonic 3% but also on measures to improve perfusion as hypothalamic ischaemia is assumed to be the underlying cause. Rapid correction of sodium levels should be avoided to prevent central pontine myelinolysis.

Analgesia

Analgesia is one of the mainstays of anaesthesia. Pain stimulation may result in vasomotor reflexes, which in turn can disturb cerebral perfusion. In aneurysm surgery a sudden rise in blood pressure secondary to painful stimuli may induce rupture of the aneurysm prior to clipping. The dura is sensitive to pain and on occasions profound bradycardia is observed and has been described to be because of the trigeminocardiac reflex (primitive reflex from amphibians) as a vagal-induced reflex from stimulation of trigeminal nerve fibres within the dura.

Haemostasis

Excessive blood loss during surgery for traumatic brain injury, especially when there is a laceration to the venous sinuses or from skull base fractures, should be promptly controlled to avoid compromise to cerebral perfusion. Similarly, during surgery to resect vascular tumours, especially intracranial meningiomas, not only is there excessive blood loss because of the tumour vascularity but there is also release of fibrinolytic factors leading to a degree of coagulopathy, aggravating the blood loss. Patients with traumatic brain injury also undergo an acute inflammatory reaction, with extensive fibrinolysis; coagulopathy is common in this group of patients. In these situations urgent attention to correct the coagulopathy, in addition to blood replacement, help to achieve control. The CRASH-2 trial showed a trend towards improved outcomes, including haemorrhage extension and new bleeding foci, in patients with traumatic brain injury given tranexamic acid. Other studies are ongoing. The use of cell savers may be considered if these situations are predicted.

Neuroprotection

The detrimental effects of hypoxia and hypoperfusion are worsened by an ongoing cascade that perpetuates further neural cell death. Surgery commonly aggravates such damage when conducted on the already vulnerable brain. Furthermore, operative manoeuvres may temporarily compromise focal cerebral blood flow, such as application of temporary vascular occlusion for proximal control in aneurysm surgery. Under these circumstances measures for neuroprotection are instituted.

The principles of neuroprotection include avoiding aggravating factors, decreasing metabolic rate/demands and possibly pharmacologically blocking mediators resulting in cell injury. In practice neuroprotection aims to break the vicious cycle initiated and aggravated by the cellular metabolic disturbances.

Hyperglycaemia should be corrected as the hypoxic brain metabolises excess glucose through anaerobic oxidation. This results in lactic acidosis, which has detrimental effects on cell membranes, causing further cellular failure. This is particularly true in cases with partial arterial occlusion or at times of reperfusion where excess glucose influxes into already damaged tissue.

Lowering of cerebral metabolic rate has protective effects and can be achieved by induced hypothermia or by pharmacological agents. Moderate hypothermia reduces the metabolic rate by 7–10% per degree centigrade reduction in temperature. Severe hypothermia is best avoided not only because of possible systemic complications including cardiac dysrhythmias and coagulopathy, but it may also result in increased apoptosis. Agents such as propofol, which is preferable for intra-operative use over thiopentone because of its shorter anaesthetic effects, at doses achieving burst suppression are neuroprotective because of lowering cerebral metabolic rate ($CMRO_2$).

Despite extensive experimental work, in practice the use of agents blocking the potential detrimental mediators that perpetuate further cell death is limited. Currently nimodipine, a calcium channel blocker, is used following aneurysmal SAH to lower the incidence of permanent neurological deficits as a result of delayed ischaemia. Similarly intravenous magnesium has been used. The clinical benefits of NMDA channel blockers and antagonists, iron chelators, free radical scavengers and other agents have not yet been established.

Special considerations

Aneurysm surgery

Multiple neurophysiological parameters may be deranged at the time of potentially complex surgery when clipping an intracranial aneurysm following SAH. The brain is

Table 17.2 Summary of strategies available for neuroprotection. Of the drugs to block mediators, only nimodipine has proven efficacy

Avoid aggravating factors	Decrease metabolic rate/ demands	Block mediators
Hyperglycaemia	Hypothermia	Nimodipine – proven in SAH
Reperfusion injury	Propofol/barbiturates	NMDA antagonists
Partial occlusion of blood supply	Terminate seizures	Magnesium
		Fe chelators/free radical scavengers

particularly vulnerable to hypoxia and hypoperfusion after the SAH insult. In addition episodes of hypertension may result in re-bleeding from the ruptured aneurysm prior to clipping with disastrous consequences. These facts are considered during intubation and induction of anaesthesia. Adequate analgesia should be insured during application of the head pins for the fixation frame and may include local anaesthetic infiltration of the pin sites on the scalp.

The precautions in positioning and observing the degree of neck rotation are applied.

There are several factors underlying the commonly encountered brain swelling following SAH, which need to be addressed to achieve brain relaxation. Factors that may contribute to brain swelling after SAH are:

- derangements in cerebral autoregulation;
- derangements in CSF circulation because of the blood resulting in communicating hydrocephalus;
- obstructive hydrocephalus from intraventricular haemorrhage;
- intraparenchymal haematoma (ICH);
- hyponatraemia.

Meticulous anaesthetic techniques are applied to prevent aggravation of brain swelling and correction of physiological abnormalities (where possible).

Almost all intracranial aneurysms are deeply located around the basal cisterns and retraction injury during access represents a major complication from this surgery. Retraction on a swollen brain results in underlying ischaemia or even contusion with detrimental post-operative swelling. Brain relaxation is imperative. Pre-operative insertion of a lumbar drain following induction greatly assists in brain relaxation by CSF drainage during the procedure. However, this would be contraindicated in the presence of a mass-producing ICH or excessive compartmental swelling. There are at least theoretical concerns that rapid lowering of the ICP in the presence of an unsecured aneurysm may induce re-bleeding because of accentuation of the trans-mural pressure across the aneurysm wall. Mannitol 20% is a commonly used agent to lower the ICP. In this particular situation it is recommended that its administration should be delayed to just before opening of the dura to avoid the potential re-rupture of the aneurysm by lowering the ICP in the presence of a closed intracranial compartment. Mannitol 20% and brief hyperventilation allow surgical access to the basal cisterns and CSF drainage, which is the most effective manoeuvre achieving brain relaxation with minimal retraction. In the presence of hydrocephalus and ventriculomegaly, a ventriculostomy is effective. Prolonged hyperventilation should not be used as it may increase the volume of ischaemic brain.

Proximal control of the aneurysm by temporary occlusion of the parent vessel is required in cases of premature rupture during dissection, or as a planned manoeuvre to aid completion of dissection of the aneurysm's neck, identification of the branches and to lessen the tension within the aneurysm sac to allow optimal clip application. Neuroprotection during this period is frequently employed. Commonly used options include a dose of mannitol 20% (which is also a free-radical scavenger), elevating the blood pressure (to promote collateral circulation), mild hypothermia and propofol in doses achieving burst suppression.

In some complex and large aneurysms it is desirable to lower the tension within the sac at the time of clip application and brief cautious induced hypotension may be an alternative to temporary clipping of the parent artery. For more complex lesions particularly with awkward access to place a more proximal temporary clip, intravenous adenosine administration resulting in brief cardiac asystole allows the optimum clip application. Clear communication between the anaesthetist and surgeon is essential.

Posterior fossa surgery

Positioning precautions are applied in the prone or the lateral/park-bench positions. Frequently cranial nerve, especially the facial nerve, and brainstem monitoring such as brainstem auditory evoked potentials (BAEP), somatosensory evoked potentials (SSEP) and motor evoked potentials (MEP) are used. For motor recordings short-acting muscle relaxants are used for endotracheal intubation, and no further doses are given. Interpretation of the recordings takes into account general parameters including the influence of anaesthesia; a total intravenous anaesthesia (TIVA) technique may be preferable. If volatile anaesthesia is chosen, the neurophysiologist must be informed, and sevoflurane at less than 1 MAC would be the agent of choice.

Exaggerated cardiovascular reflexes may occur during surgical manipulations of the floor of the fourth ventricle and frequently of the trigeminal nerve during microvascular decompressions (MVD). Profound vagal mediated bradycardia may necessitate anticholinergic administration to block the reflex activity.

Pre-existing or post-surgical lower cranial nerve deficits may result in multiple complications mainly because of aspiration from bulbar palsy and rarely stridor from bilateral involvement. Whenever these are present or anticipated a nasogastric tube is placed peri-operatively for feeding and if respiratory complications from aspiration occur or extensive bulbar dysfunction is likely to be prolonged then a temporary tracheostomy is considered.

Cardiovascular and respiratory centre dysfunction following surgical manipulations of the floor of the fourth ventricle would necessitate post-operative ventilation.

Vomiting is frequently seen following posterior fossa surgery and care for airway protection should be observed during extubation and in recovery until full consciousness is regained. The use of regular post-operative anti-emetics is considered at an early stage in addition to those given intra-operatively.

Pituitary/neuroendocrine surgery

Lesions requiring surgery may present with a wide range of metabolic disturbances from hypopituitarism or hormonal excess in cases of secretory adenomas. Pre-operative endocrinological correction of these is necessary for most cases. In urgent cases, such as for pituitary apoplexy, hydrocortisone administration covers the potential hypocorticism resulting from pituitary hypofunction and the diminished pituitary reserves to deal with the additional surgical stress.

In patients with acromegaly, growth hormone excess may cause hypertension, diabetes, cardiomyopathy and sleep apnoea. These should be identified in pre-assessment and treated where possible. Plans can be made for a potentially difficult intubation. In cases presenting with significant sleep apnoea, post-operative planning for airway management is important, particularly if nasal packs are placed following trans-sphenoidal surgery.

Patients with Cushing's disease requiring surgery may pose a particular challenge because of the associated metabolic disturbances, diabetes and cardiac complications, both intra- and post-operatively. This group in addition is more vulnerable to develop systemic infections and deep vein thrombosis.

Post-operative monitoring and correction of electrolyte disturbances, particularly the serum sodium levels, is particularly important and awareness of the fact that fluctuations frequently occur (see Table 17.3).

Table 17.3 Summary of common sodium problems in neurosurgical patients

Sodium problem	Cause	Associated with cerebral condition	Treatment	Time scale
Hyponatraemia	Cerebral salt wasting	SAH	Na replacement, consider fludrocortisone	Brief, usually resolves spontaneously over 2–4 weeks. May be longer lasting
Hyponatraemia	SIADH	Many – tumours, infections, drug side effects (carbamazepine)	Acute Na replacement, water restriction, consider diuretics	<48 hours duration
			Chronic and asymptomatic fluid restriction, Na replacement, consider vasopressin-2 receptor antagonists	
Hypernatraemia	Diabetes insipidus	Suprasellar or pituitary lesions, especially those involving the hypothalamus	Fluid administration to keep up with losses and maintenance requirements. Consider DDAVP if excessive fluid loss continues	Can occur intra-operatively or post-operatively

Awake craniotomies

Certain cases require monitoring and assessment of the neurological function during resection of intrinsic brain lesions at or adjacent to eloquent areas. In addition to the general principles of neuroanaesthesia the specific aims are to reduce the patient's discomfort. Meticulous attention to positioning is required as the procedure can be prolonged and the patient's head is fixed in place allowing minimal movement of the body. Adequate local anaesthetic infiltration of the scalp with knowledge of the regional cutaneous sensory nerve supply is one of the key elements for successful anaesthesia. Commonly the patient is anaesthetised for the first part of the procedure to allow the craniotomy to be performed, and occasionally some tumour resection. Controlled 'wake-up' then takes place. It is essential to avoid coughing, straining, gagging or vomiting at this stage as the cranium is 'open' and brain exposed. Anti-emetics are used liberally. The recognition of hypoventilation during these periods should be as early as possible and counteracted otherwise detrimental effects including uncontrollable brain swelling may be difficult to control. Most patients will respond to a request to take deep breaths and this permits control of $PaCO_2$.

The use of cortical stimulation to map the eloquent cortical, and more recently the subcortical brain regions, requires fully co-operative patients with no residual effects of muscle relaxants or sedation. Seizures are commonly associated with the intrinsic lesions that require awake craniotomy and may be induced by motor cortical stimulation intra-operatively. Therefore adequate prophylactic anticonvulsants should be administered and the therapeutic dose should be reached in those presenting with epilepsy prior to the procedure. Seizures can often be rapidly terminated intra-operatively by applying ice-cold saline to the stimulated area. This allows the procedure to continue without the need to resort to general anaesthesia.

Spinal surgery

Anterior cervical approaches involve partial retraction of the pharynx to gain access to the spine. The endotracheal tube should be securely fixed. Fibre-optic intubation to avoid manipulation of the unstable cervical spine is considered in those cases requiring surgery following trauma, degenerative disease with subluxation and some spinal tumours. In some cases, an awake fibre-optic intubation will be the method of choice.

Positioning depends on the operative approach to the spine. In the prone position, care should be taken to ensure adequate chest support and an abdomen with free movement. Both prevent compression of the major intra-abdominal vessels, which could lead to epidural venous engorgement as blood diverts away from the compressed intra-abdominal vessels to return to the heart. This also allows minimal inflation pressures to ventilate the lungs, thus minimising intrathoracic pressure.

Neuroprotection to the spinal cord is analogous to cerebral neuroprotection particularly after spinal cord injury, surgery for vascular anomalies or intrinsic cord lesions.

Monitoring both motor and sensory function is becoming standard for surgery involving intrinsic spinal cord lesions and during corrective surgery for spinal deformities. Muscle relaxants are withheld after intubation to enable MEP recordings.

Blood loss can be excessive in spinal surgery and hypotension resulting in cord hypoperfusion can cause cord infarction, especially in cases of spinal cord lesions or swelling and in the elderly. This should be predicted and corrected promptly.

Table 17.4 Summary of the differences between spinal shock and neurogenic shock

	Spinal shock	Neurogenic shock
Blood pressure	Lesions above T5 can develop autonomic dysreflexia (see text)	Decreased – loss of sympathetic tone and loss of systemic vascular resistance. Blood pools in dependent body parts
Heart rate	No change	Decreased – unopposed vagal tone, worsened by hypoxia and endobronchial suction
Neurology	Loss of sensation and motor power below the level of injury, with gradual return of reflexes. Initially flaccid paralysis, but over time spasticity and hyper-reflexia develop	Disrupted autonomic pathways
Cause	Spinal cord injury	Severe brain injury, cervical or high thoracic spinal cord injury
Treatment	Initially maintain spinal cord perfusion. Later supportive measures and rehabilitation	Exclude haemorrhage. Fluid resuscitation is first- line therapy. Vasopressors and vagolytics (atropine) may be necessary

Multi-modal analgesia intra-operatively and in the post-operative period ensures mobilisation following major procedures.

Exaggerated or obtunded spinal reflexes following cord injury may result in positional hypotension, which is particularly sensitive to hypovolaemia and may be associated with bradycardia. Corrective measures should be instituted early.

Autonomic dysreflexia is a pathological reflex that can cause profound hypertension leading to stroke and death if left untreated. Patients with a spinal cord injury above T5 are most susceptible, although it can occur in patients with lesions between T6 to T10. It is unlikely if the lesion is below T10. Cases that precipitate the hypertensive crisis are those performed below the umbilicus – most commonly urological procedures. A surge in blood pressure in patients having spinal surgery and an existing spinal injury should arouse suspicion of a blocked/kinked urinary catheter or urinary retention.

Transthoracic approaches to the spine require endobronchial intubation to allow deflation of a lung and access to the thoracic spine. Adequate ventilation to the dependent lung should be insured and post-operative chest drains are left *in situ* until full lung re-expansion (see one-lung ventilation (OLV) in Section II, Chapters 7 and 9).

AVM surgery

On a few occasions emergency surgery is required for AVM surgery in the presence of a mass-producing ICH. The general principles of anaesthesia with increased ICP are observed and if adequate brain relaxation is achieved following evacuation of the ICH, the surgery may proceed to resect the AVM, provided its anatomical configuration is favourable. As most large and high-flow AVMs are either treated conservatively or with multiple-staged endovascular embolisations surgical resection of these lesions without adjuvant embolisation is uncommon. Where surgery is performed without prior embolisation, there are cases of excessive life-threatening brain swelling after the microsurgical resection of the AVM. This occurs because of the loss of autoregulation of the circumferential feeding vessels to the AVM that were previously subjected to high blood flow. In these situations, induced hypotension counteracts the excessive blood flow. The loss of autoregulation results in elevated BP distending (rather than reflex constricting) the affected vessels. In extreme cases induced hypotension is needed to continue in the post-operative period for 24–48 hours. This is known as 'normal pressure breakthrough phenomenon'.

Extubation

Smooth extubation avoiding excessive cough or gag reflex is particularly important following procedures in which a vascular repair is performed and similarly in those in which a flap or a graft is used for repair of a venous sinus or dural defect to prevent a CSF leak.

Patients with compromised neural function are particularly vulnerable, even to brief periods of hypoxia and elevated $PaCO_2$. Adequate spontaneous ventilation and conscious level to protect the airway should be insured prior to extubation.

Immediate post-operative care

Measures undertaken during surgery to control ICP, achieve homeostasis and neural protection are to continue in the post-operative period. In particular adequate ventilation should be ensured. Airway protection may be compromised by diminished conscious level, in patients with bulbar dysfunction or following procedures resulting in local swelling. Avoidance of post-operative mechanical ventilation whenever possible is the goal. An awake patient is the best neurological function monitor. This will often require transfer to a high-dependency unit for close observation, and intervention if neurological deterioration should occur. When there is a serious risk to the airway, or when neurological recovery is poor, the patient should be transferred ventilated to the intensive care unit.

Rises in ICP detected by conventional monitoring techniques occur relatively late on the intracranial volume–pressure curve and fail to act as a warning measure of relative ischaemia. Some neurointensive care units have the benefit of multi-modal brain monitoring, permitting earlier detection and treatment of problems in the sedated, ventilated patient. These are not however in widespread use.

Further reading

CRASH-2 trial collaborators. Effects of tranexamic acid on death, vascular occlusive events and blood transfusion in trauma patients with significant haemorrhage (CRASH-2): a randomised, placebo-controlled trial. *Lancet* 2010;376:23–32.

Gupta AK, Gelb AW. *Essentials of Neuroanaesthesia and Neurointensive Care*, 2nd edn. Elsevier, 2008.

The Brain Trauma Foundation. https://www.braintrauma.org/coma-guidelines/.

Chapter 18

Trauma cases

Rhys Thomas and Wayne Sapsford

Introduction

There are few areas in medicine which have changed as much in the past ten to 20 years as the management of the severely traumatised patient, driven for the most part by the complexity and severity of the trauma in recent military conflicts. Few patients offer a greater challenge than the critically injured patient. The acuity and uncertainty of the extent of the injuries require the anaesthetist to be both vigilant and methodical as the case progresses. Rapid changes in the patient's condition occur commonly and constant communication between anaesthetist, surgeon and the rest of the team is vital. The anaesthetist should take an active lead in the operating theatre, in combination with the senior surgeon present, as he/she has the greatest situational awareness and needs to be aware of the resources at his/her disposal. Therefore, the traditional metaphorical 'blood brain barrier' or physical drape that still exists between the surgeon and anaesthetist in some elective surgery has been replaced by constant communication, supporting an integrated damage-control philosophy. There are three central tenets to the damage-control philosophy: permissive hypotension, damage-control or haemostatic resuscitation, and damage-control surgery.

The damage-control philosophy was initially conceived as a surgical approach to the multiply injured patient when it was realised that such patients lacked the physiological reserve to survive complex reconstructive surgery and restoration of anatomy. Damage-control surgery is confined to that surgery which is necessary to control haemorrhage and limit contamination. Temporary cavity closure further abbreviates the surgery and the patient is then normalised physiologically in the intensive care unit before definitive anatomical repair 24 to 72 hours later. However, such an approach to a severely traumatised patient cannot be used in isolation. Haemostatic resuscitation and permissive hypotension also contribute to the philosophy of damage control in an effort to limit the development of the 'lethal triad'. An institutional massive transfusion protocol for trauma is also required.

The 'lethal triad' is the term used to describe the vicious cycle of hypothermia, acute coagulopathy and acidosis seen in severely injured, haemorrhaging trauma patients. Haemorrhage leads to hypoperfusion and decreased oxygen delivery, a switch to anaerobic metabolism, lactate production and metabolic acidosis. Heat production is limited in an anaerobic metabolic state and this is exacerbated by exposure and the administration of cold fluid and blood. A temperature of less than 35° C is an independent predictor of mortality in trauma. Coagulopathy, once considered a result of clotting factor consumption

A Surgeon's Guide to Anaesthesia and Peri-operative Care, ed. Jane Sturgess, Justin Davies and Kamen Valchanov. Published by Cambridge University Press.

and loss (from bleeding), dilution (because of fluid resuscitation) and dysfunction (because of acidosis and hypothermia), have now been shown to be caused directly by the trauma itself. Trauma patients have an established early coagulopathy related to hypoperfusion and initiated by tissue injury. Furthermore, hyperfibrinolysis also appears to contribute to the coagulopathy of trauma. This coagulation derangement is distinct from disseminated intravascular coagulopathy and has been termed the acute coagulopathy of trauma – shock (ACoTS). It has also been shown that patients with a coagulopathy on arrival in the emergency department have a four-fold increase in mortality.

Haemostatic resuscitation is an attempt to address the problem of the coagulopathy seen in massively injured patients from whatever cause. Permissive hypotensive resuscitation, in the pre-hospital environment in particular, results from the recognition that aggressive fluid resuscitation may exacerbate blood loss by interfering with haemostatic mechanisms and dislodging clot, especially where haemorrhage is into the torso, which is not controllable with direct pressure or tourniquets. Resuscitation fluid administration is restricted until surgery when the source of the haemorrhage can be controlled. This approach is also known as balanced resuscitation. The main drawback of this approach is the acceptance of a period of sub-optimal end-organ perfusion until definitive control of the haemorrhage is achieved.

The damage-control philosophy is designed to incorporate its three central tenets concurrently. Damage-control resuscitation, incorporating balanced or hypotensive resuscitation, occurs throughout the pre-hospital, the emergency department, the operating theatre damage-control surgery phase and beyond into the intensive care management. In order to facilitate this, communication and co-operation between the anaesthetists and surgeons is vital. Regular updates between the two parties should occur at specific times and every ten minutes during the operative phase of management.

Initial assessment

A trauma patient arrives in a good resuscitation department to be received by a pre-formed trauma team consisting of emergency department physicians (the most senior of whom should lead the trauma team activation), anaesthetists, surgeons (general/trauma and orthopaedic), radiologists, nurses, operating department practitioners (ODPs), radiographers and a scribe. The ATMIST handover (see Table 18.1) is communicated and the patient transferred onto the gurney. The patient should be receiving maximal oxygen flow via a tight-fitting mask with a non-rebreathing reservoir bag, which should deliver a fractional inspired oxygen concentration (FiO_2) of 0.85, and ventilation should be achieved, if necessary, with the aid of an oropharyngeal or nasopharyngeal airway and a jaw thrust

Table 18.1 ATMIST handover

A	Age
T	Time of injury
M	Mechanism of injury
I	Injuries sustained
S	Symptoms and signs (usually the vital signs)
T	Treatment given

when indicated. If the patient is already intubated a rocuronium time or 'roc time' and the times of any subsequent boluses of muscle relaxant are relayed by the pre-hospital doctor. This conveys the duration of paralysis and the muscle relaxant used so that the anaesthetists will have an estimate of the time for the next dose of muscle relaxant.

Anaesthetic risk is often difficult to determine. The more complex, multiply injured patients afford the least time for assessment. Therefore all patients must be considered to be at risk of aspiration and for cervical spine injury, head injury, hypovolaemia, intoxication, and potentially a difficult airway. Where time permits an AMPLE history should be obtained (Allergies, Medications, Past medical history, time of Last meal, Events surrounding the traumatic event). A rapid assessment of the GCS and the movement of the four limbs is essential for predicting outcome in head-injured patients. An assessment of the ASA physical class classification may also be possible. Note that an E is added to the numerical value if the patient requires an emergency operation.

Access is a priority in life-threatening trauma. Intra-osseous needles have revolutionised access because of their speed and success rate. This is then followed by a large-volume subclavian trauma line. Confirmation of the patency of any pre-existing access is always necessary. Monitoring is also essential. Both need to be established early after the arrival of the patient in the resuscitation department. An ECG, for the pulse rate and the respiratory rate (derived from the impedance changes), pulse oximetry, non-invasive blood pressure monitoring and capnography for end-tidal carbon dioxide (CO_2), when intubated and ventilated, represent the minimum monitoring standards in the early stages of a resuscitation. End-tidal CO_2 measurement is also possible on a face mask with the correct equipment.

Airway and breathing

The primary survey is started (see Table 18.2). The anaesthetist is situated at the head and the primary concern is maintenance of the airway and cervical spine control, followed by oxygenation and ventilation.

Basic materials for airway management include bag-valve-mask (BVM) devices attached to high-flow oxygen, suction, oral and nasopharyngeal airways, laryngoscopes with a

Table 18.2 Primary survey

(C)	Catastrophic haemorrhage	Control with direct pressure using haemostatic dressings or tourniquets
A	Airway maintenance with cervical spine protection	Ensure patency of airway with in-line C-spine immobilisation and oxygen
B	Breathing	Verify breathing and address life-threatening complications
C	Circulation	Arrest external bleeding, assess for internal haemorrhage, check pulse at radial, femoral and carotid positions, blood pressure, and capillary refill
D	Disability	AVPU, GCS, pupils, limb movement
E	Exposure	Temperature, undress and examine whole body especially junctional areas, logroll and cover with warming blanket to avoid hypothermia

Table 18.3 Indications for a definitive airway

Airway protection	Unconsciousness	GCS ≤8, drug, alcohol or metabolic coma
	Maxillo-facial trauma	
	Aspiration risk	Bleeding, vomiting
	Obstruction risk	Expanding neck haematoma, laryngeal or tracheal injury, airway burns, stridor
Oxygenation		Hypoxia, cyanosis Tension pneumothorax Carbon monoxide poisoning
Ventilation	Apnoea	Unconsciousness, neuromuscular paralysis
	Inadequate respirations	Opiate overdose, respiratory fatigue, hypercarbia, severe metabolic acidosis, tension pneumothorax, flail chest, haemothorax
	Severe traumatic brain injury	GCS ≤8 to ensure optimum pCO_2
Resuscitation		Exsanguination, septic shock, neurogenic shock, cardiogenic shock

selection of blades, endotracheal tubes of various sizes, stylets, bougies and drugs for induction, analgesia and neuromuscular blockade.

The airway must be managed in stages. The tongue will occlude the airway most commonly in injured patients. This is dealt with by anterior displacement of the mandible with a jaw thrust. Beware bony fractures to the face, which may compromise the airway despite a jaw thrust. Surgical emphysema from a disrupted airway will cause significant swelling and distortion of the anatomy and an expanding neck haematoma will also obstruct the airway. Stridor, the use of the accessory musculature and paradoxical respiratory movement suggest impending airway collapse. In these situations declining pulse oximetry values, cyanosis, pallor and apnoea are late signs and mandate immediate airway intervention.

A definitive airway is the presence of a cuffed tube in the trachea. This is the best way to deliver oxygen in sufficiently high concentrations and effective ventilation. A cuffed tube also ensures protection of the lungs from aspiration and facilitates suctioning of aspirated blood and airway secretions. The indications for a definitive airway are where there is need for airway protection, a reduced conscious level, a need for oxygenation, a need for ventilation and a need to optimise resuscitation (see Table 18.3).

A definitive airway is best placed using direct laryngoscopy and orotracheal intubation. This method is rapid and has technical advantages. Blind nasal intubation is contraindicated in basal skull fractures, in the presence of expanding cervical haematomas and partial airway obstruction, because of the risk of converting a partial airway obstruction into a complete obstruction. The urgency for airway intubation often dictates the plan but it should always be preceded by a period of optimal pre-oxygenation, and assisted ventilation may be necessary as patients are often hypoxaemic and hypercapneic. Rapid sequence intubation (RSI) follows a period of a minimum of three minutes oxygenation via a face mask or bag-valve-mask (BVM) assisted ventilation, in which case it is called a modified RSI. Suction should be immediately available and cricoid pressure applied, to reduce the risk of regurgitation and aspiration of gastric contents, as well as in-line cervical stabilisation. This is especially indicated in blunt trauma. An induction agent is administered (typically ketamine, thiopentone or etomidate) and a neuromuscular blocking drug (typically suxamethonium or rocuronium) to facilitate intubation. All induction agents have the potential to produce or exacerbate hypotension and must be used with care, especially in hypovolaemic patients, and at much reduced doses. In general some fluid resuscitation is necessary during induction but should not delay the process. Some re-adjustment of the cricoid pressure and use of a rigid stylet or bougie may be required to improve intubation rates in some difficult-to-intubate patients. An 8 mm cuffed endotracheal tube is standard in adults. It may be pre-loaded with an introducer and have a 10 ml syringe attached to inflate the cuff. Videolaryngoscopy is becoming very common in trauma to try and reduce the time to first intubation and as an aid in difficult intubations. Two commonly used devices are the Airtraq® and Glidescope®.

Ease of intubation can be assessed by use of the Mallampati classification. Here, the visual appearance of the oropharynx is divided into four classes depending on the structures visualised. In Class I the soft palate, uvula and tonsillar pillars are visible, while in Class IV, only the soft palate is visible. However, the patient needs to be co-operative, upright and to open the mouth fully and protrude the tongue. This is often not possible in trauma patients. In the classification by Cormack and Lehane the appearance on laryngoscopy is graded from I to IV and it correlates to ease of intubation. The entire laryngeal aperture is visible in grade I, posterior laryngeal anatomy (arytenoid cartilages) is visualised in grade II, only the epiglottis is seen in grade III and only the soft palate in grade IV. Grades III and IV are considered difficult intubations.

The difficult airway can be a challenge in trauma as it is seldom possible to stop and return to the issue of a definitive airway later. A difficult airway is defined as one in which a trained, experienced anaesthetist experiences difficulty with mask ventilation, tracheal intubation, or both. It is imperative that it is recognised at the outset. It may either be because of intrinsic anatomic airway variability, traumatic injury to the area, or both. Awake intubations may be performed where a difficult airway is anticipated but only in spontaneously breathing, awake, co-operative and haemodynamically stable patients and with the use of a fibre-optic bronchoscope. This is contra-indicated where the airway is contaminated with blood, a so-called 'red out'. Where the patient is unco-operative, haemodynamically unstable, or anaesthetised, then spontaneous ventilation should be maintained if possible for intubation. There are five main causes of a difficult airway in trauma. They are: traumatic brain injury and intoxication, cervical spine injury, the disrupted airway, maxillo-facial trauma and airway compression. In trauma, assessment may well be difficult because of suboptimal views when cervical spine immobilisation is employed and therefore all trauma patients are considered difficult intubations. A robust plan of action on a failure to intubate must be discussed and agreed with the whole trauma team prior to intubation.

In a 'cannot ventilate, cannot intubate' emergency the use of a supraglottic airway such as a laryngeal mask may provide a temporary airway but will not prevent aspiration; this is 'plan B'. Transtracheal jet ventilation via a needle cricothyroidotomy will maintain oxygenation at the expense of hypercarbia, or an oesophageal tracheal combitube may be used as a temporising measure. These two techniques are now performed rarely because of complications associated with their use. An emergency invasive airway access technique such as cricothyroidotomy or tracheostomy is now recognised as the airway technique of last resort;

this is 'plan C'. The anaesthetist and surgeon must have discussed this potential eventuality before intubation is attempted. As a surgeon, it is better to be aware, present and prepared for this eventuality than caught off guard, so good communication is essential from the outset. In trauma patients, crew resource management is key and consideration should be given to a surgical airway early in all cases where a difficult airway is anticipated as patients are frequently unsuitable for awake intubations. When the surgery is a life-saving procedure it will not be possible to wake the patient up; failure is not an option!

Confirmation of endotracheal intubation is best done by direct visualisation of the ETT passing between the vocal cords either with a laryngoscope or a fibre-optic bronchoscope. The best indirect method is to confirm exhaled carbon dioxide by end-tidal CO_2 capnography or dye indicator. Clinical assessment of chest wall rise and fall and auscultation are prone to error and should not be relied on alone.

Life-threatening chest injuries which compromise oxygenation and ventilation need to be excluded and treated if detected. These include tension pneumothorax or haemopneumothorax, open pneumothorax, massive haemothorax or haemopneumothorax and cardiac tamponade. Treatment of a tension pneumothorax or haemopneumothorax in the emergency department is by immediate thoracostomy and subsequent placement of an intercostal chest tube connected to an underwater drain. Needle decompression is mainly reserved for prehospital management of these conditions. An open pneumothorax should be treated by the placement of a seal with a flutter-type valve that lets air egress but not enter the chest. This should be supplemented with an intercostal drain in the emergency department. A massive haemothorax (>1500 ml of blood) or haemopneumothorax should be treated with an intercostal drain in the first instance. Thoracotomy may well be required. Cardiac tamponade, often detected on FAST scanning of the pericardium, is a surgical emergency requiring immediate clamshell thoracotomy or median sternotomy, often performed in the emergency department. There is no place for needle pericardiocentesis in a cardiac tamponade of traumatic origin.

Circulation

It is in the management of the fluid resuscitation of a trauma patient that the role of the anaesthetist has most expanded and changed. Previously, it was the responsibility of the anaesthetic team to monitor and manage the circulatory system before and during surgery. This meant assessing the degree of shock and treating it with an appropriate volume of crystalloid or colloid solution. Nowadays, in a well-organised resuscitation the anaesthetist will manage the damage-control resuscitation of the patient. This consists of permissive hypotension and haemostatic resuscitation. Permissive hypotension refers to the maintenance of a palpable radial pulse (effectively a systolic pressure of 90 mmHg) and limiting fluid boluses to 250 ml until control of haemorrhage is achieved. Haemostatic resuscitation refers to the very early use of blood and blood products as primary resuscitation fluids to replace lost blood with blood, to treat the intrinsic acute traumatic coagulopathy (ACoTS) and to prevent the development of a dilutional coagulopathy. The age-old debate about crystalloid or colloid fluid resuscitation has finally been resolved: neither is suitable in severe trauma. Damage-control resuscitation proceeds concomitantly with damage-control surgery rather than delaying the surgical phase until the patient has been adequately resuscitated.

In order to permit damage-control resuscitation a massive transfusion protocol must be established. Ideally, the need for blood and blood products should be identified in the prehospital phase and relayed to the receiving hospital. The massive transfusion protocol is then activated and warm blood made available to the haemodynamically unstable patient on arrival in the emergency department. A blood sample should be drawn and sent to the haematology laboratory for a group and cross-match before a significant transfusion has occurred which may obfuscate the blood typing. Initially, group O blood should be transfused (O –ve or +ve to males and O –ve blood to females) and group AB +ve fresh frozen plasma until a group or group and cross-match is available when a more targeted blood transfusion can be commenced.

Permissive hypotension

There is no doubt that in haemorrhagic shock, the interruption of oxygen delivery leads to cellular ischaemia, progressive organ dysfunction and eventually, irreversible organ failure. However, it has now been recognised that aggressive fluid resuscitation, especially with crystalloids and colloids, interferes with haemostatic mechanisms and results in further haemorrhage, cellular ischaemia and organ failure. Permissive hypotension – or balanced resuscitation – defers or restricts the fluid resuscitation to maintain a palpable radial pulse or a systolic pressure of 80 mmHg in the younger, fitter trauma population (higher in the elderly) until haemorrhage can be controlled. Haemorrhage control may simply entail a pressure dressing, supplemented by digital pressure or a tourniquet, where appropriate in the case of extremity bleeding, but will require intracavity surgery when the blood loss is into the torso. This strategy carries the inherent risk of suboptimal end-organ perfusion but it is arguably preferable to uncontrolled haemorrhage when the first, and best, clot is dislodged by a combination of higher arterial pressures and a coagulopathy. This strategy is contra-indicated only in the isolated head injury patient as attempts must be made to maintain an adequate cerebral perfusion pressure and this necessitates the maintenance of a mean arterial pressure of 90 mmHg.

The benefits of a hypotensive resuscitation strategy in trauma is difficult to demonstrate scientifically. However, a few studies have shown a modest reduction in mortality or, at least no difference between groups in those treated with immediate or delayed resuscitation. In general, victims of penetrating trauma in these studies would appear to benefit most. A Cochrane review of the literature pertaining to immediate and delayed resuscitation in trauma showed no difference in mortality. It is worth pointing out that it is a widely accepted practice to limit fluid resuscitation in ruptured abdominal aneurysm patients until control of the aorta is obtained proximal to the leak. Hence, it would not be unreasonable to utilise this strategy in penetrating trauma, which is likely to involve major vessels and where the haemorrhage cannot be externally controlled. Its use in blunt trauma should not adversely affect the patient and may be beneficial. Indeed, despite the lack of evidence, guideline recommendations for clinical practice advocate judicious administration of fluid resuscitation and the National Institute for Health and Clinical Excellence (NICE) endorses a strategy of no fluid administration in the pre-hospital phase in patients without head injury if a radial pulse is palpable. This strategy should be coupled with expert and timely haemostatic resuscitation.

Haemostatic resuscitation

Haemostatic resuscitation is the use of blood and blood products early in the resuscitation of a trauma patient. In particular, this strategy is directed towards the early coagulopathy of the 'lethal triad' and this is central to improving outcomes. Not only are packed red blood cells

(PRBCs) used to replace lost blood but also fresh frozen plasma (FFP), platelets, cryoprecipitate, tranexamic acid, calcium replacement and even recombinant activated factor VII are used to address the deficiencies in both the trauma patient and in the PRBC transfusion. In essence, the combination of the blood and blood products effectively reconstitutes whole blood; indeed, warm whole blood can also be used when an emergency donor panel is convened. The use of FFP in this way has been shown to reduce absolute mortality in those trauma patients requiring a massive transfusion in both penetrating and blunt trauma. A 'shock pack', consisting of four units of PRBCs and four units of thawed FFP should be immediately available when the massive transfusion protocol is implemented.

Platelets should also ideally be administered in a 1:1 ratio with PRBCs. Again, studies have demonstrated improved survival with a 1:1 ratio compared to lower ratios. Giving PRBCs, FFP and platelets in this way approximates to the use of whole blood. In practice this involves the administration of one pool of platelets (four to six individual donor units) for every four to six units of PRBCs. The current British and US military practice is to administer PRBCs, FFP and platelets in a ratio of 1:1:1.

More recently donated RBCs are preferable to older units in patients who have a massive transfusion. Transfusion of older units has been associated with higher rates of infective complications and organ failure. This effect is thought to be mediated by passenger leucocytes and a significantly increased odds ratio of death has been associated with PRBCs stored for over two weeks, despite leucodepletion, in patients who received over six units of PRBCs. Therefore, where possible, the youngest stored PRBCs should be utilised first in the haemostatic resuscitation of these severely injured patients.

Fibrinogen replacement is also required in trauma patients undergoing a massive transfusion. Fibrinogen deficiency develops early and is a factor in the development of a coagulopathy. Fibrinogen can be replaced with cryoprecipitate, which contains fibrinogen, factor VIII, von Willebrand factor, and factor XIII. Guidelines recommend fibrinogen supplementation when plasma fibrinogen levels fall below 1.5–2.0 g/l. Tranexamic acid is an antifibrinolytic agent. Hyperfibrinolysis has been shown to occur in ACoTS and contributes to a coagulopathy. Tranexamic acid has been extensively used in, and has been shown to reduce blood loss after, elective surgery. The evidence for the use of tranexamic acid in trauma is the CRASH-2 study, a large multicentre, randomised controlled study with a 30% reduction in mortality in patients who were actively bleeding and with few adverse effects. It is recommended in the European guidelines as an adjunct in the management of traumatic haemorrhage.

There are yet other factors that must be borne in mind when managing a massive transfusion in haemostatic resuscitation. Not only is hypocalcaemia common in critically ill patients, citrate, used as an anticoagulant in many blood components, chelates calcium and exacerbates the problem. Ionised calcium levels of <1.0 mmol/l will lead to coagulation defects and it is recommended that the level of ionised calcium be kept at a level of ≥ 1.0 mmol/l. Care must also be taken to monitor and treat hyperkalaemia when a patient receives a massive transfusion as potassium is released by lysis of red blood cells in stored blood and patient serum levels can rapidly rise to dangerous levels resulting in potentially fatal arrhythmias. Serum potassium should be kept below 6.0 mmol/l. Factor VII is a vital component of the coagulation cascade. It acts in the presence of tissue factor (exposed when the endothelium is breached) to initiate local haemostasis at the site of injury. It is this clot which is regarded as the best clot in trauma and hypotensive resuscitation is directed at preserving this haemostatic mechanism. Recombinant activated factor VII has been advocated as a pharmacological haemostat. However, studies to date have failed to demonstrate any evidence of an improvement in survival. Two parallel multicentre randomised controlled trials have shown a statistically significant reduction in blood transfusion requirements in blunt but not penetrating trauma. The product is very expensive, it loses its efficacy in acidotic patients and the early use of FFP and platelets in haemostatic resuscitation may render its use increasingly unnecessary.

Once haemorrhage control is achieved, the goal of fluid resuscitation is to optimise oxygen delivery, improve microcirculatory perfusion and reverse tissue acidosis. The optimum systolic blood pressure will be one that results in an acceptable urine output and a normalisation of the lactate and base deficit. It is often possible to have normal parameters by the end of the surgical phase with aggressive haemostatic resuscitation.

Disability and exposure

The anaesthetist is in the best position to assess the conscious level of the trauma patient. A simple AVPU score or a GCS (the most important component of which is the motor score) is vital before intubation and ventilation, where they can be obtained. The assessment of the size and reactivity of the pupils is also best performed by the anaesthetist. This is particularly the case in traumatic head injury as a blown pupil may be the only indication of severe head injury, which requires emergency treatment in an unconscious patient.

Hypothermia is one arm of the lethal triad. Major injury reduces the production of body heat but patients should be brought in to the emergency department with clothing cut off to better assess all the injuries and 'bubble wrapped' up to insulate them against the elements. The competing priorities of exposure and maintenance of body temperature can be difficult to reconcile. Prevention of heat loss and hypothermia is better than re-warming a cold patient. Heat preservation strategies must be adopted from the outset and continued through the patient's journey until the patient can thermoregulate again. There are several strategies to mitigate heat loss, which are supported by NICE guidelines on the management of peri-operative hypothermia (see Table 18.4). The detrimental effects of hypothermia on coagulation, platelet function and metabolism are well recognised. A core temperature of $<34^\circ$ C significantly affects enzyme activity, coagulation and platelet function compared to trauma patients with a temperature $>34^\circ$ C. Hypothermia also causes decreased thromboxane production resulting in further platelet dysfunction, microvascular bleeding and a prolonged bleeding time. Other problems seen in hypothermia include a reduced cardiac output and arrhythmias, a shift of the oxygen dissociation curve to the left, further impairing oxygen delivery to the tissues, and shivering which increases oxygen

Table 18.4 Hypothermia prevention and treatment

Hypothermia prevention and treatment
Limit exposure and 'bubble wrap' patients in transport
Warm all blood, blood products and intravenous fluids before administration
Use forced air warming devices
Use heating mattresses Warm the emergency department and operating theatre Head warmer Warm humidified breathing circuit

consumption and lactataemia. A core temperature of <32° C in an exsanguinating trauma patient is usually fatal.

In the operating theatre there is a further conflict between the need to reduce heat loss and appropriate surgical exposure of the patient. For severe trauma the patient should be placed supine on the operating table, on a warming mattress in a very warm theatre and, in torso injury, exposed from the neck to the knees in order to allow the surgeon access to both the chest and abdomen and the junctional areas. The arms should be out on arm boards so that the patient is in a crucifix or trauma 'T' position. This allows the surgeon better access to the chest and the anaesthetist access for arterial and venous line placement. A forced air warming device should be placed over the head, neck and arms where appropriate, and another over the legs. In more minor trauma some compromise can be made and more of the torso may be covered by forced air warming devices.

Monitoring

Basic non-invasive monitoring (the ECG, pulse rate, the impedance-derived respiratory rate, pulse oximetry, non-invasive blood pressure and end-tidal CO_2 capnography) and peripheral venous access will already have been established in the emergency department. In all but the most severely injured patients who need a resuscitative thoracotomy or laparotomy there is usually time for the anaesthetists to establish additional lines and monitoring in the ED or in the operating theatre before the surgery starts. Occasionally, there must be concurrent activity in the operating theatre and, in that case, adequate surgical exposure of the patient in the trauma 'T' position must also allow the anaesthetists to work on the arms, neck and supraclavicular regions. The anaesthetist will wish to gain central venous access with a large single or double lumen line or preferably the introducer sheath of a Swan–Ganz catheter, usually into the subclavian vein. Access to the internal jugular vein is usually hindered by cervical spine immobilisation and it tends to collapse more than the subclavian vein in hypovolaemic patients, making cannulation more hazardous. This access is used for rapid blood and blood product transfusion using infusers specifically designed for this purpose, which can rapidly transfuse warm (38° C) fluid. The Level 1® or Belmont® infusers are examples of such devices. Arterial access for the continuous measurement of the blood pressure and for the intermittent measurement of arterial blood gases is usually obtained in the arm, either at the wrist or in the antecubital fossa. Arterial line placement must not delay the surgery and is only necessary for deciding when to stop the resuscitation process. Other monitoring devices that will usually be utilised include a central temperature probe and a transoesophageal echo probe to estimate cardiac output. Measurement of the central venous pressure (CVP) is less common now but may be easily applied to one lumen of the central line. Systolic pressure variation software can also be used in lieu of a CVP trace to estimate filling of the capacitance vessels. Most anaesthetic equipment will also display the FiO_2, the inspired anaesthetic gas concentrations and the hysteresis loop of the respiratory cycle. A urinary catheter should be placed to decompress the bladder and to monitor the urine output. A nasogastric tube (or orogastric if there is suspicion of a base of skull fracture) will help reduce the risk of aspiration and empty the stomach and both tubes help to increase surgical access at laparotomy.

Knowledge of the temperature, pH and coagulation status of the patient is vital if the 'lethal triad' is to be avoided. During the damage-control resuscitation and surgery regular blood samples will be sent for point-of-care testing. Modern analysers will return the partial pressure of oxygen in the sample, the acid–base status, lactate, haemoglobin, ionised calcium, potassium and other variables within a few minutes. These are necessary results to tailor the haemostatic resuscitation of the patient appropriately. The authors believe the best point-of-care testing of coagulation to be the ROTEM®. This is a development of thromboelastography. This in vitro point-of-care test provides a quantitative and qualitative indication of the coagulation state of a blood sample. The system records the kinetic changes in a sample of citrated whole blood during clot formation as well as when the sample clot retracts and/or lyses. Different parameters of the clotting are measured, analysed, monitored, interpreted and charted and presented in a graphical format which reflects the various physiological results. Analysis of the shape of the curve, and comparison of the results obtained through the application of specific reagents and reference values will result in a better understanding of complex disorders of haemostasis. A ROTEM® should be sent approximately every hour and the result takes at least ten to 20 minutes to process. The ROTEM® result will detect all relevant alterations in haemostasis which may have an impact on coagulation such as coagulation enzyme activity and the overall degree of coagulability, platelet function, fibrinolysis, consumptive coagulopathy and anticoagulant therapy. This diagnostic point-of-care test assesses the components of coagulation in an integrated fashion and facilitates targeted blood component therapy. Care must be taken in interpreting the result when the patient is hypothermic as the ROTEM® analysis takes place at 37 degrees centigrade.

Drugs in trauma anaesthesia

The anaesthetic armamentarium in trauma includes induction (hypnotic) agents, amnestics, analgesics, muscle relaxants and inhalational gases. Caution must be exercised as the therapeutic indices of these drugs are reduced in trauma patients and they can all have a significant haemodynamic impact. The commonly recommended induction agents include ketamine and thiopentone. The amnestics used are benzodiazepines and the opioid analgesics include morphine, fentanyl and its congeners (remifentanil, alfentanyl and sufentanyl). The neuromuscular blocking agents most used are suxamethonium, rocuronium, vecuronium and atracurium. Inhalational agents for the maintenance of general anaesthesia include isoflurane, desflurane and sevoflurane.

Ketamine is a rapidly acting intravenous anaesthetic that produces a functional and electrophysiological dissociation between the cortex and limbic system, producing anaesthesia and unconsciousness in larger doses. Ketamine has sympathomimetic effects that support the heart rate and blood pressure, making it a desirable induction agent in trauma. Ketamine increases the cerebral metabolic rate and, historically, this has been regarded as a relative contraindication in head-injured patients. However, it is now recognised to maintain cerebral perfusion at a level that more than compensates for this metabolic rate increase. It also increases myocardial oxygen demand, produces copious airway secretions and is associated with emergence delirium in adults. Its versatility and cardiovascular stability have made it a favourite drug in the pre-hospital environment where smaller doses are used for analgesia and sedation and it is rapidly becoming the drug of choice for induction in trauma. *Etomidate* is cardiovascularly stable and a useful induction agent in haemodynamically unstable trauma patients. It also reduces cerebral blood flow, cerebral oxygen consumption and ICP while maintaining cerebral perfusion pressure, so it has particular utility in head injured patients. It is associated with adrenal suppression which is marked for 24–48 hrs and has deterred its use. *Propofol* is a useful sedative-hypnotic agent that can be used for induction when given by bolus and maintenance of anaesthesia when infused continuously. However, its cardiovascular depressant effect precludes its use in severe trauma.

Midazolam is the most frequently used benzodiazepine in trauma. Benzodiazepines are anxiolytics and produce amnesia; they are cardiovascularly stable and do not depress respiration in smaller doses. Midazolam is often given with ketamine to reduce the emergence delirium. However, they also act synergistically with opioids and volatile anaesthetic agents and can cause apnoea and hypotension.

Opioids reduce the trauma and surgically induced stress response. *Fentanyl* is considered cardiovascularly stable; morphine is not as it causes a dose-dependent release of histamine. They will tend to produce hypotension in larger doses, especially in underfilled patients. This effect is used to promote rapid filling in the patient who is cardiovasculary empty but still in a profoundly vasoconstricted state brought on by shock. These agents are respiratory depressants and decrease both the hypercarbic and hypoxic drive to breathe. They also decrease gastrointestinal motility and promote nausea and vomiting. *Remifentanil* is unique among opioids in that it undergoes ester hydrolysis in blood and tissues (as opposed to hepatic metabolism) and has a very short half-life. Therefore, it may be administered as an infusion.

Neuromuscular blocking agents relax skeletal muscle, facilitating endotracheal intubation, mechanical ventilation and surgical exposure. *Suxamethonium*, a neuromuscular junction agonist, is the only depolarising agent. It has a rapid onset of action of about 45 seconds and a short duration of action or paralysis of five to eight minutes as the drug diffuses away from the junction to be metabolised. It is used in conjunction with induction agents to secure the airway by passing an endotracheal tube in a rapid sequence induction (RSI). Suxamethonium use has its drawbacks. It may cause anoxic brain injury and death in the 'cannot ventilate, cannot intubate' situation. It can cause arrhythmias, rhabdomyolysis and masseter muscle spasm (hindering intubation) and it may trigger malignant hyperthermia. It can also cause a transient and usually insignificant rise in serum potassium levels but in some patients with up-regulated acetyl choline receptors and with severe trauma, burns, and major crush injuries the efflux of potassium from damaged skeletal muscle may be deleterious and even lead to cardiac arrest. Suxamethonium also causes rises in intraocular pressure and intracranial pressure and so it should be used with caution in eye and head injured patients.

Rocuronium is a competitive antagonist at the neuromuscular junction and a non-depolarising muscle relaxant. It is a rapid-onset and short-acting neuromuscular blocking agent and may be used in lieu of suxamethonium and when the airway is believed to be manageable, especially if sugammadex is available (*vide infra*). Its onset time is about two minutes and its duration of action is 30–35 minutes. *Vecuronium* and *atracurium* are considered to be of intermediate duration and are used mainly in the operating theatre; while *pancuronium*, a long-duration muscle relaxant, is probably used best in the pre-hospital environment in trauma. The non-depolarising muscle relaxant compounds are relatively cardiovascularly stable but the benzylisoquinoline group (the –curiums) produce histamine release, which can cause bronchospasm and hypotension in larger, rapidly administered doses. These drugs (with the exception of atracurium, which breaks down spontaneously), together with the aminosteroid group (the –oniums), are metabolised in the liver and may persist in the presence of hepatic and renal dysfunction. *Sugammadex* is a new drug, which is used to reverse the non-depolarising muscle relaxants if necessary.

Inhalational halogenated anaesthetic agents produce unconsciousness, amnesia, analgesia and a degree of muscle relaxation. Their mechanism of action is incompletely understood. *Desflurane* is the least soluble and its effects diminish most rapidly on discontinuation. Desflurane and *isoflurane* are excreted by the lungs, while *sevoflurane* is metabolised a little bit more. They are all vasodilators and have cardiac depressant effects in larger doses with isoflurane being the most cardiovascularly stable. They all increase cerebral blood flow but decrease cerebral oxygen consumption. These agents are widely used in severe trauma but at greatly reduced dosages as part of a balanced anaesthetic technique. Nitrous oxide is a potent analgesic but does not cause unconsciousness alone. It is also insoluble and high concentrations (50–60%) are required for its effect. This causes the gas to diffuse into air-filled spaces such as an untreated pneumothorax or pneumocephalus and so this agent is avoided in trauma anaesthesia. The gases used for ventilating the trauma patient are oxygen or a combination of oxygen and air to reduce the FiO_2.

Anaesthetic considerations in trauma to specific areas

Head injury

Most potentially preventable head injury morbidity is caused by a delay in recognising and treating an intracranial haematoma by evacuation or the failure to correct hypoxia/hypercarbia, hypotension or hyperglycaemia. The anaesthetist is well placed to assess the neurological status of the patient (AVPU and GCS) and the pupils, and to inspect and palpate the scalp for lacerations, haematomas, depressed fractures, and evidence of base of skull fractures such as Battle's sign, raccoon eyes, scleral haemorrhage without a posterior limit, haemotympanium, cerebrospinal fluid rhinorrhoea or otorrhoea.

The fundamental aim in traumatic brain injury (TBI) is to maintain cerebral perfusion and oxygenation in order to limit the region of ischaemic secondary brain injury. Autoregulation, the ability to maintain a constant blood flow over a range of perfusion pressures, may be lost in this region so cerebral blood flow will change with perfusion pressure. Cerebral blood flow is lowest in areas affected by secondary brain injury in the hours immediately after the injury. Furthermore, any rise in the intracranial pressure (ICP) will reduce the cerebral perfusion pressure and the cerebral blood flow. In order to limit rises in ICP, special care must be given to cardiovascular stability and maintaining cerebral blood flow. Neuromuscular blockade is necessary to prevent coughing or 'bucking' which substantially increases ICP. Rocuronium may be preferable to suxamethonium as it does not cause fasciculations. Propofol may be used as an induction and also as a sedation agent. It is preferred to halogenated volatile anaesthetic gases for sedation as the latter tend to increase cerebral blood flow as they are vasodilators, despite decreasing cerebral oxygen consumption. Care must be taken to maintain cervical spine immobilisation as spinal injuries commonly occur following head trauma. The ventilation should be adjusted to maintain a pCO_2 between 4–4.5 kPa and an oxygen saturation of >97%. Hypotensive resuscitation is contraindicated in head injuries and haemostatic fluid resuscitation should be directed towards a mean arterial blood pressure of 90 mmHg. Other strategies used by anaesthetists to reduce the ICP in addition to sedation and paralysis include the use of mannitol, hypertonic saline and furosemide, short periods of manual hyperventilation, head up positioning, barbiturate coma and modest hypothermia. The anaesthetist may also be called upon to manage seizures.

Spinal injury

Meticulous care must be taken to maintain cervical spine immobilisation to prevent secondary injuries to the spinal cord. This may lead to intubation difficulties as in this position up to 20% of patients will have a grade III view of the larynx. Fibre-optic bronchoscopy may be the best way to intubate such patients but direct laryngoscopy is not contraindicated, despite the movement it produces between the cervical vertebrae.

Spinal, neurogenic shock because of loss of vasomotor tone, can be expected with injuries above the T6 level. However, beware of attributing hypotension to spinal shock as hypovolaemia is more likely to be the cause of hypotension even in cord-injured patients. A bradycardia may be present in the high thoracic injuries because of interruption of the sympathetic cardiac accelerator fibres. Hypotension and bradycardia may require fluid resuscitation, vasopressors and atropine. The principles of management of head injuries apply to an injured spinal cord and cord perfusion should be maintained and hypoxia avoided. In conscious patients a detailed neurological examination is required. Any sensory or motor function below the level of the spinal injury indicates an incomplete injury. A CT scan of the head, cervical and thoracolumbar spine provides the clinician with sufficient information to rule out or define the nature and extent of the spinal injury.

Burns

The airway is particularly at risk in burned patients. Burns to the head and neck may rapidly cause airway obstruction from massive oedema and the airway above the larynx may already be injured because of the inhalation of hot gases and smoke. Signs of potential airway compromise include singed nasal hairs, a hoarse voice, a brassy cough, erythema and swelling of the mucous membranes and soot in the sputum. A decision to intubate must be made early as the oedema will continue to increase for 12–36 hours. The main reasons for intubation of patients are listed in Table 18.3. In burned patients intubation may be required for unconsciousness as a result of trauma or carbon monoxide poisoning, developing acute respiratory failure from smoke inhalation, cyanide poisoning, or blast injury and the need for extensive fluid resuscitation. There is a theoretical risk of life-threatening hyperkalaemia following the use of suxamethonium in this patient group but its use is safe in the initial 24 hours. Circumferential burns to the chest may require escharotomies to permit chest expansion and ventilation. Limbs may also benefit from escharotomies if the circulation is impaired.

Intravenous access is essential and may be difficult to obtain. Cannulae should be inserted through intact skin where possible. Intravenous fluid resuscitation should be started where the burn is >15% total body surface area (TBSA) in adults and >10% in children. Hartmann's solution is the preferred crystalloid fluid and the volume to give is 2 ml/kg/%TBSA in adults and 3 ml/kg/%TBSA in children with half given in the first eight hours following the burn and the second half in the subsequent 16 hours in addition to maintenance fluids. Fluid resuscitation should be guided by the urine output. Thermoregulation is lost with loss of skin integrity and with general anaesthesia. Cooling of the burn with cold water and cold fluid resuscitation may also exacerbate the hypothermia. All available means of maintaining normothermia must be employed (see Table 18.4).

Beware carbon monoxide poisoning especially in patients burned in confined spaces such as house fires. Carbon monoxide binds to haemoglobin as carboxyhaemoglobin (COHb) and reduces the oxygen carrying capacity of the blood. It also binds other haem-containing compounds including the cytochrome system. Pulse oximetry cannot distinguish between oxyhaemoglobin and COHb and it will overestimate the oxygen saturation in the presence of COHb, so a co-oximeter is needed. Oxygen therapy reduces the half-life of COHb from 250 minutes to 40 minutes and hyperbaric oxygen therapy can reduce it further to 15–30 minutes. Oxygen therapy is the mainstay of treatment in the early treatment of patients with carbon monoxide poisoning. Other toxic compounds of combustion include cyanide, ammonia, phosgene, hydrogen chloride, fluorides and bromides as well as other organic chemicals. These compounds may produce a chemical burn to the respiratory tract, interstitial lung oedema, impaired gas exchange and acute respiratory distress syndrome, systemic acid–base disturbances and other metabolic abnormalities.

Conclusion

The successful resuscitation and treatment of a severely injured trauma patient is a challenge for the pre-hospital system, the emergency department physicians, the anaesthetists, the surgeons and the entire major trauma centre. Permissive hypotension, haemostatic resuscitation and damage-control surgery offer clinicians the best chance of salvaging these patients but the potential for massive transfusions of blood and blood products necessitates an institutional recognition of the need for a co-ordinated protocol to mobilise large quantities of blood and blood derivatives in a timely manner. Keeping some of these patients alive may often depend on every cog in the system working seamlessly from the portering staff, who may be needed to ensure the blood is available in the right place at the right time, to the willingness of hospital managers and politicians to mobilise sufficient resources in support of trauma.

Further reading

Bickel WH, Wall MJ Jr, Pepe PE, *et al.* Immediate versus delayed fluid resuscitation for hypotensive patients with penetrating torso injuries. *N Engl J Med* 1994; **331**: 1105–9.

Boffard KD, Riou B, Warren B, *et al.* Recombinant factor VIIa as adjunctive therapy for bleeding control in severely injured trauma patients: two parallel randomized, placebo controlled, double-blind clinical trials. *J Trauma* 2005; **59**: 8–15.

Borgman MA, Spinella PC, Perkins JG, *et al.* The ratio of blood products transfused affects mortality in patients receiving massive transfusions at a combat support hospital. *J Trauma* 2007; **63**: 805–13.

Brohi K, Singh J, Heron M, Coats T. Acute traumatic coagulopathy. *J Trauma* 2003; **54**: 1127–30.

Brohi K, Cohen MJ, Gunter MT, *et al.* Acute coagulopathy of trauma: hypoperfusion induces anti-coagulation and hyperfibrinolysis. *J Trauma* 2008; **64**: 1211–7.

CRASH-2 Trial Collaborators. Effects of tranexamic acid on death, vascular occlusive events, and blood transfusion in trauma patients with significant haemorrhage (CRASH-2): a randomised, placebo-controlled trial. *Lancet* 2010; **376(9734)**: 23–32.

Rontondo MF, Zonies DH. The damage-control sequence and underlying logic. *Surg Clin N Am* 1997; 77: 761–76.

Chapter 19

Orthopaedic cases

David Tew and Alan Norrish

Introduction

Orthopaedics involves a variety of treatments on both bones and joints, and also the soft tissues around them. Common procedures might include fracture fixation, joint replacement, joint arthroscopy, repair of injured tendons and muscles as well as correction of limb deformities. The patient's age ranges from the neonate to the elderly.

Pre-operative assessment

While many procedures are planned as elective admissions, a significant proportion of orthopaedic surgery is performed emergently. The timing of the pre-operative assessment for elective procedures should be about one month before the date of the planned surgery. This allows medication review, investigation and treatment of unstable co-morbidities, and correction of conditions such as anaemia and hypertension (Table 19.1). Drugs commonly modified in the peri-operative period include rheumatoid biologic agents, anticoagulants, oral hypoglycaemics, NSAIDs, MAOI (monoamine oxidase inhibitors) and lithium. Most other medications are continued up to the day of surgery.

Where patients require emergent treatment, delaying surgery may not be an option. Careful modification of peri-operative care is needed, balancing the risks of threat to limb and life.

- *Example 1*: the patient presents with both a femoral neck fracture and a recent myocardial infarction. A multi-disciplinary approach to treatment options may include proceed with surgery, conservative management, surgery after a delay to allow some degree of scar formation in the new infarct (weeks), lesser surgery to temporise the fracture with a plan for more definitive surgery after a suitable time period (months). In this scenario, a key factor will be the presence of decompensating heart failure.
- *Example 2*: the trauma patient presenting with an open fracture with vascular compromise (requiring emergent surgery) who has had a recent meal and has a full stomach. The same discussion of life versus limb takes place but a suitable anaesthetic plan needs to be formulated to minimise the risk of aspiration.

Often anaesthetists require documentation that a patient is at serious risk of losing limb function before attempting to provide anaesthesia in such circumstances.

A Surgeon's Guide to Anaesthesia and Peri-operative Care, ed. Jane Sturgess, Justin Davies and Kamen Valchanov. Published by Cambridge University Press.

Table 19.1 Aims of pre-assessment for elective orthopaedic surgery

Medication review/advice	Reduces on the day cancellations, aids enhanced recovery and intra-operative management
Fasting guidance	Reduces cancellations or excessive fasting 6 hours for solid food and particulate drinks (tea with milk); 2 hours for clear fluids. Explains that fasting is to prevent aspiration of stomach contents on induction or maintenance of anaesthesia, not to prevent nausea and vomiting Some enhanced recovery programmes are encouraging pre-operative carbohydrate loading
Physiotherapy (pre-habilitation)	Aids enhanced recovery
Managing patient expectation	Aids enhanced recovery
Consent (especially for regional anaesthetic procedures)	Good medical practice, and allows for informed consent Permits discussion between surgeon and anaesthetist, e.g. if a regional technique is/is not appropriate in the patient with severe respiratory disease
Identify and optimise co-morbidities	Aids appropriate surgical timing, e.g. delaying surgery until after cardiology review of unstable angina or respiratory review of brittle asthma Allows planning of intra-operative management, e.g. the unstable neck in a rheumatoid arthritis patient having shoulder surgery, or the difficult intubation in the patient with ankylosing spondylitis
Risk scoring (see risk scoring)	Allows assessment of risk and discussion with patient Patients may choose conservative treatment options Alternatively post-operative ITU/HDU can be prepared Most common risk scoring relates to cardiovascular health This population also requires an assessment of memory to predict post-operative cognitive dysfunction

Co-morbidities most commonly complicating peri-operative care in orthopaedic patients are:

- cardiovascular disease (hypertension, ischaemic heart disease, rhythm disturbance, valvular heart disease, peripheral vascular disease)
- respiratory disease
- diabetes
- musculoskeletal disease (rheumatoid arthritis and ankylosing spondylitis are of particular concern to the anaesthetist)
- neurological disease including cerebrovascular disease

Cardiac disease

The general principle is that patients do not receive treatment for this disease (just because they are scheduled for surgery) unless such treatment is justified on purely cardiac grounds. Interventions such as myocardial revascularisation or valve repair/replacement will take place when clinically indicated (e.g. meeting European Criteria) and not necessarily

Table 19.2 Advice for elective surgery on anti-platelet/anticoagulation

Low-dose aspirin	Coronary stents, AF	Continue
Other anti-platelets, e.g. clopidogrel	Coronary stents (take advice, see text)	Stop seven days before surgery
Warfarin	Low risk of thrombotic complications, e.g. atrial fibrillation	Stop five days before surgery Check INR on day of surgery
	Medium or high-risk of thrombotic complications, e.g. valve replacement	Stop five days before surgery Bridging therapy with LMWH (based on body weight) starting two days after warfarin stopped. Stop LMWH on the morning of the day before surgery. Allow 24 hours between last dose of LMWH and surgery Check INR on day of surgery

expedited prior to surgery. This can cause problems when patients fail to meet the criteria for safe surgery (e.g. severe aortic stenosis) yet have a disease severity that does not meet the criteria for valve replacement. A discussion between patient, surgeon, anaesthetist and cardiologist can often guide the safest method and timing for elective orthopaedic surgery. Most cardiac medication (except anticoagulants) is continued up to and including the day of surgery. Being nil by mouth is not a reason to omit common medications. Surgery may be cancelled if patients omit their regular cardiac (e.g. anti-anginal) medication on the day of surgery. This information must be reinforced at the pre-operative assessment.

Anticoagulation and antiplatelet therapy

Many centres use the indication for warfarin therapy to define such patients as low, medium or high risk with respect to the likelihood of thrombotic complications on stopping their warfarin and publish guidelines on suggested courses of action. Where local guidelines are published haematological advice is not normally required (unless there are special features) and this can be organised through the pre-assessment process. Where warfarin is stopped an INR should be checked immediately prior to surgery (Table 19.2).

Special consideration is required for patients with stents in their coronary arteries, as they present a particular hazard. Stents come in two varieties, bare metal stents (BMS) and drug-eluting stents (DES). Patients with BMS are put on double anti-platelet therapy for three months following stent insertion and should not have any elective surgery during this period. They are at risk of intra-stent thrombosis until vascular epithelium grows over the bare metal. This epithelialisation takes several months to complete. At that point, clopidogrel may be stopped and single therapy with aspirin continued for life. The BMS may be complicated by proliferative overgrowth of epithelium, which causes re-stenosis of the stent (through fibrosis and thrombus formation). For this reason, stents were designed which elute drugs (e.g. paclitaxel or sirolimus derivatives) to inhibit this epithelial overgrowth. For DES, a minimum of one year is required for epithelialisation during which time patients take double anti-platelet therapy and elective surgery is generally forbidden. Any patient with any stent(s) will remain on lifelong anti-platelet therapy to reduce the risk of stent thrombosis (there may still be some bare metal present years after insertion) and this will include the peri-operative period so aspirin should be continued. Peri-operative stent thrombosis outweighs the risk of bleeding for most orthopaedic surgery. Patients intolerant of aspirin may be maintained on alternative anticoagulants (e.g. clopidogrel), presenting a management challenge. In such complex cases the multi-disciplinary team approach with surgeon, anaesthetist and cardiologist is needed to make the safest peri-operative plan (e.g. to use LMWH).

Pacemakers

Patients with pacemakers will normally have annual checks of function and battery life. They should be questioned to ensure these are on schedule. They should also carry a pacemaker card giving details of the model. They should bring this with them to hospital as anaesthetists will check this as part of their assessment. Many newer pacemakers do not respond favourably to a magnet being placed over them in a crisis. Orthopaedic surgery using bipolar diathermy is best for patients with pacemakers (see physics and diathermy). If monopolar diathermy is unavoidable then the plate should be placed as far away as possible from the device and diathermy carried out in short bursts. If a patient has an implanted defibrillator this will require special treatment and need to be turned off. The device may interpret the use of diathermy as ventricular fibrillation and internally shock the patient every time diathermy is used. Implantable defibrillators need to be turned off just before surgery and turned back on again shortly afterwards by pacing technicians from the cardiology department. It must be organised in advance at the pre-operative assessment.

Respiratory disease

Patients with severe respiratory disease present a sizeable anaesthetic challenge and for many patients a regional technique will be preferable. A regional or central neuraxial blockade is not always feasible as some patients will not countenance local anaesthesia and in others it may not be technically possible. In the clinic, assessing whether respiratory patients can lie flat and still for the expected duration of surgery is important when considering spinal anaesthesia. If severely compromised, respiratory patients may require general anaesthesia and high-dependency post-operative care. In some instances, it may be possible to perform surgery (e.g. knee replacement or foot surgery) with the patient in a much more upright position than normal using a regional anaesthesia technique. Respiratory patients may be unable to tolerate the diaphragmatic paresis that comes with interscalene brachial plexus blocks (e.g. for shoulder surgery) and many supraclavicular blocks (e.g. for elbow, forearm and hand surgery). These complex patients require a joint anaesthetic and surgical plan, made before the day of surgery, which can be discussed with the patient.

Other drugs

1. Oral hypoglycaemic drugs (particularly metformin) should be stopped for 24 hours before elective surgery.
2. Some hospitals advise withholding one dose of lithium on the day before surgery.

3. Non-steroidal anti-inflammatory (NSAIDs) drugs are often stopped for seven to ten days prior to surgery to modify their anti-platelet effects. An alternative pain relief plan may need to be established for this period.
4. Patients taking non-reversible monoamine oxidase inhibitors (MAOI) should stop these drugs for at least four weeks before surgery as they seriously interact with a variety of anaesthetic drugs. Stopping these medications brings problems in itself and should only be done in liaison with the primary care physician. These patients need alternative antidepressants, as MAOI are often last resort drugs for patients with severe, suicidal depression previously unresponsive to conventional, safer treatment.
5. Patients with inflammatory arthritis are often on treatment with anti-TNF medication or other biologic agents. These should be stopped for one week before the surgery and for two weeks after in order to minimise the chance of infection.
6. Rheumatoid and other patients may be on long-term steroids and require an increase in the post-operative period to allow them to respond to the stress of surgery.

Special medical considerations

Haemophilia – patients with haemophilia often require knee surgery. Close liaison with haematologists in the peri-operative period is key to ensure that levels of clotting factors are optimal.

Sickle cell disease – sickle cell patients often require orthopaedic surgery and careful liaison with the haematologists is needed and may involve exchange transfusion (for severe homozygous disease).

Ankylosing spondylitis – these patients present difficulties with airway management, restrictive respiratory disease and cardiac defects (pump and valves). They may require post-operative intensive care, and should be discussed with the anaesthetist.

Post-transplant surgery, particularly renal and liver transplants – these patients are often on immunosuppressive agents. It is important to avoid modifying any of their medication without discussion with the transplant physicians. In addition, certain medications may need to be avoided or the doses altered in the presence of renal and liver transplants. It is advisable to ask the transplant physicians looking after these patients if they should be transferred to that centre for surgery (there may not be time if the surgery is emergent). The answer will often (but not always) be yes, especially for patients with liver and multivisceral transplants.

One of the pillars of orthopaedic surgery is to aim for mobilisation and rehabilitation as rapidly as the surgery will allow (Table 19.3). Most orthopaedic surgery allows for immediate mobilisation, but this aim may not be realised because of post-operative pain. One of the key aspects of successful orthopaedic peri-operative care is the control of pain. There are many aspects involved in controlling pain and they can be categorised as pre-operative, peri-operative and post-operative.

There are some analgesic medications to be avoided in certain orthopaedic patients.

Example Prolonged use of NSAIDs in patients with fractures that have features that make them less likely to heal. These fractures rely on the inflammatory response to heal which may be diminished by the prolonged use of anti-inflammatories.

Table 19.3 Techniques to enable early mobilisation and rehabilitation

Timing	Technique	Action/problem
Pre-operative	Information – what to expect on the day of surgery including anaesthesia and surgery, time to mobilisation and expected length of stay	Reduces anxiety and sets expectations. Often performed in pre-op classes
	Pre-emptive analgesia, paracetamol, NSAID, gabapentin	Some evidence it may reduce post-operative pain
Peri-operative opioid-sparing analgesia	Ketamine – also anaesthetic	Can be used to help position patients with fractures before performing regional techniques. Care with hallucinations
	Gabapentin	Drowsiness, gastrointestinal symptoms
	Magnesium	Recent evidence to show reduced opiate consumption post-operatively
Peri-operative regional anaesthesia	Epidural or spinal – with or without ultra-low-dose opiate	Potential hypotension. Potential decreased mobility. Important to time anti-thrombotic therapy to reduce risk of spinal/epidural haematoma
	Peripheral	Possible reduced mobility
Peri-operative	Normothermia	Reduce shivering and increased energy and oxygen demand
Peri-operative/ post-operative	Anti-emesis	Dual agent for high-risk patients
Post-operative	On-going oral analgesia	Multimodal and opiate-sparing

Venous thromboembolism (VTE)

Many patients undergoing orthopaedic surgery have a significant risk of venous thromboembolism (VTE) as a factor of the major surgery coupled with the reduction in mobility. The risk of VTE is minimised by the use of mechanical devices such as graduated compression stockings and calf or foot pumps. Maintaining optimal hydration and achieving early mobilisation further reduce the risk of VTE.

In many orthopaedic operations a significant amount of equipment is needed, including simultaneous fluoroscopy. For this reason close liaison with theatre scrub staff is important to ensure that all equipment is available or 'loaned in' to allow the operation to proceed in a timely manner. The need for X-rays during the procedure must be taken into account when selecting an operating table and positioning the patient. Often complex positions are used with patients elevated up high or turned prone where airway, venous and other access may be more complex. Care must be taken to ensure these risks are controlled prior to prepping and draping the patient, when it becomes much more difficult.

Intra-operative management

Blood loss

Pre-operative haemoglobin can be optimised and blood can be grouped and saved or cross-matched to allow rapid access if blood products are needed. Where a significant amount of blood loss is routine, e.g. hip replacement, a 'cell saver' is used to recycle blood lost through the wound by a surgical suction catheter. Tranexamic acid is also used routinely to minimise blood loss in lower limb joint replacement surgery (its use is contra-indicated in patients with a personal history of thromboembolic disease and some centres avoid using it in patients with coronary stents).

Infection control

Whenever surgical implants are used, it has been shown that prophylactic antibiotics can reduce the risk of infection. The timing of these antibiotics is very important. The antibiotic should have reached peak tissue concentration at the time of the incision. The exact pharmacological agent used is often determined by local policy, but it will be effective against gram-positive organisms such as *Staphylococcus aureus*. Because this is the most common organism causing post-operative infection in orthopaedic surgery, patients should be screened prior to admission for MRSA and where possible this should be eradicated prior to surgery. If the surgery is urgent, e.g. a fracture, and the MRSA status is suspicious (e.g. from a nursing home) but unknown, then vancomycin prophylaxis should be given unless contraindicated. It is generally accepted that many cephalosporins are contraindicated in patients over the age of sixty because of the risk of developing *Clostridium difficile* infections. Post-operative infection is more common where there is a focal area of sepsis elsewhere on the patient, particularly distal to the proposed surgical area (e.g. leg ulcer on the same side in a patient waiting for a hip replacement). For this reason, where possible, surgery should be delayed until concomitant infections are fully resolved. There is no consensus on the duration of prophylactic antibiotics, but typical local protocols suggest a single pre-operative dose or one pre-operative and three post-operative doses (or 24 hours, whichever is the sooner).

Common hip surgery cases

The hip is one of the most common anatomic sites for surgery, particularly in children, the retired and the elderly. In retired patients the surgery is most often elective hip replacement surgery and in the elderly urgent hip fracture surgery.

Hip fractures are very common in the elderly with around 120,000 occurring every year in the UK.

Key points for the anaesthetist

- Mechanical fall or syncope
- Cause of syncope (is there underlying severe aortic stenosis/rhythm disturbance/MI?)
- Hypothermia or rhabdomyolysis
- Confusion – acute, acute on chronic or chronic – take history from carers/next of kin
- Nottingham hip fracture score given the risk of 30-day mortality

Involvement of a geriatrician in the pre-operative as well as the post-operative phase is a marker of best practice. Routine pre-operative investigations in hip fractures include: FBC,

U&E, G&S, ECG and chest X-ray. Where suspicion arises around a non-mechanical fall, serial ECGs and troponin levels may also be included. Evidence has shown that proceeding to surgery within the first 36 hours from admission is associated with a better outcome and for this reason tests that may delay surgery, such as echocardiogram for a heart murmur, are not performed unless they can be done rapidly. The general principle with hip fractures is that they need to be fixed as soon as possible and tests that will not make immediate surgery safer should be delayed until the post-operative period. Often senior anaesthetic input is needed to make these delicate decisions on a patient by patient basis – for example, when echocardiography is not rapidly available, by assuming that a patient with an uncharacterised systolic murmur may indeed have aortic stenosis, and providing care (intra-operative and post-operative) based on that assumption: invasive monitoring, peri-operative inotropes and high-dependency post-operative care.

Two types of anaesthesia are used for hip fractures: regional or general. Regional anaesthesia may be either a spinal or an epidural. No definitive evidence has shown that either regional or general anaesthetic is better, but the Scottish Intercollegiate Guidelines Network (SIGN) suggest using a regional anaesthetic unless contraindicated. This remains a topic of national interest with current multicentre studies set up to try and provide therapeutic suggestions.

Hip fracture patients anticoagulated with warfarin should be given vitamin K unless contra-indicated. This should be done with care, using small doses (0.5 to 1 mg) after taking haematological advice (indiscriminately giving high-dose vitamin K causes difficulties in re-warfarinising post-operatively, often for many weeks). Fresh frozen plasma should not be routinely administered, but only considered when vitamin K is contraindicated. Where circumstances are unusually complex (e.g. very high INR or serious bleeding) prothrombin complex concentrates (PCC, e.g. beriplex) may be needed. Prescribed on haematological advice, PCC can resolve clotting problems very quickly (e.g. in minutes). Hip-fracture patients taking anti-platelet medication (e.g. clopidogrel) should not have their surgery delayed for longer than 36 hours, but general anaesthesia may be advisable as placing central neuraxial block needles (spinal or epidural) in the presence of deranged clotting is a risk factor for devastating epidural haematomas.

Prophylaxis for VTE should be routinely used in hip fracture patients. Chemical prophylaxis may include LMWH or fondaparinux. It should be given six hours after surgery and continue for 28 days unless contra-indicated. Mechanical prophylaxis with graduated compression stockings and foot or calf pumps should also be considered. The timing of VTE prophylaxis is important as insertion of a central neuraxial block needle in the 12 hours following a prophylactic dose of LMWH or fondaparinux is contraindicated. After a CNB has been placed, two hours must elapse before chemical prophylaxis can be given. 6 pm daily is recommended as the best time to prescribe LMWH (the anaesthetist can always delay that evening's dose if placing CNB at the end of the day after 4 pm).

Both hip fracture patients and elective hip replacement patients should receive prophylactic antibiotics. There is also an indication for the use of tranexamic acid, particularly in hip arthoplasty. It has been shown to reduce the need for post-operative blood transfusion. In hip arthroplasty, bone cement is often pressurised inside the intramedullary canal to secure the prosthesis. There is the risk that emboli or possibly a reaction to the cement may cause a systemic effect that can, in rare circumstances, be fatal. Adequate cleaning and preparation of the canal may help to avoid this and in very fragile patients over-pressurisation of the cement should be avoided. In certain types of hip fracture a long intramedullary femoral nail may be needed and this may involve reaming the intramedullary canal. This can lead to the complication of fat emboli and the respiratory compromise that follows. Instrumenting and, in particular, reaming of the intramedullary canal should be avoided in elderly frail patients unless no alternative is available. Where hip fractures are pathological, secondary to multiple femoral metastases, consideration should be given to venting the femur distal when instrumenting the canal to avoid systemic emboli.

Elective hip surgery offers the advantage of allowing a comprehensive pre-operative assessment. The FBC, U&E, G&S, chest X-ray and ECG can all be arranged. Particular attention is paid to the state of the skin on the affected limb, looking for signs of infection or active psoriatic plaques. Assessment of blood pressure, urine analysis and multisite swabs to identify MRSA are also carried out. Liaison with any relevant specialties can also be carried out depending on the co-morbidities. Common supplementary tests include the echocardiogram and lung function tests.

As mentioned above, a key element of the pre-operative assessment is the mental preparation of the patient for surgery. Many hospitals have introduced 'enhanced recovery programmes' (ERP) where every step of the patient's pathway has been optimised to allow early, but safe, discharge. Key elements of ERP include: patient education and support, primary care engagement, pre-operative physiotherapy and occupational therapy, surgical, anaesthetic and analgesic techniques to facilitate early mobility, intensive post-operative physiotherapy and early discharge with appropriate support. Enhanced recovery programmes for joint replacement have seen a high level of patient satisfaction and have resulted in significantly reducing the average length of stay after hip replacement.

The specific type of anaesthetic chosen for hip replacement should aim to minimise post-operative nausea and pain, but leave motor function intact to allow day of operation mobilisation whenever possible. With these principles, the choice of anaesthetic is down to the patient's and anaesthetist's choice. Common combinations include general anaesthesia with selective regional block (e.g. femoral or lumbar plexus using low doses of local anaesthetic drugs) or short-acting spinal anaesthetic with local infiltration of anaesthetic (field block) or a combination. Elastomeric pumps with continuous intra-articular infusion of low-dose local anaesthetic may contribute to effective multimodal post-operative pain relief after hip replacement and have the possible advantage of reducing morphine consumption.

Common knee, foot and ankle surgery cases

One unique factor of operating on the knee, foot and ankle areas is the common use of a tourniquet. Tourniquets may be elastic or pneumatic. The use of pneumatic tourniquets is recommended because the pressure can be directly controlled. The tourniquet time should always be kept to a minimum. If the tourniquet is left up for more than two hours an appreciable rate of permanent neurological damage occurs. The pressure of the tourniquet should not exceed more than 150 mmHg greater than that of the systolic blood pressure. When the tourniquet is let down, there is a potential for systemic complications. This may be because of a reperfusion injury or an embolic phenomenon. It is important that the surgeon and anaesthetist communicate clearly when the tourniquet is to be let down. After major operations, such as knee replacement, unless contra-indicated, tranexamic acid should be administered as the tourniquet is let down. If the tourniquet time threatens to significantly exceed two hours then a tourniquet break can be arranged at a suitable time for the surgeon, the tourniquet is deflated briefly (15 minutes) to allow temporary reperfusion of the limb and then re-inflated to provide improved operating conditions.

When operating around the knee, tibia, ankle and foot there is a higher possibility of developing compartment syndrome of the leg during some types of surgery (particularly fracture fixation). For this reason, a pre-operative discussion between the anaesthetist and surgeon needs to take place to identify the risk of compartment syndrome and to determine whether or not a regional block is advisable. A regional block may mask the symptoms of an evolving compartment syndrome and when the risk is high, many centres avoid the use of such blocks. The severe pain of compartment syndrome may breakthrough peripheral nerve blockade and, if clinically suspected, direct compartment pressure monitoring or alternative tests (e.g. arterial blood gas estimation) may be useful as late compartment syndromes are often associated with marked acidosis and hyperkalaemia. Where there is any doubt fasciotomy is advised.

One of the most common operations in orthopaedic surgery is knee arthroscopy. Where patients are expecting to go home a few hours after their operation, there is an imperative for immediate post-operative mobilisation. Consideration needs to be given to the type of anaesthesia to achieve this. A common choice is a general anaesthetic and local infiltration of anaesthetic around the wounds in the knee (field block).

For most knee, foot and ankle operations a combination of local anaesthetic infiltration in the wound or localised blocks (e.g. ankle block or ray block) together with a general anaesthetic allow rapid discharge without pain. To avoid VTE complications, most patients are given prophylaxis as for hip surgery, but the chemical prophylaxis is limited to 14 days.

Total knee replacement is an example of a very common orthopaedic operation where patients are normally kept in for two or three days after the operation. They should undergo a thorough pre-operative assessment, as for total hip replacements. However, even more emphasis is placed on the pre-operative exercise regime and the prehabilitation in order to achieve early range of movement. Day of surgery mobilisation has been shown to be key to enabling enhanced recovery. Minimising loss of motor function around the knee and post-operative nausea, while keeping pain fully under control, are the aims of a successful anaesthetic in knee replacement surgery.

Common choices include general anaesthetic or spinal anaesthetic with a high-volume, low-concentration, local anaesthetic infiltration field block. If peripheral nerve blocks are used they are focused on the sensory supply of the knee or designed to have short enough duration, to allow early mobilisation. Physiotherapy on the day of surgery is very important, both for hip and especially knee replacement surgery. This can be in the bed and ideally includes mobilising around the room.

In an attempt to reduce the use of opioid-based patient-controlled analgesia (PCA) many ERP protocols use twice daily slow-release oral opioid analgesia with oxycodone or morphine (e.g. oxycontin or MST), supplemented with normal doses of these drugs for breakthrough pain (e.g. oxynorm or oramorph) with a step-down to tramadol, codeine or meptazinol prior to discharge. Sometimes PCA is required for patients to control post--operative pain. It is very effective at pain relief, but does have the side effects of post--operative nausea and does make mobilising more complicated. However, it may be useful in some patients. A continuous intra-articular infusion of high-volume, low-concentration local anaesthetic (e.g. 0.1% bupivacaine) is often used in joint replacement surgery. It provides effective pain relief and does allow early mobilisation. However, some surgeons have concerns about the risk of infection. This can be alleviated somewhat by using closed elastomeric pumps that can be loaded by the surgeon in the sterile field, sealed and left for two to five days and then removed on the ward. Other cited disadvantages include the possibility of reduced mobilisation because of being encumbered by lines. This is less so again with elastomeric pumps because they do not require a power supply and are small. It is likely that we will see increasing use of elastomeric intra-articular infusion pumps after both hip and knee replacement surgery in the future.

Common upper limb cases

Pre-operative tests for surgery on the upper limb are similar to that for the lower limb. In shoulder and elbow surgery there may be a choice of suitable anaesthetics. A typical combination would be a regional block with or without a general anaesthetic. For the shoulder, an interscalene brachial plexus block is often used and for the elbow, forearm and hand, the supraclavicular brachial plexus block. The axillary plexus block is less predictable but may be useful in certain circumstances (less risk of pneumothorax and almost no diaphragmatic paresis). For shoulder surgery in patients with respiratory disease some anaesthetists may use a combination of suprascapular and axillary nerve blocks to avoid the risk of diaphragmatic paresis. Because the blocks can be long lasting, liaison between surgeon and anaesthetist regarding the risk of compartment syndrome is important. In addition, patients discharged home with an active block must be warned to be very careful with the affected limb which is at risk of injury (e.g. cooker burns or car door entrapment). The best strategies to avoid this are using a sling where appropriate and teaching the patient to control the blocked arm by using the non-blocked limb to hold it.

Continuous infusion pumps, particularly elastomeric pumps, have an important role in post-operative pain relief in shoulder and elbow surgery. The continuous infusion is similar to that for hip and knee replacements, but it is not typically intra-articular, but rather into the area where the block is placed around the plexus or in the subacromial space. This gives excellent pain relief, but may cause a profound motor block as well. For this reason, its use is often limited to the first 24–48 hours.

Patient positioning is important in all surgery, but particularly so in surgery of the shoulder and elbow. The operating field is very near to the airway and care must be taken to avoid disturbing the airway during the operation.

Surgery to the hand is often undertaken in the supine position with a tourniquet. Many of the common operations in the hand can be done under a local anaesthetic. Often a mixture of a fast-acting and longer acting local anaesthetic are used (e.g. prilocaine and levobupivacine or ropivacaine). Patients can normally tolerate a tourniquet, without an anaesthetic for a limited period (e.g. up to ten mins). If the tourniquet is required for longer, e.g. in Dupytren's surgery, either a regional technique is chosen which includes the area of the tourniquet, or a general anaesthetic is given. Many patients will find it difficult to tolerate lying still in one position for more than about an hour without experiencing aches or pain in their neck, back, knees and shoulders. The operative area remains numb but they end up having systemic opioids for their positional discomfort, increased sedation or even general anaesthesia in order to cope. For surgery on the fingers a ring block can be used. Adrenaline is never mixed with local anaesthetic for a ring block as it may cause irreversible digital ischaemia.

As for lower limb surgery, aiming for rapid rehabilitation after surgery is the norm. This involves a multi-disciplinary team of hand therapists and physiotherapists. The shoulder, elbow and hand joints are particularly prone to post-operative stiffness. This can be minimised by pre-operative patient education classes similar to those used in knee and hip replacement, to explain to patients the post-operative rehabilitation exercises and to start prehabilitation.

Other post-operative considerations

Some surgery on the limbs can result in significant fluid shifts. In the immediate post-operative period, care must be taken to maintain an accurate fluid balance and maintain vital organ function through adequate tissue perfusion and oxygenation. Where major surgery is contemplated, or any surgery on particularly fragile patients, it is recommended that high-dependency care be used in the post-operative period to allow close monitoring.

For major surgery, it is common in the post-operative period to request a FBC to look for anaemia and U&Es to check for acute kidney injury. There is no consensus as to the best time to do these tests post-operatively, but most surgeons favour between 24–48 hours after surgery. In high-risk patients, it may need to be sooner and more often. Individual trusts may have transfusion guidelines, but it is generally recommended that if a patient is not clinically compromised and has a post-operative haemoglobin of 60% or greater of their pre-operative haemoglobin, they do not need a transfusion. Where a patient is symptomatic (e.g. with chest pain, tachycardia or dizziness) or has a significant history of vascular insufficiency, a haemoglobin above 10 g/dl should be maintained.

It is common for orthopaedic patients to have dizziness and nausea after surgery when they first sit and stand up after surgery. This is related to postural hypotension. It is important to ensure they are well hydrated and that any antihypertensive medication is only given if needed (it may be necessary to omit antihypertensive treatment for a day or two after lower limb arthroplasty).

During surgery on the limbs, there is potential for damage to nerves and vessels. Careful pre- and post-operative examination and documentation needs to be made of the distal sensory and motor function as well as distal pulses and perfusion. Often bandages and casts are used, and these run the risk of being too tight and causing an effective compartment syndrome. In the post-operative period any unexpected pain or poor perfusion should result in loosening to bandages and splitting of tight casts, followed by reassessment. Occasionally, a compartment syndrome is not relieved by removing tight bandages. A low threshold for returning to theatre is required if there is a clinical suspicion of compartment syndrome.

After surgery on both the upper and lower limbs, swelling can be an important negative factor. Swelling should be minimised where possible and techniques to achieve this include elevation, ice or cold packs and encouraging movement in the distal limbs where possible.

Summary

In conclusion, successful orthopaedic surgery requires close surgical and anaesthetic collaboration in the peri-operative period. Where patients are well prepared pre-operatively, from both the medical and psychological perspective, their peri-operative period will have a higher chance of going smoothly. Enhanced recovery programmes are now commonplace in orthopaedics and have made a big difference in the patient experience, reducing length of stay and mortality.

Further reading

Evidence, methods & guidance. Pre-operative tests: the use of routine pre-operative tests for elective surgery. National Institute for Health and Clinical Excellence. June 2003. http://www.nice.org.uk/nicemedia/live/10920/29094/29094.pdf

Gerstein NS, Schulman PM, Gerstein WH, Petersen TR, Tawil I. Should more patients continue aspirin therapy peri-operatively? Clinical impact of aspirin withdrawal syndrome. *Ann Surg* 2012; **255(5)**: 811–9.

Management of hip fracture in older people. Sign Guideline No. 111, ISBN 978 1 905813 47 6, June 2009, http://www.sign.ac.uk/pdf/sign111.pd.

McClelland DBL. *Handbook of Transfusion Medicine*. 4th edn. United Kingdom Blood Services, 2007. http://www.transfusionguidelines.org.uk/docs/pdfs/htm_edition-4_all-pages.pdf.

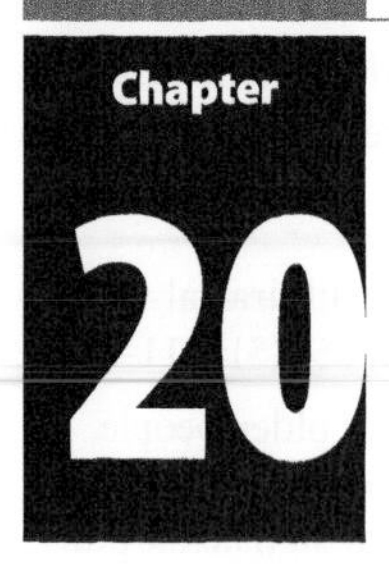

Urology cases

Hemantha Alawattegama and Manit Arya

The challenges for the anaesthetist in urological surgery arise from the complex nature of some of the surgical procedures and the population that require intervention.

Urological surgery has evolved and surgical approaches have changed considerably over the last few years, introducing new challenges to the anaesthetist. For example open prostatectomy, a relatively common procedure previously, has been slowly superseded by laparoscopic, and more recently, robotic prostatectomy. In its place is a two- to four-hour laparoscopic/robotic procedure with its associated risks and physiological insults. This has resulted in a reduction in blood loss, smaller incisions and a significantly shorter length of stay.

As with all types of medicine and surgery, anaesthetic practice has progressed to accommodate and compliment these new approaches and techniques. The patients needing urological surgery tend to be either the very young or the elderly. The latter group present with a variety of co-morbidities. The importance of pre-assessment and physiological optimisation is paramount in ensuring good clinical care. This should be accepted as common ground for both anaesthetist and surgeon alike.

Pre-operative management

Pre-assessment

Many centres now have anaesthetic led pre-assessment clinics to review patients who have complex pre-morbid conditions, patients who are undergoing complex surgery, or both. See (Table 20.1).

Table 20.1 Suggested benefits of an anaesthetic led pre-assessment clinic in urology

Reduced cancellations on day of surgery	Medication advice, especially anticoagulation, antihypertensives
Permit specialist investigations to be ordered	ECHO, CPET
Optimisation of medical conditions	Cardiology review for aortic valve disease Review of medical therapy for respiratory disease Review of medical therapy for ischaemic heart disease Review of medical therapy for diabetic control and diabetic disease Renal advice if dialysis is required

A Surgeon's Guide to Anaesthesia and Peri-operative Care, ed. Jane Sturgess, Justin Davies and Kamen Valchanov. Published by Cambridge University Press.

Renal failure

Patients undergoing various urological procedures have a higher incidence of renal failure compared to the general population. These are primarily because of renal and post-renal (obstructive) causes. Patients with renal failure present a specific group of problems in the peri-operative period – fluid balance, anaemia, electrolyte balance, changes in the way drugs act on and are handled by the body.

Fluid balance

It is important to know whether the patient produces urine and can tolerate a fluid load. For anuric, dialysis-dependent patients, pre- and post-operative dialysis may be required.

Some patients, depending on the severity of their renal impairment, require additional work-up to prepare them for surgery and potentially increased input post-operatively. An extreme case is that of a patient undergoing a nephrectomy with a non-functioning second kidney. These patients would require some access to be placed intra-operatively to allow dialysis in the immediate post-operative period.

For nephrectomy patients it is vital to maintain adequate organ perfusion of the remaining kidney with appropriate volume replacement and cardiovascular support. A urine output of 0.5 ml/kg/h is presumed to indicate a functioning, well-perfused kidney. This can be challenging when an epidural is used intra- and post-operatively.

For patients undergoing urinary diversion procedures it is difficult to estimate urine output and fluid losses once the urinary system has been 'opened' and urine no longer drains into the urometer.

Anaemia

Patients with chronic renal failure are usually anaemic and blood transfusion to correct this, pre-operatively, can cause heart failure because of volume overload. These patients can have their haemoglobin increased by using erythropoietin in the weeks preceding their procedure if required.

Electrolyte balance

Potassium is of particular importance, and should be measured regularly before, during and after the procedure.

Pharmacokinetics

Table 20.2 The pharmacokinetic changes observed in renal failure

Clearance	Decreased
Half-life	Increased
Protein binding	Decreased – low albumin levels, especially important for highly bound acidic drugs, e.g. warfarin
Accumulation kinetics	Repeat dosing may need dose adjustment, e.g. gentamicin

Pharmacodynamics

Table 20.3 The pharmacodynamic changes observed in renal failure. CNS = Central nervous system

CNS	Increased sedation with morphine/codeine as it has an active metabolite that is renally cleared
Respiratory system	Increased respiratory depression with morphine/codeine
Renal function	Care needed with nephrotoxic drugs
Haematological system	Care needed with anticoagulation

Table 20.4 Drugs used in anaesthesia and renal failure

Induction agents	Possible need for reduced dose
Muscle relaxants	Suxamethonium – care with potassium, may be contra-indicated Vecuronium/rocuronium renally excreted and relatively contra-indicated Atracurium/cis-atracurium – broken down to inactive compounds by plasma esterases and alkaline degradation. Usually drug of choice
Analgesics	Morphine and codeine have active opiate metabolite that has a long half-life that is dependent on renal clearance. Relatively contra-indicated Fentanyl – drug of choice

Drugs in anaesthesia and renal failure

Many drugs will have a decreased clearance and an increased half-life (see Tables 20.2, 20.3 and 20.4).

Drugs used during anaesthesia can have prolonged and greater effect in patients with renal dysfunction. This is because of a combination of factors including impairment of metabolism, clearance and reduced protein binding (reduced albumin). Most drugs are excreted by the kidney either unchanged or as a metabolite, which may or may not have activity. Initial, one-off doses of drugs generally have their effect terminated by redistribution. However, care has to be taken with drugs that are to be infused over a period of time. For example, muscle relaxants such as vecuronium and rocuronium are renally excreted and infusions of these should be avoided. Cis-atracurium and atracurium, on the other hand, are enzymatically metabolised by ester hydrolysis and non-enzymatically by alkaline degradation.

The use of opiates is not restricted, but again caution needs to be applied. Morphine is metabolised by the liver to the more active morphine-6-glucuronide, which is renally excreted. Their use in a patient-controlled analgesia system is still possible, but with reduced dosing and increased time interval between boluses. Fentanyl is metabolised to an inactive product by the liver, and some centres advocate fentanyl PCAs over morphine. It is important to note over time that this, too, will accumulate.

Suxamethonium, a depolarising muscle relaxant, can increase serum potassium levels by 0.5 mmol/l and must be used with care in patients with renal failure. This occurs because of muscle fasciculation resulting in release of K^+ from muscle cells.

The use of volatile anaesthetic agents such as isoflurane and desflurane is not affected by renal function as they are excreted by the respiratory system.

Peri- and intra-operative management

Peri-operative checklist

It is standard practice to run through a list of pre-operative safety checks using the World Health Organisation surgical safety checklist. Not only does this promote safer anaesthetic and surgical practice but it also improves communication among the team thus reducing the risk of adverse events intra- and post-operatively. Identification of correct surgical site is essential, for example when a non-functioning kidney or diseased kidney is to be removed while the healthy organ is to remain. Removing the wrong kidney has occurred with subsequent death of the patient.

Patient warming

This reduces the risk of hypothermia in prolonged surgical cases and can also decrease blood loss and incidence of surgical infections. A heated flexible carbon polymer sheet on the operating table is often used for this purpose. Additionally, during endoscopic urological procedures, irrigating fluid can be run through a fluid warmer.

Deep venous thrombosis prophylaxis

The guidelines for prevention of thromboembolic episodes in surgical patients have been formulated by the Thromboembolic Risk Factor Consensus Group. The mainstay of prophylaxis is early mobilisation when possible and compressive stockings. Intra-operative pneumatic calf compression and low molecular weight heparin are necessary in higher risk patients although the latter is avoided in lower urinary tract resections (e.g. TURP, TURBT) are the risk of post-operative bleeding in these cases outweighs the risk of thrombosis.

Anaesthesia

Many urology cases can be undertaken under regional anaesthesia and, in some situations, this has distinct benefits. It is important to note, however, that a regional anaesthetic does not mean that it is without risk. Full monitoring and continuous vigilance are imperative.

a) Local anaesthesia/nerve block

- Penile block (either a ring block or blocking the right and left dorsal penile nerves) – useful for circumcision, dorsal slit, penile biopsy, reduction of paraphimosis
- Genitofemoral nerve block – scrotal and labia majora surgery
- Ilio-inguinal and ilio-hypogastric nerve block – scrotal, testicular and hydrocoele surgery

b) Neuroaxial block as for local anaesthesia format

There are three types of blocks that come under this title, a spinal anaesthetic (subarachnoid), caudal anaesthesia and an epidural.

A **spinal** anaesthetic, where the dura is punctured by a small-gauge needle (usually 25G) and local anaesthetic injected intrathecally, provides predictable surgical anaesthesia for procedures on the T10 dermatome down. This is ideal in patients who are having procedures on the lower abdomen and have respiratory compromise or in whom neurological assessment would be beneficial (see later). The use of this technique does not preclude respiratory or cardiovascular complications. A 'high' spinal, in which the spread of the local anaesthetic moves cephalad, can result in severe respiratory depression, cardiovascular collapse (vasodilatation and inhibition of cardiac accelerator fibres) and in its most severe form, loss of consciousness and respiratory drive (total spinal).

Caudal anaesthesia is used predominantly in children. This involves injecting local anaesthetic into the caudal space, which is a continuation of the epidural space, via the sacral hiatus. It provides analgesia in the perineal area and is usually used as an adjunct with a general anaesthetic.

An **epidural** is predominantly used for post-operative analgesia and rarely as a stand-alone anaesthetic technique, although this is possible.

c) General anaesthetic

On the whole this is the most common form of anaesthesia used and, depending on the case, may be in tandem with a regional technique for post-operative pain control. It is the technique of choice for patients undergoing prolonged procedures, intra-abdominal and/or thoracic operations, with cardiac instability (or expected instability – blood loss, fluid shifts etc.). Patients can be spontaneously breathing or ventilated. The monitoring used depends on the complexity of the case and the premorbid history of the patient, and may include invasive monitoring such as central venous access, invasive arterial monitoring and cardiac output monitoring.

General complications of laparoscopic/robotic surgery

Many surgical cases are now performed with either laparoscopic or robotic assistance. In urology these now commonly involve radical/partial nephrectomies and robotic-assisted radical prostatectomy (including robotic-assisted radical cystectomy in some centres). The benefits surgically are well documented and include a reduced length of stay, reduced post-operative pain and quicker recovery. From the anaesthetic point of view, the major issue is the management of the pneumoperitoneum.

Physiological effects of a pneumoperitoneum

Cardiovascular

Initial insufflation of CO_2 can cause a vagal bradycardia because of peritoneal distension, with potential asystole – low initial flows of CO_2 with good communication between the surgeon and anaesthetist is important. The increased intra-abdominal pressure causes an increased venous return from pooled blood in the splanchnic circulation with an expected increase in cardiac output. However, a reduction in venous return and cardiac output follow as the sustained increased pressure compresses the vena cava. This is offset by an increase in systemic vascular resistance by two factors: the increase in the intra-abdominal pressure and the release of catecholamines causing vasoconstriction. It is not uncommon to see patients during this period with higher blood pressures than normal with an increased heart rate. These result in increased myocardial workload and oxygen consumption and may be sufficient to cause cardiac decompensation with cardiogenic shock in patients with severe cardiac disease.

Respiratory

The insufflation of CO_2 pushes the diaphragm up, causing splinting of the diaphragm and reduction in pulmonary compliance. In tandem with the supine position and potential Trendelenburg position, the functional residual capacity (FRC) of the lung is considerably reduced. This can happen to such an extent (depending on the intra-abdominal pressure and degree of Trendelenburg) that the FRC falls below closing volume, resulting in atelectasis, V/Q mismatch, potential hypoxaemia and hypercarbia. It is important to take these factors into account when determining the intra-abdominal pressures to be used and the extent of positioning. This is particularly important in the patient with severe respiratory disease, neuromuscular disease or morbid obesity.

Effects of CO_2

Constant insufflation of CO_2, a gas that is 20 times more soluble in plasma than O_2, results in a rapid and sustained increase in $PaCO_2$ and a respiratory acidosis. This can, to an extent, be compensated by an increase in minute ventilation, but in prolonged cases this may not be possible. The CO_2 causes tachycardia and increased myocardial contractility, which puts more pressure on the heart.

Other risks

Inadvertent bowel or vascular trauma during port insertion. Newer, blunt and optical ports have reduced the risk but it remains a potential catastrophic complication. Care on insertion and a high index of suspicion is necessary.

Venous gas embolism is rare, but again potentially catastrophic. It can occur by either direct injection of gas intravascularly or by gas being drawn into an open vessel. These result in a reduced venous return, fall in cardiac output and cardiovascular collapse. At any suspicion of a venous gas embolism, gas insufflation must be stopped immediately with release of the pneumoperitoneum and lateral decubitus and head down positioning of the patient. This position is adopted in an attempt to prevent the gas bubble progressing into the pulmonary vessels. A central line may allow some of the embolism to be aspirated. Cardiovascular support is the mainstay of management. As CO_2 is highly soluble in plasma, the absorption of the embolism and hence physiological effects are less than with an air embolism.

The changes in cardiovascular and respiratory physiology are more pronounced in robotic surgery (when compared to laparoscopic surgery) because of the steep Trendelenburg position required. Patients listed for robot-assisted surgery require stringent cardio-respiratory assessment to ensure they can tolerate these stresses.

Specific urological procedures and complications

With the advent of Holmium laser enucleation of the prostate (HoLEP), the specific risks associated with transurethral resection of the prostate (TURP), particularly monopolar TURP, are avoided. The former, however, is not available in every centre and even in those that undertake it, monopolar TURP still remains the mainstay and, arguably the gold-standard treatment, for symptomatic benign prostatic hyperplasia/acute urinary retention.

TURP

The complication of TURP syndrome that can occur during TURP surgery is related to the use of 1.5% glycine as the non-ionic medium for intra-operative irrigation. The 1.5% glycine is hypotonic, and when absorbed through prostatic venous sinuses in large volumes results in TURP syndrome which is characterised by volume overload, a dilutional drop in the plasma sodium (hypo-osmolarity syndrome) and potential glycine toxicity. Glycine is directly cardiotoxic, resulting in bradycardia, and retino-toxic, which can result in blurred vision – glycine is an inhibitory neurotransmitter in the retina. Additionally, absorbed glycine is metabolised in the liver to ammonia and glycolic acid – the ammonia may result in increased confusion.

The effects of glycine toxicity are difficult to distinguish from that of hyponatraemia.

The amount of irrigating fluid absorbed depends on several factors including:

- duration of surgery (ideally not more than 60 minutes)
- height of irrigation fluid (ideally <60–70 cm above the symphysis pubis)
- the presence of prostate capsular breaches during surgery

TURP syndrome, in its worst presentation, includes symptoms of cerebral oedema (headache, irritability, confusion, fitting etc.), dyspnoea, cardiac failure and cardiovascular collapse.

It is as a result of this potential life-threatening complication that spinal anaesthesia is the mainstay of anaesthetic management; it allows early detection of cerebral oedema by allowing direct monitoring of patients' level of consciousness. Under general anaesthesia, the only indication of an evolving TURP syndrome may be an initial bradycardia and hypertension.

Management centres on immediate cessation of irrigation, haemostasis and support of the respiratory (supplemental oxygen and sometimes intubation and ventilation) and cardiovascular system. A blood gas gives the plasma sodium concentration and serum osmolarity should be checked. Administration of a loop diuretic will aid loss of free water (although sodium loss is also promoted, this is proportionally less that for water). The administration of hypertonic saline (3%) to correct hyponatraemia needs to be undertaken cautiously as rapid sodium correction can lead to central pontine myelinolysis. Haemolysis because of hypotonic irrigation can cause a significant drop in haemoglobin, and potential renal failure because of acute tubular necrosis.

Patients should be referred to a high-dependency/intensive care environment for observation, fluid management and cautious titrated sodium replacement. Patients who have a seizure should be intubated and ventilated.

Patients with a pre-morbid medical history of cardiac failure should be considered very carefully before proceeding with TURP – and alternative surgical approaches offered.

HoLEP

HoLEP surgery makes use of laser rather than electrocautery, and can therefore use normal saline as the irrigation fluid rather than the electrically inert glycine. Saline absorption during HoLEP is less of a problem than during TURP as the laser performs tissue resection and coagulation at the same time. This procedure is favoured for patients who require large resections and/or have risk factors for TURP syndrome. Bipolar TURP is another alternative in which normal saline can be used as the irrigating fluid.

TURBT

Although this initially appears to be a relatively straightforward procedure and most patients have multiple anaesthetic charts from repeated surgeries, it is important to ascertain the location of tumour resection. The obturator nerve runs along the outside of the lateral wall of the bladder and resection over this can result in stimulation of this nerve. This in turn causes the obturator "kick" – sudden adduction of the leg on the side of resection.

This can result in bladder perforation. If there is a potential for lateral tumour wall resection, it is prudent to undertake a general anaesthetic as opposed to a spinal, as this would allow muscle relaxation intra-operatively if needed. Using a lower diathermy current and under-filling of the bladder can also lessen the risk of an obturator 'kick'. More recently, obturator nerve blocks have been used by some to prevent this phenomenon.

Radical cystectomy

This is a complex procedure which is often coupled with the formation of an ileal conduit or a neobladder (+/- Mitrofanoff). Open surgery requires a long mid-line incision. Extensive bowel handling, large fluid shifts into the '3rd space' and major blood loss are not uncommon. See Table 20.5 for the common problems during cystectomy surgery. These procedures warrant central line, arterial line and large-bore intravenous cannulation. Positioning varies from supine with arms by the side to crucifixion position with episodes of lithotomy. Regardless of the position used, care must be taken to ensure adequate padding, and care on moving legs into lithotomy. The crucifixion position is associated with the risk of post-operative brachial plexus injury and it must be ensured that there is no tension in the arm and neck on initial positioning and that regular checks are made throughout the procedure.

Post-operative pain can be controlled either with an epidural (low thoracic) or patient-controlled analgesia. Non-steroidal analgesia can be used, as long as good renal function is maintained. These patients are managed in a high-dependency unit/area in the immediate post-operative period, with close monitoring of renal function.

Table 20.5 Common problems during radical cystectomy

Problem	Solution
Fluid balance/blood loss	Invasive cardiovascular monitoring and large-bore intravenous access are usually required (CVP and arterial line)
Nerve damage from positioning	Brachial plexus in crucifixion position Common peroneal, femoral and sciatic in lithotomy. Attention during positioning
Pain relief	Low thoracic epidural often required, or PCA
Post-operative care for pain relief and fluid balance	Patients often cared for in a high-dependency unit
Post-operative renal dysfunction	HDU care for cardiovascular support where necessary. Regular monitoring of renal function, medication review, liaison with nephrology

Radical/partial nephrectomy

These cases are performed either as an open procedure or robotically/laparoscopically.

If the tumour has extended to the inferior vena cava, the anaesthetist and surgeon must plan for caval manipulation, clamping and possible resection/reconstruction. Any occlusion of the inferior vena cava can result in a significant reduction in venous return and cardiac output. On occasion the reduction in cardiac output can be so severe that complete cardiovascular collapse occurs. If the patient does not tolerate caval clamping, regardless

Table 20.6 Major problems encountered in the kidney position

Kidney position with 'broken table'		
Respiratory problems	V/Q mismatch – reduced ventilation in lower lung, but increased blood flow Reduced compliance	Hypoxia and atelectasis
Cardiovascular problems	Inferior vena cava obstruction (especially right lateral) and decreased venous return	Decreased cardiac output and hypotension, with resultant decrease in end-organ perfusion (brain and kidney)
Nerve injury	Stretching at the neck and shoulder	Brachial plexus, ulnar nerve
Tissue injury	Compression of the lower arm circulation	

of whether this is to control blood loss during resection or to resect and replace a segment of cava, veno-venous bypass will be necessary. In those cases where there is an anticipated caval reconstruction, good communication between the anaesthetist and surgeon allows adequate patient and theatre preparation. This will include large-bore intravenous access, insertion of bypass lines and discussion with the transfusion and bypass service. The perfusionist and bypass machine should be present in theatre.

Patients are positioned supine or in the 'kidney position' (lateral, or semi-lateral with a support). This position can cause specific problems as shown in Table 20.6. The latter results in a V/Q mismatch because of a reduction in ventilation of the lower lung but, paradoxically, an increase in its blood flow. This is compounded by a decrease in compliance and lung volumes and a resultant atelectasis. Added to this is a potential 'break' in the table to open up the space between ribs and pelvis for surgical access. This can cause inferior vena cava compression (especially in right lateral) and a reduction in venous return and cardiac output. Other issues that require vigilance are the potential for neuropathies as a result of stretching of the neck and shoulders, compression of the lower arm circulation and ensuring the patient is well secured on the table.

Radical prostatectomy

The advent of robotic surgery has improved morbidity and mortality figures in prostatectomy. Patients undergoing robotic-assisted procedures have a significantly improved recovery, reduced length of stay, reduced blood loss and a lower requirement for analgesia as compared to open prostatectomy. The specific anaesthetic issues are:

- difficulty of access to the patient once the robot is in position
- prevention of gastric contents pooling in oropharynx – insertion of nasogastric tube with free drainage is recommended
- nerve injury, so careful positioning is required. The peroneal nerve is at particular risk
- risk of cerebral oedema because of prolonged steep Trendelenburg position.

Judicious use of fluid in the initial stages makes the surgical anastomosis of the bladder and urethra easier, as large volumes of urine from the bladder neck make visualisation harder.

This has to be balanced, however, with ensuring good perfusion and the cardiovascular effects of the positioning.

The open procedure, when necessary, is undertaken as a major case, requiring central line and arterial monitoring, with the potential for sudden, large volume blood loss. The mid-line incision warrants the use of an epidural or patient-controlled analgesia.

Perforated bladder

With the majority of cases involving the use of scopes and distension of the bladder, there is always a risk of inadvertent bladder perforation. This may or may not be realised intra-operatively. Perforations can be extraperitoneal, giving rise to suprapubic pain, or intra-peritoneal with generalised abdominal pain and signs of peritonism, and ultimately progressive signs of shock. Early recognition and surgical management is important to prevent severe shock. The use of spinal/epidural may mask the pain of such events, and obtund the normal compensatory responses to shock. This can lead to a delayed diagnosis and profound hypotension that is difficult to treat.

Post-operative care

Many of the major open cases performed in urological surgery require high-dependency care for the first 24 hours. This level of care will provide cardiovascular support, careful fluid balance, monitoring of renal function and pain relief.

After this initial period many patients are transferred to the ward.

The advent of laparoscopic and robotic surgery has transformed the recovery of patients having even the most major of urological surgeries, with many being transferred straight to the ward.

Enhanced recovery programmes have been introduced for prostatic surgery, and are likely to be introduced for renal and bladder surgery.

Summary

In summary, the close interactions between anaesthetist and surgeon in urology are invaluable to ensure a smooth and uncomplicated patient journey. Urology patients often present in the extremes of age and with many co-morbidities. Therefore thorough pre-operative assessment and careful post-operative planning are mandatory.

Further reading

Acute kidney injury: prevention, detection and management of acute kidney injury up to the point of renal replacement therapy. *NICE Clinical Guideline 169*, August 2013. guidance.nice.org.uk/cg169.

Bettelli G. High-risk patients in day surgery. *Minerva Anestesilogica* 2009; **75**: 259–68.

Gainsburg DM. Anesthetic concerns for robotic-assisted laparoscopic radical prostatectomy. *Minerva Anestesiologica* 2012; **78**: 596–604.

Jensen V. The TURP syndrome. *Can J Anaesth* 1991; **38**: 90–6.

Bariatric cases

Michael Margarson and Christopher Pring

Introduction

The words 'obesity' and 'bariatric' are not found in the current surgical syllabus. The terms are sometimes used interchangeably, but obesity is generic, whereas bariatric is generally held to refer to weight-loss surgery.

Obesity, and specifically morbid obesity, is endemic in our population and morbidly obese patients undergo many types of surgical procedures. The greatest experience of managing the morbidly obese patient peri-operatively is among those surgeons and anaesthetists regularly performing bariatric operations. This chapter is written by consultants with a special interest in bariatric surgery, but the following comments and learning points are applicable to any obese patient, undergoing any type of surgery.

Anaesthesia, obesity and bariatric surgery

Although lagging behind the US, Britain is the 'fat man'of Europe, with over 25% of adults having a BMI of >30. The relentless rise in the prevalence of obesity over recent years has placed a significant health and cost burden on our health system. Bariatric surgery has become the recognised treatment of choice for morbid obesity worldwide, with some 10,000 surgical procedures performed each year in the UK. However, there are hundreds of thousands of non-bariatric surgical procedures performed on morbidly obese patients, and these patients are a high-risk surgical group, that all doctors will have to deal with.

Morbid obesity shortens life span by 8–10 years. Mortality ratio increases with increasing BMI because of the increased risks of disease states that are associated with obesity (diabetes, hypertension, dyslipidaemia, sleep apnoea, many cancers).

When considering the peri-operative risks of surgery for morbid obesity (bariatric surgery), one needs to consider the health risks of other treatment options. Clearly, doing nothing about treating morbid obesity has significant health risks, which are cumulative. Best medical treatment, consisting of dietary, exercise and psychological programmes, has limited health benefit in the long term, as demonstrated by The Swedish Obese Subjects Study. This was a prospective case controlled study of over 4,000 adults whose BMI was greater than 34 for men or 38 for women. Half of this group underwent surgery and half underwent best medical treatment. The cohorts were followed up for an average of 11 years. One of the main findings from this study was that surgery had a 0.76 mortality ratio

A Surgeon's Guide to Anaesthesia and Peri-operative Care, ed. Jane Sturgess, Justin Davies and Kamen Valchanov. Published by Cambridge University Press.

compared to medical treatment (i.e. – patients had a 24% greater chance of being alive if they underwent surgery).

We can state, therefore, that morbid obesity presents a significant health risk and that surgery for morbid obesity presents the most effective treatment option. However, in order to minimise peri-operative risk, we need to understand more about the physiology and pathology of excess fat.

BMI and shape

Although morbid obesity is defined as a BMI of >40, it is not the BMI of the patient that determines the number and severity of co-morbidities. There are many young patients with BMI >50 who have excellent exercise tolerance and no co-morbidities. The term 'morbid obesity' is a bit of a misnomer and it is perhaps better to think in terms of obesity with morbidity, asking oneself what co-morbidities each obese individual has. The ASA status tells one far more about peri-operative risk than the BMI.

Although obesity is undoubtedly associated with a shortening of lifespan in the long term, paradoxically it appears that being overweight or obese is associated with better short-term outcomes in many disease states: patients have a significantly better chance of surviving ICU stay with a BMI of 30–40 compared with the normal BMI. This phenomenon has been described for a number of interventions and conditions, and has been entitled the Obesity Paradox. Although the mechanism of protection is unclear, it is clearly a genuine effect.

Good fat and bad fat

The most important factor associated with the development of co-morbidities and long-term damage is the fat distribution, and more specifically the mass of metabolically active central adipose tissue.

Peripheral fat, on the thighs, buttocks and outside the abdominal wall, is relatively inert and benign. This is the classical female or gynaecoid fat distribution, also described as the pear-shape.

It is the intra-abdominal fat (metabolically active 'bad fat or toxic fat') that is particularly associated with the development of significant co-morbidities. It is also patients with this pattern of central deposition, i.e. those patients with a large mass of intra-abdominal fat, who are the most challenging in terms of both surgical access, and also where the physical presence of this fat impacts most upon cardio-respiratory mechanics, by splinting the diaphragm and impairing venous return in the anaesthetised patient. This fat distribution is typically seen in males and is referred to as the 'apple'-shape. Apples are unhealthy.

Morbidly obese males have a much higher incidence of peri-operative death than females. The development of end-organ damage is associated with male gender, the presence of central fat and the duration of obesity, and thus usually directly reflected by age. This is behind the widely used adage 'beware the older apple'.

Obesity with central fat deposition is characterised by a chronic inflammatory state. Intra-abdominal adipocytes secrete pro-inflammatory cytokines, which themselves demonstrate antioxidant properties, thereby promoting physiological stress. This physiological stress manifests itself as the metabolic syndrome.

Body mass index is a crude way of estimating visceral fat. Waist/hip ratio would be a more accurate way of determining visceral fat. However, historically BMI has been used and this has formed the basis of most of the academic literature.

Co-morbidities of obesity

Metabolic syndrome

The presence of insulin resistance and then overt diabetes, together with hypertension and a degree of dyslipidaemia is termed the 'metabolic syndrome'. It is the longer-term effects of this diabetes and hypertension that lead to significant heart disease and have such an effect in terms of shortening life. The development of the full syndrome may take some 10 to 15 years, but a degree of insulin resistance is found early in most obese patients.

The secondary effects of insulin resistance and diabetes upon the microvascular tissues, and the secondary effects upon wound healing and infection rates are well recognised. The 'stiffening' of tissues with long-term diabetes is also of specific concern in anaesthesia, as this is associated with a higher incidence of airway problems.

Another problem is peripheral and autonomic neuropathy – the two go hand-in-hand – which can markedly impair autonomic responses. The patient with symptoms of postural hypotension will lack the normal vasoconstrictor responses to hypotension, which are already obtunded by anaesthesia, and will be much more cardiovascularly unstable, especially when put into the reverse Trendelenburg (head up) posture. Patients with the combination of long-term diabetes and antihypertensive medication, especially ACE-inhibitors, tend to have very unstable blood pressures at the time of anaesthesia induction.

Sleep apnoea

Significant and untreated sleep apnoea is one of the biggest risk factors for unexpected peri-operative death and an understanding of the condition is essential for all involved in the management of obese patients. It is the most common of a group of sleep-disordered breathing conditions, all associated with obesity, which are of importance to the anaesthetist.

Sleep apnoea is a condition of intermittent upper airway collapse and hence obstruction, occurring during sleep. Most patients with the condition are unaware that they have it, but it has an incidence closely related to BMI – so around 50% of patients with a BMI of 50 will have sleep apnoea of some degree. Like all diseases there is a spectrum of severity.

The condition has two main effects:

1. Individual episodes of airway obstruction are associated with oxygen desaturation episodes, these in turn being associated with catecholamine release. This puts a long-term strain on the heart and many patients develop hypertension, both systemic and pulmonary, leading to biventricular heart dysfunction and ultimately cardiac failure. Patients with significant sleep apnoea have impaired exercise tolerance and are often limited by shortness of breath on fairly minimal exertion, reflecting poor cardiac reserve. It is heart failure, i.e. the presence of poor ventricular function and hence poor reserve, and the inability to compensate appropriately by increasing cardiac output in response to peri-operative stresses, that leads into the cycle of organ hypoperfusion and the development of multiple organ failure and death.

2. Sleep apnoea resets the body's hypoxic and CO_2 response levels. By this blunting of the normal responses, many patients with significant sleep apnoea are particularly sensitive to the respiratory-depressant effects of opioids and sedative agents. This can lead to CO_2 retention in the early post-operative period, and at higher levels of arterial CO_2 cause further sedation and further respiratory depression, a vicious cycle leading ultimately to hypoxia and what the Americans succinctly describe as a 'dead in bed' event. Having an understanding of the condition and screening pre-operatively to identify those at-risk patients is an essential part of the care of morbidly obese patients. The avoidance of longer-acting anaesthetic agents, and the use of co-analgesics to minimise opioid usage, is a key part of reducing risk to this patient group, and is covered in more detail later in the chapter.

Fatty liver

Fatty infiltration of the liver is a direct consequence of calorie overload and hence common in the morbidly obese. In its more extreme form the patient develops hepatic steatosis, but unless there is marked liver dysfunction bordering on cirrhotic changes, this seems to be of little significance in the peri-operative period for bariatric surgical patients. This may in part be because of the use of 'liver diets'– very low calorie diets of 10 to 14 days duration, utilised with the specific intention of losing 5–10 kg in the immediate pre-op period. These cause fat stores to be used up, and a large amount of this is from the liver. Liver function, especially with regard to drug metabolism and clearance, seems to be rarely affected and is not considered a problem in clinical practice.

The causes of peri-operative mortality and morbidity

Cardiac

Heart failure, that is impaired baseline function that does not have adequate reserve to improve cardiac output in the peri-operative period, is the biggest contributor to peri-operative death in the obese patient. Thus hypertensive heart disease as the marker and the associated cardiac failure is the condition to watch for. In the bariatric surgical population, acute myocardial infarction is unusual, but as the age demographic of patients presenting for obesity surgery changes, an increasing number of patients with known ischaemic heart disease are presenting. In particular the peri-operative management of patients with coronary stents *in situ* who are still requiring anti-platelet therapy is problematic, as obese patients have a particular risk of stent thrombosis (see below).

Thromboembolic

Obesity is an inflammatory and pro-thrombotic condition. The adipocyte releases inflammatory cytokines ('adipokines') and additionally oestrogens and plasminogen activator inhibitor (PAI). The baseline incidence of venous thrombosis is therefore elevated in the obese – meta-analyses would suggest by a factor of approaching two-fold – and delays in post-operative mobilisation because of the difficulties in getting such patients safely out of bed further increase the risk of stasis and DVT formation.

Historically thromboembolism was the biggest killer following bariatric surgery, but with the routine use of mechanical compression devices, higher doses of low molecular weight heparin, and particularly with the early mobilisation allowed by modern enhanced recovery techniques, it occurs much less frequently today. National guidelines from the UK Haematology and Thrombosis Group that recommend higher doses of heparins as thromboprophylaxis may have also helped, as in the past these patients may have been relatively under-dosed.

Timing of commencement and duration of treatment with heparins is contentious. Many haematologists would suggest that the stress response of surgery starts to significantly affect fibrinolysis within a few hours of the commencement of surgery, and that for effectiveness the first dose of heparin should be given soon after surgery. If the likelihood of ongoing surgical bleeding is high, or the effects potentially catastrophic (a small volume bleed in an enclosed space, e.g. after plastic, ophthalmic or neurosurgery) then clearly the start of heparin administration should be delayed, but against this must be balanced the significantly increased risk of thrombosis in the morbidly obese as opposed to the non-obese population.

Following uncomplicated bariatric surgery most clinicians advise heparins to be administered at around four hours post-operatively. Some centres are happy to give doses pre-operatively, but this is an area where good evidence to support practice is lacking.

The risk of DVT formation remains elevated for several weeks after intermediate surgery, and within the sphere of bariatric surgery the majority of units use around two weeks of post-operative pharmacological prophylaxis after anything other than gastric bands.

The role of invasive anti-thromboembolic devices, in particular IVC filters, is unclear. UK haematological guidelines suggest they should only be considered in patients with known DVT who cannot receive anticoagulant agents in the peri-operative period, and who are at high risk of pulmonary embolism. There is no good evidence to support their use as prophylaxis in routine practice.

Multiple organ failure

The stress of uncomplicated bariatric surgery is modest and most patients, even with poor cardiac reserve, can get through 24–48 hours of moderately increased cardiac demand. However, it is the development of a 'second hit' – usually some surgical complication or myocardial event, occasionally a chest infection – which pushes the patient beyond their cardiac reserve and can lead first to organ hypoperfusion and then down the slippery slope into the development of multiple organ dysfunction and then multiple organ failure. It is the presence of degrees of heart failure, i.e. an inability to increase cardiac output to match levels required, that is most strongly associated with mortality.

Anastomotic breakdown

The most significant surgical complication in the high-risk patient is leakage of bowel contents. The most frequent presenting sign of leak is an unexplained post-operative tachycardia that persists. Imaging to demonstrate and confirm a leak is difficult, as many morbidly obese patients simply do not fit within the bore of a standard CT scanner, and clinical signs of localised pathology are extremely difficult to elicit. Of all patient groups, it is probably the higher-risk morbidly obese patient in whom early exploratory re-laparotomy or re-laparoscopy is worthwhile, and experienced bariatric surgeons and anaesthetists know this well. One of the golden rules of obesity surgery is that unexplained post-operative tachycardia should be considered to indicate leak until proven otherwise, and in this situation early clinical review by a senior surgeon is indicated.

Anastomotic and/or staple-line bleeding is another relatively common occurrence. Obese patients will rarely become unstable as they have larger circulating volumes compared to patients of normal weight, but the presence of a large intra-abdominal haematoma (something in excess of 2–3 units of blood, i.e. a 3–4 g fall in haemoglobin) would by many surgeons be considered an indication for re-laparoscopy and washout. Intra-luminal bleeding tends to be managed conservatively. The decision-making as to when endoscopy and re-laparoscopy is indicated is complex and beyond the scope of this chapter.

Pre-operative assessment

Multi-disciplinary teams

Key to the successful management of any group of complex patients is the availability and the utilisation of expert input from an early stage in the process. Cancer MDTs have led the way, but this model has been successfully transferred into bariatric surgery, albeit with different areas of focus. In many ways these MDTs are more important in bariatric surgery, as the operation is not essential, and a clear and accurate assessment of peri-operative risk, versus likely benefit, allows a full and frank discussion with the patient before decisions are made. It also allows for maximum input to identify areas where optimisation should take place prior to the operation.

Successful outcomes for bariatric procedures demand patient understanding, and the ability to comply with the change in diets required for sustained weight loss. In the UK, guidelines produced by the National Institute for Health and Clinical Excellence strongly supported the role of dieticians to assist all patients to manage these changes, but also to assess and screen out those patients who will struggle to cope. A bariatric specialist dietician is also invaluable to clarify eating patterns and thus advise the suitability of restrictive versus malabsorptive bariatric procedures.

Psychologists are another group of considerable value in the pre-op assessment phase. They may help to identify patients with addictive behaviours, who may frequently transfer their addictions to another area (e.g. alcohol or drugs). There is a cohort of morbidly obese patients with significant underlying psychological disorders who are at high risk of worsening of their mental state if the 'prop' of food is removed. Several long-term follow-up studies of bariatric surgery have shown a significantly increased incidence of suicide and violent death among the patient groups who received surgery.

Finally, the input of the multi-disciplinary team is essential to get the best estimate of risk for any individual patient. Quoting surgical risks for entire populations is not appropriate and both potential risk and benefit should be tailored to the specific individual; this is a powerful part of the MDT process. Patients seeking bariatric surgery often have unrealistic expectations and in some the risks of surgery will far outweigh the potential benefits. Identifying and quantifying the risks (failure, medical or psychological), before the patients are offered a procedure will almost certainly improve outcomes.

Obesity surgery mortality risk score

The Obesity Surgery Mortality Risk Score (OS-MRS) published by DeMaria in 2007 was the first scoring system for risk assessment and stratification in bariatric surgery. It is the only system that has been validated independently by multiple centres worldwide. The OS-MRS assigns one point for the presence of each of the following five categories:

- Age >45 years
- Male gender
- BMI >50
- Hypertension
- Known risk factors for pulmonary embolism (i.e. previous PE, presence of IVC filter, history of right-sided heart failure or pulmonary hypertension, obesity hypoventilation syndrome)

Patients with a score 0–1 are low risk (class A); 2–3 intermediate risk (class B); 4–5 high risk (class C).

Other risk stratification systems do exist, such as the Longitudinal Assessment of Bariatric Surgery (LABS) Consortium Metabolic Acuity Score. The LABS data provide a continuous risk scale and do not stratify patients into discrete groups, making it a more complex system to use for stratifying risk. Broadly however, the LABS data demonstrated four risk factors associated with adverse outcome: extreme BMI, history of venous thrombo-embolism, obstructive sleep apnoea and inability to walk 200 ft.

The OS-MRS score was based on primary gastric bypass surgery. It has not yet been validated or extended to revision surgery or sleeve gastrectomy, but it remains a pragmatic method of stratifying risk. Class C patients can be identified pre-operatively and medical optimisation can be directed appropriately. However, only BMI can realistically be altered pre-operatively.

The OS-MRS may assist in planning peri-operative management for higher-risk patients, and certainly allows a degree of risk stratification when comparing outcomes between centres.

Principles of anaesthesia

Airway safety

Safe ventilation of morbidly obese patients requires a secure airway, which usually means a correctly placed endotracheal tube. This is because the weight of the chest wall, together with the abdominal contents plus any additional effects of the pneumoperitoneum of laparoscopic surgery pressing on the diaphragm, require high ventilatory pressures. Laryngeal masks and other similar devices do not provide a proper seal, and attempts to ventilate patients using these devices will often lead to air being forced into the stomach, both distending bowel and affecting surgery, and introducing a significant risk of causing reflux and aspiration of gastric contents.

Some anaesthetists will attempt to manage patients without intubation because of perceived difficulties in intubation. Obesity alone is a relatively weak risk factor for difficult intubation. It is the presence of associated sleep apnoea, long-term diabetes and particularly a very thick neck that predict difficulty.

What is significantly more difficult for anaesthetists – and for anybody who finds themselves trying to support breathing in these patients – is bag mask ventilation. Patients do not die from failed intubation, they die when basic face-mask ventilation and oxygenation cannot be maintained.

Monitoring

The level and invasiveness of peri-operative monitoring depends upon patient factors and upon the magnitude of the surgery being undertaken. Oximetry, ECG and blood pressure measurements are a standard for any general anaesthetic. There are specific practical difficulties in monitoring morbidly obese patients in the operating theatre, particularly in obtaining reliable blood pressure measurement. Blood pressure cuffs on an upper arm, which can be very fat and sometimes even conical in shape, may be unreliable, particularly if there is an associated cardiac rhythm disturbance such as atrial fibrillation. For this reason the threshold to place arterial lines is lower, as once in place these give a very reliable measurement, and also in those patients who will require significant post-op opioids, allow arterial blood sampling in the first post-operative night for early identification of developing CO_2 retention.

Drug dosing in the obese

Dosing of drugs in the morbidly obese, whether anaesthetic, antibiotic, or any other class, can be difficult. It is very important to distinguish between total body weight, lean body weight and ideal body weight when calculating drug doses, or the danger of significant under-dosing or overdosing may occur.

Ideal body weight is predicted from gender and height, and comes from a perceived 'ideal' weight that is associated with healthiest and longest life – it was originally derived from information collated by the life insurance industry, applicable to populations. A male of height 180 cm has an ideal body weight of around 72 kg, based on having a 'normal' fat content of around 15%. But this does not take build into account. Obviously a heavily built and muscular individual will have an ideal body weight that is greater than a much less heavily built individual of the same height.

Lean body weight is easier to understand: it is the body mass of an individual if they were to have no adipose tissue. As a healthy male should have around 15% body fat, the lean body weight of the same 180 cm male is 15% less than the 72 kg 'ideal' body weight, so around 58 kg. A normal healthy female would typically have around 18% body fat.

A patient weighing 200 kg could typically have 70 kg of lean body weight and 130 kg of excess body fat; this patient does not require drug dosing based on total body weight. As an example, a dose of gentamicin would usually be given at 4–5 mg/kg, but this is of *lean body weight* – a dose of 280–350 mg would be acceptable – but a dose of 800–1000 mg (4–5 mg/kg of total body weight) would clearly be totally inappropriate, highly toxic and indefensible.

This principle holds true for all drugs, but some substances are more fat soluble and so it is appropriate to increase doses – but very rarely by more than 50%.

It is an excellent rule of thumb to assume no obese male has a lean body mass greater than 90 kg and no obese female a lean body mass greater than 70 kg, and to base drug doses even in the most massive patients on these weights.

Positioning the patient

One of the key concerns with the obese patient is the increased risk of pressure injuries during surgery and a lack of specific equipment often exacerbates the problem. The effect of a greatly increased body mass, often coupled with prolonged duration of surgery (over two hours) makes pressure ischaemia more prevalent, and peri-operative hypotension will exacerbate tissue hypoperfusion and hence ischaemia. Elevations in creatine phosphokinase, a marker of rhabdomyolysis, are seen in many patients and in studies performed, significant rises (20-fold or greater) occur in perhaps 5–10% of patients. At its most extreme, muscle damage – classically of the gluteals – causes significant release of myoglobin, leading to renal tubular necrosis and acute renal failure.

Nerve injuries with poor positioning are another well-recognised complication and are usually indefensible (see Section III, Chapter 30 Nerve injury). Again these are because of a combination of direct pressure and reduced tissue blood flow, which may be from local pressure effects or from global hypotension with a low cardiac output state.

The pneumoperitoneum

It is an enlightened anaesthetist and surgeon who understand and can intelligently discuss how best to manage the pressures and volumes in the pneumoperitoneum to achieve the best outcome for the patient. Both must understand the concerns of the other, and the limits of what can be achieved, in order to find a compromise in the difficult cases.

Clearly the surgeon requires a good view, and the greater the workspace and better the view, the faster the surgery and the less the likelihood of surgical error. Against this must be balanced the problems of very high intra-abdominal pressures with its direct and indirect potential to cause tissue hypoperfusion, and organ dysfunction or failure, and the risks and problems associated with very deep anaesthesia and/or neuromuscular blockade.

It is generally suggested that for upper abdominal surgery in the adult patient, around 3 litres of pneumoperitoneum is required to give a good view. However, depending on anatomical factors of the individual patient, which area of the abdomen is being operated upon, and the degree of head up or head down tilt that the patient can tolerate, this volume may change.

There is a huge variation in abdominal compliance among patients, such that in some patients good volumes and good operating conditions can be achieved at relatively low pressures (maybe 10–12 mmHg), whereas in others both volumes and views may be limited even with considerably higher pressures (e.g. 16–18 mmHg). It is noteworthy that in gynaecological cancer surgery several European centres start at pressures of 8 mmHg – this has been influenced by studies suggesting that the likelihood of peritoneal seeding is greater at higher levels of peritoneal pressure and stretch.

At high intra-abdominal pressure, organ perfusion may be significantly compromised as pressures approach 20 mmHg, which by many is considered the definition of an abdominal compartment syndrome.

Compliance is defined as the change in volume (measured in 100s of ml) for a change in pressure (measured in mmHg), i.e. the ease of stretch. Precise figures are unimportant, but the concept is. A poorly compliant abdomen in the obese patient is affected by several factors, the most important factor being tension at baseline: this relates primarily to the current visceral (i.e. intra-abdominal) fat mass and whether the abdomen has previously been even more distended. It is fairly evident that if the abdomen has previously been stretched, but the patient has now lost a significant amount of weight from within the abdomen, that the compliance will be improved. This is the reason for the frequently better compliance of women, especially multiparous women who have carried a baby to term, and of those who have lost considerable fat mass through dieting.

The patient who under anaesthesia in the supine position has a flattened abdominal wall is likely to have a compliant abdomen. The patient who in the supine position maintains a 'fullness' i.e. a rotund abdomen (typically the apple-shaped male) will have a poorly compliant abdominal wall and will be a challenging laparoscopy.

Muscle relaxants

Muscle relaxants do not always improve the compliance of the abdomen. In some patients muscle tone may limit pneumoperitoneal stretch, in which case relaxants can increase compliance and improve views, but other factors also come into play, e.g. previous laparoscopy, weight loss and pregnancy as described above.

Different muscle groups have very different sensitivities to relaxant administration. Skeletal and abdominal wall musculature have intermediate sensitivity. The diaphragm is extremely difficult to block completely. Ophthalmic muscles and upper airway/pharyngeal musculature are very sensitive, and it is particularly this latter area, with the risks of inadequate airway tone leading to partial or complete obstruction post-extubation, that concern anaesthetists when residual blockade exists. A less well-recognised side effect of residual blockade, but of possibly greater importance, is the risk of dysfunctional swallowing and aspiration of pharyngeal secretions and refluxed gastric contents into the lungs, predisposing to lung infection in the high-risk patient.

It is almost impossible to block the diaphragm completely, so if there is central respiratory drive the diaphragm is likely to move. Respiratory effort is driven by high CO_2 concentrations in the blood, and suppressed by opioids. It is often inter-breathing and respiratory efforts that disrupt surgery, and a balance must be found between driving down the blood CO_2 levels by aggressive ventilation, using opioids to suppress ventilator drive, and muscle relaxant use to 'soften' respiratory movement. The situation is further complicated with surgeries where the peritoneum is breached and large volumes of CO_2 find their way into the tissues and are absorbed in large quantities, pushing the arterial CO_2 levels up. During normal laparoscopy, there is perhaps an additional 10–40 ml of CO_2 absorbed each minute that has to be cleared over and above the metabolic production of some 150–200 ml – a load increasing required ventilation rates by around 10–20% only. However, particularly during procedures around the oesophageal hiatus and in inguinal herniorrhaphy, this absorption may be massive, needing much greater ventilation and potentially causing real problems with an acute acidosis.

Deep versus standard neuromuscular blockade

The dilemma facing the anaesthetist is to balance the potential improvement in surgical operating conditions from deep neuromuscular blockade versus the risks described above. Reversal agents are never 100% effective, and a great deal of the reversal effect is because of metabolic clearance of the administered relaxant. Inappropriately high dosing of relaxants can lead to significant residual paralysis despite the use of reversal agents.

Reversal of neuromuscular blocking agents is usually performed in UK practice but less so in Europe. The historical standard is to use neostigmine to increase concentrations of acetylcholine at the neuromuscular junction. But there can be paradoxical effects with neuromuscular transmission worsening with relative overdose. In addition parasympathetic activation can cause bradycardias and excessive salivation.

Recently a new agent, sugammadex, has been introduced which has a direct effect in binding and hence inactivating a certain family of steroidal neuromuscular blocking agents. In theory this may allow higher doses of the specific muscle relaxants (rocuronium and vecuronium) and hence a deeper level of relaxation to be used throughout the surgical procedure; but the reversal agent is very expensive, has a degree of anaphylaxis associated, and may have effects on bleeding rates. For these reasons, at the time of writing, this agent is still awaiting approval by the US regulatory authorities. However it does show great promise.

Post-operative care

Monitoring

The level and duration of monitoring required following bariatric surgery is clearly a function of the risk of surgical complications, of anaesthetic complications and of the patient's overall vulnerability to these complications. Procedures that are technically very challenging, where there is intra-operative bleeding and/or concerns around the development of leak, will require closer observation in the first 12–24 hours. Patients with significant co-morbidities and risk factors are best observed in a high-care or HDU environment, but the need for true ICU facilities is very low.

Appropriate pre-op assessment for bariatric surgery will identify the high-risk patients and in established units the need for HDU admission can be as low as one bed day per 100 procedures. In less experienced units it is better to play safe and the benefits of arterial line monitoring may mandate larger proportions of patients going through the critical care unit. Availability of beds plays a major role in determining the threshold for admission. Again it is vital to look at the ASA status and the particular co-morbidities that may benefit from these higher levels of care, and not to base a decision on the need for HDU care upon BMI alone.

Analgesia

Obese patients are a group where early post-operative mobilisation and the ability to move independently is of great benefit, both to the patient in terms of minimising thrombosis risk, but also to the nursing staff in reducing their workload, and to the hospital in reducing lengths of stay. Central to this is good analgesia, and adoption of the principles of enhanced recovery techniques. Nausea associated with the use of opioids prevents mobilisation and thus multimodal analgesic techniques, utilising regular paracetamol, non-steroidals and other co-analgesic agents to minimise opioid requirements, are the preferred approach.

The other major concern is of opioid-mediated respiratory depression, particularly among patients with degrees of sleep apnoea and the related condition of obesity hypoventilation syndrome. Respiratory depression is most common on the first night following surgery, and particularly with the use of longer-acting opioids, and especially morphine. The American Society of Anesthesiologists has produced practice guidelines on the management of patients with known sleep apnoea. These are currently undergoing revision, but the central tenet of these guidelines is that patients who receive longer-acting opioids by intra-muscular, intravenous or epidural routes must be monitored for a period of some 12 hours in a higher level (HDU or Level 1 high-care unit) with continuous oximetry as a minimum. However, following laparoscopic bariatric surgery, the combination of regular paracetamol and early non-steroidal analgesia, together with a prepared and motivated patient, means that the vast majority require nothing more than oral opioid analgesia once they leave the recovery area. Given that a significant proportion of patients with sleep apnoea are undiagnosed, a systems approach that utilises short-acting opioids intra-operatively, then significant doses of co-analgesics and thus aims to avoid parenteral opioids, is safest for the bariatric surgical population.

Mobilisation

There is not a single group of patients who are more likely to benefit from enhanced recovery techniques than the morbidly obese. The use of short-acting agents, minimisation of the intra-operative time period (so that as little anaesthetic as possible is absorbed into fat), and early and vigorous encouragement and assistance to mobilise should be the norm for the vast majority of patients. In only a few should the need for nasogastric tubes, catheters and various other lines (i.e. the HDU/ICU cohort) delay this process. Motivating and informing the patient prior to surgery, another key part of the MDT role, is central to achieving this goal.

Summary

Anaesthesia and peri-operative care of the morbidly obese patient is challenging and there are many traps for the unwary. However if the major areas of risk, particularly related to sleep apnoea and its implications, and drug dosing are understood, and there is recognition and appropriate selection of the high-risk patient ('beware the older apple'), then there is no reason that morbidly obese patients cannot be offered the same surgical options as those of normal weight.

References

Adams TD, Gress RE, Smith SC, *et al.* Long-term mortality after gastric bypass surgery. *New England Journal of Medicine* 2007; **357**: 753–61.

Blackstone RP, Cortes MC. Metabolic acuity score: effect on major complications after bariatric surgery. *Surgery for Obesity and Related Diseases* 2010; **6**: 267–73.

Dakin JD, Margarson MP. Sleep-disordered breathing and anaesthesia in the morbidly obese. *Current Anaesthesia & Critical Care* 2010; **21**: 24–30.

DeMaria EJ, Portenier D, Wolfe L. Obesity surgery mortality risk score: proposal for a clinically useful score to predict mortality risk in patients undergoing gastric bypass. *Surgery for Obesity and Related Diseases* 2007; **3**: 134–40.

Flum DR, Belle SH, King WC, *et al.* Peri-operative safety in the longitudinal assessment of bariatric surgery. *New England Journal of Medicine* 2009; **361**: 445–54.

Gross JB, Bachenberg KL, Benumof JL, *et al.* Practice guidelines for the peri-operative management of patients with obstructive sleep apnea: a report by the American Society of Anesthesiologists Task Force on Peri-operative Management of patients with obstructive sleep apnea. *Anesthesiology* 2006; **104 (5)**: 1081–93.

At a glance

Scoring systems

Jane Sturgess and Justin Davies

This chapter will consider scoring systems for surgical patients. They aim to assess the risk of death and peri-operative complications for patients undergoing elective or emergency surgery.

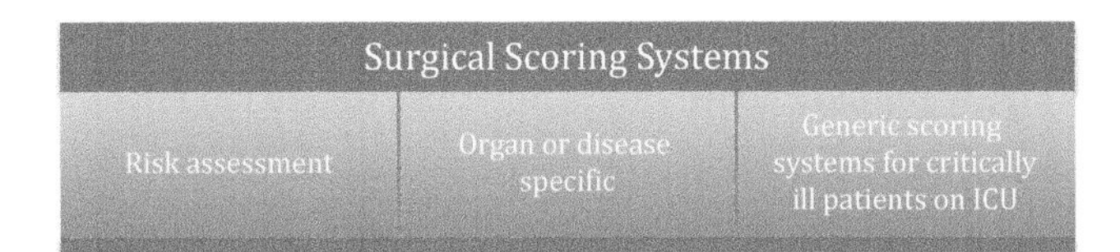

Figure 22.1 Categories of scoring systems for surgical patients.

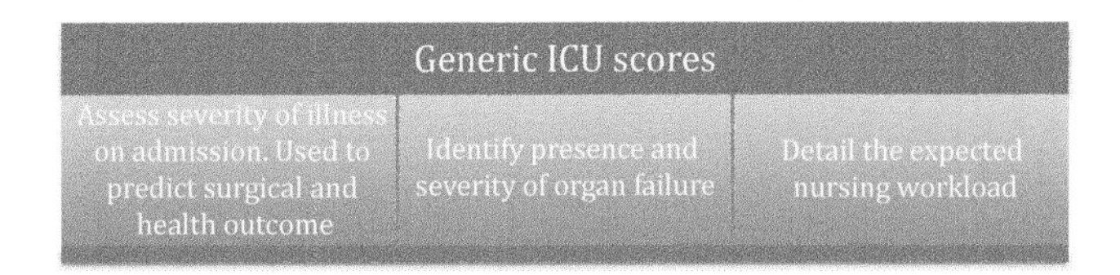

Figure 22.2 Three broad types of ICU scoring systems.

As well as being used for clinical assessment of patients, surgical scoring systems are becoming more frequently introduced into clinical trials as a comparator.

Risk assessment

ASA – American Society of Anesthesiology physical status classification system

ASA I	Fit, healthy patient
ASA II	Mild systemic disease with no functional limitation, e.g. smoker with well-controlled hypertension
ASA III	Severe systemic disease and definite functional impairment, e.g. stable diabetes and stable angina but requiring medical therapy/intervention

A Surgeon's Guide to Anaesthesia and Peri-operative Care, ed. Jane Sturgess, Justin Davies and Kamen Valchanov. Published by Cambridge University Press.

ASA IV	Severe systemic disease that is life threatening, e.g. diabetes, angina and congestive heart failure. The patient is symptomatic with breathlessness and chest pain on minimal exertion.
ASA V	Moribund patient not expected to survive 24 hours with or without the operation
ASA VI	New classification – Brain-dead organ donor
E	Emergency operation
Problems	Does not take into account operative risk, inter-observer and intra-observer variability

NYHA – New York Heart Association classification of heart failure symptoms

Class I	No limitations. Ordinary physical activity does not cause undue fatigue
Class II	Slight limitation of physical activity, but comfortable at rest. Ordinary physical activity results in fatigue, palpitation, breathlessness or angina
Class III	Marked limitation of physical activity. May still be comfortable at rest but less than ordinary physical activity leads to symptoms
Class IV	Symptoms at rest or on minimal physical activity. Unable to carry out any physical activity

Canadian Heart Association Angina Classification is much the same as NYHA but uses angina for the symptom rather than breathlessness.

CCS – Canadian Cardiovascular Society grading of angina pectoris

Class I	No limitation – angina only during strenuous physical activity
Class II	Slight limitation – angina during vigorous physical activity
Class III	Moderate limitation – angina during normal living activities
Class IV	Severe limitation – angina at rest, or increasing frequency

Goldmann

Risk	Score
Third heart sound	11
Elevated JVP	11
MI in last 6 months	10
Premature atrial contractions or non-sinus rhythm	7
>5 premature ventricular beats per minute	7
Age >70	5

(cont.)

Risk	Score
Emergency procedure	4
Intrathoracic, intra-abdominal or aortic surgery	3
Poor general status, bedridden	3

Class	Points	Risk incidence
I	<6	0.2% death
		0.7% severe cardiovascular complications
II	6–25	4% death
		17% severe cardiovascular complications
III	>26	56% death
		22% severe cardiovascular complications

Detsky's Modified Cardiac Risk

Risk	Score
Age >70	5
MI within the last 6 months	10
MI more than 6 months ago	5
Canadian Heart Association Angina Class III Angina	10
Canadian Heart Association Angina Class IV Angina	20
Unstable angina within the last 6 months	10
Pulmonary oedema in the last week	10
Pulmonary oedema ever	5
Suspected critical aortic stenosis	20
Rhythm other than sinus, or sinus + premature atrial beat	5
More than 5 premature ventricular beats	5
Emergency operation	10
Poor general medical status	5

Class	Points	Cardiac risk
I	0–15	Low
II	20–30	
III	>31	High

Lee's Modified Cardiac Risk Index

(please see *Circulation* 1999;100:1043–9)

Score one point for each risk factor identified.

1. High-risk surgical procedure	Intra-peritoneal Intrathoracic Suprainguinal vascular
2. History of ischaemic heart disease	MI Positive exercise test Current ischaemic chest pain Use of nitrate therapy Pathological Q waves identified on ECG
3. History of congestive cardiac failure	History of congestive cardiac failure Pulmonary oedema Paroxysmal nocturnal dyspnoea Gallop heart sounds or bibasal crepitations CXR with upper lobe blood diversion
4. History of cerebrovascular disease	TIA or cerebrovascular accident
5. Pre-operative insulin therapy	
6. Pre-operative creatine >2.0 mg/dl	

Points	Class	Risk
0	I	0.4%
1	II	0.9%
2	III	6.6%
3 or more	IV	11%

The Lee Score predicts the risk of a major cardiac event – MI, pulmonary oedema, ventricular fibrillation, primary cardiac arrest, complete heart block.

It can be seen that patients with 0–1 points are low risk.

Functional Status Assessment/Duke Activity Status Index

Excellent (>7 METs)	Moderate (4–7 METs)	Poor (<4 METs)
Squash	Gardening	Slow walking (2 mph)
Jogging	Climbing 1 flight stairs	Writing
Scrubbing floors	Golf	Light housework
Singles tennis	Walking 4 mph	Dressing/bathing

One MET (metabolic equivalent) represents an oxygen consumption of 3.5 ml/kg/min

Possum and P-POSSUM

Physiological And Operative Severity Score for the enumeration of mortality and morbidity.

Developed in 1991 by Copeland. Considers 12 physiological and six operative parameters for calculation. Adjusts risk for a surgical procedure based on the patients physiological condition. Tends to over-predict death for low-risk patients. The P-POSSUM equation is a modified POSSUM equation using the same variables to attempt to reduce the over-prediction of POSSUM.

The POSSUM score has been revised to consider subspecialty surgery. CR-POSSUM (colorectal), O-POSSUM (oesophagogastric) and V-POSSUM (vascular) now exist. V-POSSUM is further divided into V(p)-POSSUM, RAAA-POSSUM and RAAA(p)-POSSUM.

(p) = physiology only. RAAA = ruptured abdominal aortic aneurysm

POSSUM formula:

Ln R/1-R = -7.04 + (0.13 x physiological score) + (0.16 x operative severity score)

P-POSSUM formula:

Ln R/1-R = -9.065 + (0.1692 x physiological score) + (0.1550 x operative severity score)

Where R = predicted risk of mortality

On-line risk calculators:

- http://www.riskprediction.org.uk/op-index.php
- http://www.vasgbi.com/riskscores.htm

Organ-disease specific

Neurological

GCS – Glasgow Coma Score (3–15)

Eyes	Open spontaneously	4
	Verbal command	3
	Pain	2
	No response	1
Best verbal response	Oriented in time, person, place	5
	Disoriented	4
	Inappropriate words	3
	Incomprehensible sounds	2
	No response	1
Best motor response	Obeys verbal command	6
	Localises to pain	5
	Withdraws to pain	4
	Abnormal flexion	3
	Extension posturing	2
	No response	1

Glasgow Outcome Scale

Score	Definition	Explanation
1	Dead	
2	Vegetative state	Unable to interact with environment; unresponsive
3	Severe disability	Able to follow commands/unable to live independently
4	Moderate disability	Able to live independently; unable to return to work or school
5	Good recovery	Able to return to work or school

(From Jennett B, *et al.* Disability after severe head injury: observations on the use of the Glasgow Outcome Scale. *J Neurol, Neurosurg, Psychiat* 1981;44:285–93.)

WFNS Subarachnoid Haemorrhage Grading Scale

Grade	GCS	Motor deficit
I	15	-
II	14–13	-
III	14–13	+
IV	12–7	+/-
V	6–3	+/-

(From Teesdale GM, *et al.* A universal subarachnoid hemorrhage scale: report of a committee of the World Federation of Neurosurgical Societies. *J Neurol Neurosurg Psychiatry* 1988;51(11):1457.)

Hunt and Hess Scale

Introduced in 1968 to determine the severity of the subarachnoid haemorrhage based on the patient's clinical condition. Mortality increases from a score of 1 through to 5.

1	Asymptomatic, mild headache, some neck stiffness
2	Moderate to severe headache, neck stiffness, may have a cranial nerve palsy but no other neurological deficit
3	Mild neurological deficit, drowsiness or confusion
4	Stupor, moderate to severe hemiparesis
5	Coma, decerebrate posturing

(See Hunt WE, Hess RM. Surgical risk as related to time of intervention in the repair of intracranial aneurysms. *J Neurosurg* 1968;28(1):14–20.)

Cardiac

Parsonnet Additive Risk Stratification Model (for cardiac surgery)

Tends to over-predict mortality and has generally been superseded by the EuroSCORE.

Risk		Score
Female sex		1
Morbid obesity	BMI > 35	3
Diabetes (any type or duration)		3
Hypertension	>140/90 on two occasions	3
LV ejection fraction	>50%	0
	30–49%	2
	<30%	4
Age	70–74	7
	75–79	12
	>80	20
Re-operation	2nd operation	5
	3rd or more	10
Pre-operative IABP (not prophylactic)		2
Left ventricular aneurysm for aneurysmectomy		5
Failed operation within the last 24 hours		10
OR >24 h but during the same admission		5
Dialysis		10
Catastrophic state, e.g. cardiogenic shock, acute renal failure		10–50
Other co-morbidity – severe asthma, pacemaker, paraplegia		2–10
Mitral valve surgery	PA pressure <60 mmHg	5
	PA pressure >60 mmHg	8
Aortic valve surgery	AV gradient <120 mmHg	5
	AV gradient >120 mmHg	7
CABG and valve surgery		2

Score	Risk	Mortality
0–4	Low risk	1%
5–9	Elevated risk	5%
10–14	Significantly elevated risk	9%
15–19	High risk	17%
>19	Very high risk	31%

(See *Circulation* 1989; **79**: Suppl I:3–12.)

EuroSCORE – the European System for Cardiac Operative Risk Evaluation additive risk stratification model

Developed in the late 1990s to provide risk assessment at the bedside. Validated in Western society. Predicts complications, duration of ICU stay and use of resources. Has had a number of iterations: EUROscore II was launched in 2011 and has superseded earlier versions.

Risk	Score
1 point for every 5 years >60	1
Female sex	1
Long-term bronchodilators or inhaled steroids	1
Extra-cardiac arteriopathy, e.g. carotids >50%, aorta, limbs	2
Neurological dysfunction affecting daily life	2
Previous cardiac surgery opening pericardium	2
Pre-operative creatinine >200 micromol/l	2
Current treatment for active endocarditis	3
Rest angina on i.v. nitrates immediately pre-induction	2
One or more of: VT/VF/cardiac massage/ventilation/inotropes/IABP/acute renal failure	2
Moderate LV dysfunction (EF 30–50%)	1
Poor LV function (EF <30%)	3
MI within the last 90 days	2
Pulmonary hypertension (PA pressure >60 mmHg)	2
Emergency operation	2
CABG + other major cardiac procedure	2
Surgery to thoracic aorta	3
Post-infarct septal rupture	4

(See http://www.euroscore.org/calc.html for on-line scoring.)

Generic ICU scores

Severity of illness on admission and outcome prediction scores

APACHE – Acute Physiology and Chronic Health Evaluation (0–71)

As the name suggests this score is based upon current illness severity and chronic health (including age). The first version was published in 1981. It is now on its 4th version. The APACHE IV considers 12 physiological variables. The worst score for each in the first 24 hours of ICU stay is entered. The maximum achievable score is 71.

It is used to predict outcome – mortality, length of stay and as a performance indicator when benchmarking ICUs.

SAPS – Simplified Acute Physiology Score (0–217)

Originally designed and validated in 1984 (France), it is now on its 3rd version. The SAPS3 considers three main categories, based on a total of 20 variables. The categories are patient characteristics before admission, circumstance of admission and physiological derangement in the first hour of admission (SAPS2 looked at the first 24 hours).

SAPS3 has been adapted and there are seven separate models to predict mortality for seven geographical regions.

Organ failure scores

LODS – Logistic Organ Dysfunction Score (0–22)

Organ systems – respiratory, cardiovascular, renal, hepatic, haematological, neurological.

Developed over 12 countries and more than 13,000 patients. The organ score is weighted, i.e. max score for respiratory and coagulation is 3, liver is 1 and other organs 5. The worst score in the first 24 hours after admission is recorded. It can be used to predict mortality as well as indicate the severity of organ dysfunction. It can be used to characterise the progression of organ dysfunction over the first week of admission.

MODS – Multiple Organ Dysfunction Score (0–24)

Organ systems – respiratory, cardiovascular, renal, hepatic, haematological, neurological.

Based on a literature review of 30 publications. Developed with 336 patients in a single surgical ICU and validated with a further 356 patients. Each system is given a score 0–4 (no dysfunction – maximum dysfunction). The score is recorded as the first variables of the day.

MODS score is correlated with outcome but cannot be used to predict ICU mortality. The difference between admission and maximum score MODS (delta MODS) can be more predictive of outcome than any individual score.

SOFA – Sequential Organ Failure Score (0–24)

Organ systems – respiratory, cardiovascular, renal, hepatic, haematological, neurological.

Developed during a consensus conference in 1994 and subsequently validated in a number of mixed medical-surgical ICUs. Organs are scored 0–4, with 0 for normal function, and 4 most abnormal function. A SOFA score >15 (or 13 in patients >60 yrs) is correlated with high mortality. The SOFA scores are a marker of organ dysfunction, but can also be used to predict mortality, and to assess ICU performance.

Early warning scores

Modified Early Warning Score (MEWS)

Used to quickly notify nursing and medical staff to the clinical deterioration of a patient in hospital. A score of 4–6 will trigger a call for the patient to be reviewed, a score of greater than 7 indicates a severely unwell patient. As with all scores it is important to look for the trend rather than just the number, to determine whether the patient's condition is improving or deteriorating. The score has been shown to indicate the sickest patients, and improve timely referral to critical care teams.

Score	3	2	1	0	1	2	3
Systolic BP	<45%	30%	15% down	Normal for patient	15% up	30%	>45%
Heart rate (BPM)	—	<40	41–50	51–100	101–110	111–129	>130
Respiratory rate (RPM)	—	<9	—	9–14	15–20	21–29	>30
Temperature (°C)	—	<35	—	35.0–38.4	—	>38.5	—
AVPU	—	—	—	A	V	P	U

National Early Warning Score (NEWS)

A national, standardised modification of the MEWS, developed by The Royal College of Physicians in 2012, to promote standardisation of the early warning system across the NHS. Aggregate scores then trigger levels of clinical risk/deterioration.

Score	3	2	1	0	1	2	3
Respiration rate	<8		9–11	12–20		21–24	>25
Oxygen saturation	<91	92–93	94–95	>96			
Any supplemental oxygen		Yes		No			
Temperature (°C)	<35.0		35.1–36.0	36.1–38.0	38.1–39.0	>39.1	
Systolic BP	<90	91–100	101–110	111–219			>220
Heart rate	<40		41–50	51–90	91–110	111–130	>131
Level of consciousness				A			V, P or U

Expected nursing workload scores

TISS – Therapeutic Intervention Scoring System (0–78)

Originally developed in the 70s and revised in the 80s. It considered 76 variables and was thought too cumbersome to be of real use. The TISS-28 (1996) reduced the number of nursing work variables to 28 items. These are grouped into basic activities, ventilatory support, cardiovascular support, renal support, neurological support, metabolic support and specific interventions.

It is used to plan manpower on the ICU, and assess/benchmark amount (not complexity) of care given.

NEMS – Nine Equivalents Of Nursing Manpower Use Score (0–56)

Derived from TISS-28 to be easier to use. Validated in large ICU cohorts.

Used to classify amount of care (not complexity) provided.

Chapter 23

Modes of mechanical ventilation

Kamen Valchanov

Mechanical ventilation is used during surgery or respiratory failure to optimise gas exchange until the end of surgery or while waiting for the improvement of the underlying respiratory disease.

Modern mechanical ventilation involves positive pressure insufflation of gas into the lungs rather than negative pressure generated by the respiratory muscles, and is therefore harmful by default. However, short spells of mechanical ventilation during anaesthesia and surgery seem to be well tolerated by the majority of patients without major side effects.

Positive pressure ventilation of the lungs causes a number of undesirable side effects which can lead to lung injury, even in healthy lungs. These can sometimes lead to multi-organ dysfunction or failure (Figure 23.1).

For this reason the least harmful mode of mechanical ventilation until the end of surgery or respiratory failure recovery is likely to yield most patient benefit.

Mechanical ventilation can be non-invasive (through face masks or hoods), or invasive (through tracheal or bronchial tubes, or tracheostomy).

Both modes of mechanical ventilation employ the same principles, but non-invasive ventilation:

- Does not require sedation
- Can be done at home
- Does not impair the mucociliary apparatus

Continuous positive airways pressure (CPAP) is not per se a mode of mechanical ventilation, but often used as such. It involves administration of positive pressure throughout the respiratory cycle (inspirium and expirium) but the patient has to generate negative pressure to inflate the lungs. This mode is least invasive, and efficient for:

- Improving pulmonary oedema (by increasing the intra-alveolar pressure during expirium and reducing the work of breathing)
- Improving oxygenation
- Improving lung collapse and atelectasis

It is seldom efficient for treatment of hypercarbia, as it does not directly increase the minute respiratory volume.

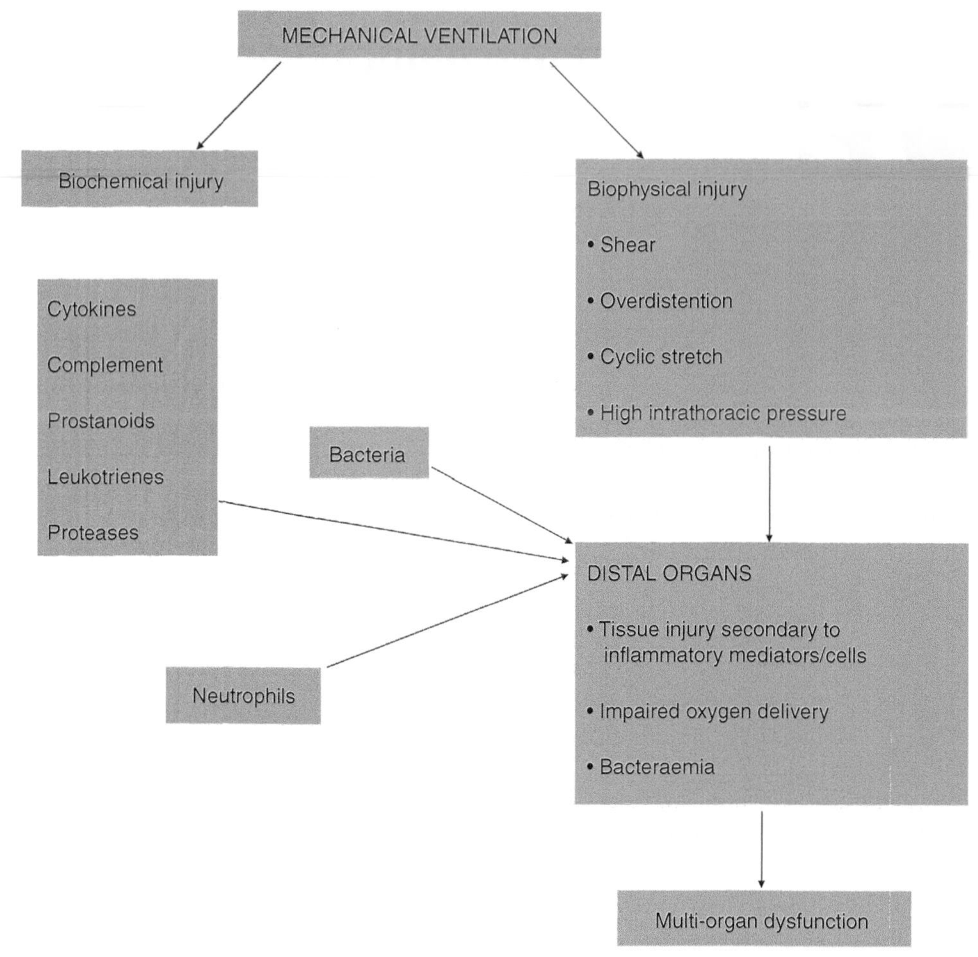

Figure 23.1 Mechanism of mechanical ventilation injury.

Non-invasive mechanical ventilation is beneficial for patients with:

- Hypercarbia
- Respiratory muscle weakness
- Immunocompromised state (as it avoids the more harmful effects of invasive ventilation)

Invasive mechanical ventilation

This involves three parts:

- interface with the patient (tracheal, bronchial, or tracheostomy tube)
- connecting tubing
- ventilator

The positioning of these tubes is traumatic in its own right. Anaesthesia and sedation are required because of stimulation of laryngeal and pharyngeal reflexes from the foreign body.

Mechanical ventilation is traumatic to the lungs. The best ventilation strategies aim to avoid:

- Pressure trauma – use the minimal inflation pressure required to avoid severe lung injury
- Volutrauma – closely related to the minimal inflation pressures. It is known from critically ill patients that tidal volume ventilation with 6 ml/kg is less harmful than 12 ml/kg. Whether these numbers apply to general anaesthesia is not known yet, but there has been a drive for low tidal volume ventilation during thoracic surgery
- Atelectotrauma – extreme deflation of distal parts of the lung results in atelectasis. Supraphysiological pressure is required to open these parts of the lung again. Each tidal breath should keep the lung 'open' and avoid atelectotrauma
- Biotrauma – the stretch of the alveoli triggers an inflammatory mediators cascade. The lowest stretch produces the least biotrauma

Positive pressure ventilation is the modern type of mechanical ventilation.

The common modes of positive pressure ventilation of the lungs include:

- Volume control ventilation (VC): Tidal volume and respiratory rate are set by the operator, and the ventilator will deliver these at any pressure or flow needed.
- Pressure control ventilation (PC): The peak airways pressure and respiratory rate are set by the operator, and the ventilator will deliver them with whichever flow, and whichever tidal volume.
- Intermittent positive pressure ventilation (IPPV): This encompasses both VC and PC but the term implies that there is a minimum number of breaths per minute set by the operator.
- Synchronised intermittent mandatory ventilation (SIMV): This mode can be used with VC or PV ventilation and only delivers mandatory breaths but also supports spontaneous breaths triggered by the patient. It is a common mode in ITU where muscle relaxation is seldom used for a long time. Anaesthetic ventilator modes usually involve muscle relaxation and hence the patient does not trigger breaths.
- Pressure support (PS): This mode of ventilation is only used in spontaneously breathing patients, and hence common in ITU, rather than operating theatres.
- Continuous positive airway pressure (CPAP): Spontaneously breathing patients are administered constant flow of gas at a constant pressure. The patient needs to generate negative pressure to generate a breath. Exhalation is against the set positive pressure.
- Positive end expiratory pressure (PEEP): Positive pressure is applied during the expiratory phase to prevent collapse of lung segments. Pressure is not permitted to drop to 0. It is suitable for mechanically ventilated patients.

Low tidal volume ventilation:

There is sufficient evidence that large tidal volume (12 ml/kg) ventilation for a long time in ITU is harmful. However, there is not yet sufficient evidence to suggest that these make a difference intra-operatively. Intuitively, the lowest tidal volumes avoiding hypoxia and hypercarbia intra-operatively are likely to produce less harmful effects on the lungs. In addition, the use of adequate muscle relaxation is likely to reduce the peak airway pressures intra-operatively and hence alveolar stretch and pressure trauma.

Further reading

Gatinoni L, *et al.* Towards ultraprotective mechanical ventilation. *Curr Opin Anesthesiol* 2012; 25.

Gatinoni, *et al.* Ventilator-induced lung injury: anatomical and physiological framework. *Crit Care Med* 2010; **38**: S539–48.

Section III

At a glance

Chapter 24

Fluids

Jane Sturgess

Fluids

Table 24.1 Crystalloid solutions

	Osmolarity	pH	Na	K	Ca	Cl	Other
Normal saline	300	5.0	154	-	-	154	Risk of hyperchloraemic metabolic acidosis when given in large doses 9 g Na
Ringer's lactate	278	6.5	131	5	2	111	Some concern about giving to diabetics or those with high lactate Hypo-osmolar so some would not recommend if raised intracranial pressure 6 g Na, and 29 mmol of lactate
4% dextrose 0.18% saline		4.0	30	-	-	30	Contains 40 g of dextrose
2.5% glucose 0.45% saline	293	3.5-6.5	77	-	-	77	Contains 25 g of glucose, and 4.5 g of Na
5% dextrose		4.0	-	-	-	-	Contains 50 g dextrose
8.4% bicarbonate	2000	8.0	1000				HCO_3 1000
5% saline	1711	5.0	565			565	Hypertonic, can cause vein damage Should be given via a central vein 3% solutions also available

A Surgeon's Guide to Anaesthesia and Peri-operative Care, ed. Jane Sturgess, Justin Davies and Kamen Valchanov. Published by Cambridge University Press.

Table 24.2 Colloid solutions

	Osmolarity	pH	Na	K	Ca	Cl	Molecular weight	Other
Gelofusine	274	7.4	154	<0.4	<0.4	125	30,000 Daltons	40 g gelatin Proposed volume expansion 4 hours duration
Hetastarch	308	4.0–5.5	154	-	-	154	130,000 Daltons	60 g starch
Haemaccel	301	7.4	145	5	6.25	145	30,000 Daltons	35 g gelatin
Pentastarch	326	5.0	154	-	-	154	63,000 Daltons	100 g starch
Albumin 4.5%		7.4	<160	<2	-	136	66,000 Daltons	40–50 g albumin

Daily requirements

Water	30 ml/kg/24 h
Sodium	1 mmol/kg/24 h
Potassium	0.5–1 mmol/kg/24 h

Fluids for resuscitation

When there are large insensible losses the deficit loss should be replaced with a similar fluid – NG loss requires isotonic fluid and electrolytes as does diarrhoea.

Massive blood loss should trigger blood and blood product replacement (see Section II Chapter 18 'Trauma cases').

It is important to realise that there are as many strongly held views on which fluid to use in resuscitation as there are fluids available to prescribe. As such a number of papers and systematic reviews are published searching for the perfect answer. As with so many areas of medicine and especially critical care, it becomes obvious that there is no simple answer. Critical illness is the result of a multitude of cellular reactions and inter-linking cascades occurring in a sequence that cannot be completely predicted. Neither can we determine which patients will have an exaggerated response of one cascade, and suppression of another. The following recommendations are the response of one group of intensivists. Another group may come up with a completely different opinion. Throughout the debate it should be remembered that a number of key investigators, upon whose papers many of the systematic reviews depend, have had their research credentials discredited.

Special circumstances based on recommendations from the European Intensive Care Society Task Force

- Severe sepsis (or risk of acute kidney injury) – hydroxy-ethyl starch (HES) with molecular weight > 200 k Daltons, 6% HES 130/0.4 or gelatin are **not** recommended
- Head injury – colloids are **not** recommended
- Organ donors – hyperoncotic solutions are **not** recommended

Fluids to rescue raised intracranial pressure

- Mannitol 0.5 g–1 g/kg. Usually presented as either 10% (100 mg/ml) or 20% (200 mg/ml) solutions. The 20% solution can crystallise
- **Or** hypertonic saline 5% 250 ml as a bolus in adult patients. It is important to observe serum sodium levels and serum osmolality

A consensus statement from the European Intensive Care Society does NOT recommend the use of colloids in patients with head injury

Estimating free water deficit in hypernatraemia

- 0.6 x patient weight x (patient sodium/140 – 1)
- 0.6 x weight = estimated body water and 140 = desired sodium concentration

Fluids in burns

Parkland formula:

Fluid required in the first 24 hours = (4 × patient weight kg) × % body surface area burned.

Half the total amount should be given in the first eight hours since the burn, with the remaining amount over the following 16 hours.

Ringer's lactate fluid is recommended in this formula, which serves as a guide. The amount of fluid is the MINIMUM required. Individual fluids should be titrated to maintain a urine output of at least 0.5 ml/kg/h.

The Cochrane review 2011 on fluids for resuscitation found no difference in risk of death between colloids and crystalloids in burns or trauma. The debate continues among intensivists and traumatologists.

Fluids in children

Resuscitation fluids

Ringer's lactate 20 ml/kg as a bolus repeated up to three times. After this, will need blood product replacement.

Maintenance fluids

Usual choice is 0.45% saline/2.5% dextrose OR 5% dextrose, especially in the very young with small intrinsic glucose reserves:

4/2/1 rule:

4 ml/kg for the first 10 kg, 2 ml/kg for the second 10 kg, 1 ml/kg for subsequent kgs

Examples:

44 kg child = 40 + 20 + 14 = 74 ml/h

20 kg child = 40 + 10 = 50 ml/h

Further reading

Perel P, Roberts I. Colloids versus crystalloids for resuscitation in critically ill patients. *Cochrane Database Of Systematic Reviews* 2011, Issue 3. Art No: CD000567.

Reinhart K, Perner A, Sprung CL, *et al.* Consensus statement of the ESICM task force on colloid volume therapy in critically ill patients. *Intensive Care Medicine* 2012 Mar; **38**(3): 368–83.

Section III At a glance

Chapter 25

Coagulation

Jane Sturgess

Methods used to aid clot formation

Agents derived from blood products

Fresh Frozen Plasma (FFP)

Contains factors II, V, VII, IX, and XI: useful in acute active haemorrhage.

Cryoprecipitate

Replacement of fibrinogen in the acutely bleeding patient (especially in DIC – fibrinogen consumption): also useful for von Willebrands, and factor VIII and XIII replacement.

Prothrombin complex concentrate – Octaplex, Beriplex

Used for rapid reversal of warfarin anticoagulation pre-operatively or during haemorrhage. Derived from human plasma and contains factors II, VII, IX and X. Effects last six to 12 hours.

Recombinant Factor VIIa

Originally used in the treatment of haemophilia, but use has transferred into the management of major haemorrhage from trauma and surgery.

It enhances thrombin generation on platelet surface at the site of injury, thereby inducing clot formation via tight fibrin plug and haemostasis.

Drugs

Vitamin K

Useful for reversal of warfarin but it has a slow onset and long duration of action, which can cause problems in those patients that require anticoagulation after major bleeding has been terminated.

Tranexamic acid

Antifibrinolytic, which competitively inhibits activation of plasminogen, reducing conversion of plasminogen to plasmin – the enzyme that breaks down clots.

A Surgeon's Guide to Anaesthesia and Peri-operative Care, ed. Jane Sturgess, Justin Davies and Kamen Valchanov. Published by Cambridge University Press.

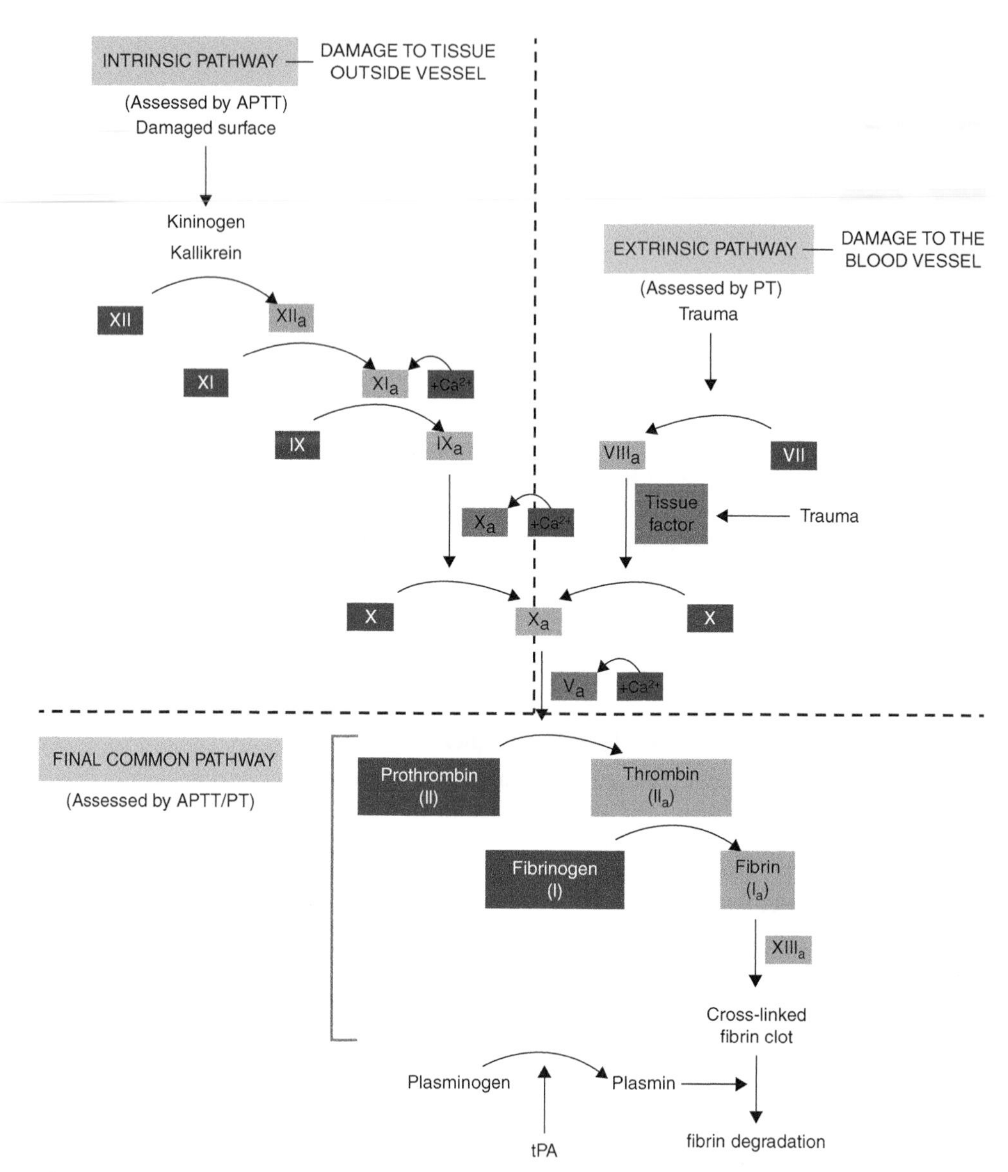

Figure 25.1 Figure to summarise the clotting cascade showing the intrinsic, extrinsic and final common pathways.

Protamine

Positively charged molecule used to reverse the anticoagulant actions of heparin. Initial heparin reversing dose is traditionally 10 mg per 1,000 U heparin.

Heparin

Large negatively charged molecule, used to block the intrinsic pathway. Used as an infusion or a bolus during vascular or cardiac surgery. Usual doses for cardiopulmonary bypass are 300 U/kg.

Haemostatic agents used during surgery

Fibrin sealants, e.g. Tisseel ™

These are usually a two-component system that is mixed together and applied to tissues to promote clot formation. It acts to replicate the final pathway of the clotting cascade. The two components are i) concentrated fibrinogen and factor XIII and ii) solution of thrombin and calcium. Available in liquid form.

Gelatin matrix/thrombin sealants, e.g. FloSeal ™

The product is a two-component system of thrombin and gelatin matrix that is reconstituted with 0.9% sodium chloride. It has a granular nature and will conform to the shape of the bleeding area. It acts when in contact with blood. The thrombin acts on i) platelets, ii) promotes the formation of fibrin and iii) on factors V, VII and XII. Available in liquid form.

Oxidised regenerated cellulose, e.g. Surgicel ™

Causes contact activation of the clotting cascade via the intrinsic pathway, leading to contraction of small vessels. Available in a fabric or sheet form.

Technology to ensure haemostasis (see also Section I Chapter 6)

Electrocautery

A heated electrode is applied to the tissue surface to cause very localised tissue destruction and therefore haemostasis. The heat is produced by the application of a direct electrical current (DC) across a resistant metal wire electrode.

Electrosurgery

Tissue destruction is caused by the passage of high frequency AC electrical current through living tissue. It can be used in a unipolar (needs a diathermy pad to receive the current) or bipolar (current passes between two forceps tips) fashion. Bipolar 'diathermy' is safer in patients with implanted cardiac devices as the current is localised and does not pass through the patient's body. As a rule of thumb, a continuous waveform (cutting diathermy) generates more heat than an intermittent waveform (coagulation diathermy). The use of electrosurgery can interfere with implanted medical devices.

Both electrocautery and electrosurgery can interfere with monitoring signals, e.g. ECG. *Ligasure*™ and *argon beam* are examples of electrosurgical technology developments.

Laser coagulation

The most commonly used lasers for coagulation are the neodym laser (Nd:YAG), the thalium laser (Tm:YAG) and the holmium laser (Ho:YAG).

HoLEP: this technology can be used for cutting and coagulation of tissues in prostate surgery.

Ultrasound activated scalpel, e.g. Harmonic Scalpel™

Rather than relying on thermal electrical energy, ultrasound relies on transferring ultrasonic high-frequency mechanical vibration energy to the tissues to denature the proteins, thereby sealing bleeding vessels. The vibration causes friction energy and heat, but the amount of heat generated is less than that in either electrosurgery or laser surgery.

Agents to prevent clot formation

The clotting cascade can be therapeutically targeted at any stage and gives rise to drugs that can be considered under the broad categories of thrombolytic, anticoagulant or anti-platelet.

Table 25.1 Mechanism of action of antithrombotic drugs.

Anti-platelet drugs	COX inhibitors	Aspirin, NSAIDs
	ADP receptor/P2Y12 inhibitors	Thienopyridines – clopidogrel, ticlopidine Nucleotide analogues – ticagrelor
	Phosphodiesterase inhibitors	Dipyridamole, triflusal
	Glycoprotein IIb/IIIa inhibitors	Abciximab, tirofiban
	Prostaglandin analogues	Prostacyclin, iloprost, trepostinil
	Thromboxane inhibitors	Thromboxane synthase inhibitors – dypyridamole, picotamide Receptor antagonist – terutroban
	Other	Clocricromen, ditazole
Anticoagulant drugs	Vitamin K antagonists – inhibition of II, VII, IX, X	Warfarin Coumarins – dicoumarol, acenocoumarol 1,3-indandiones – phenindione
	Factor Xa inhibitors	Heparin Low molecular weight heparin – dalteparin, enoxaparin, tinzaparin Oligosaccharides – fondaparinux Heparinoid – danaparoid
	Direct Xa inhibitors	Xabans – rivaroxiban
	Direct thrombin inhibitors – IIa	Hirudin, dabigatran
	Other	Antithrombin III, Protein C (no longer used)
Thrombolytic drugs/fibrinolytics	Plasminogen activators	r-tPA – alteplase, reteplase UPA – streptokinase, urokinase
	Other	Serine endopeptidases – fibrinolysin
Other		EDTA, citrate, oxalate

Pre-operative echocardiography

Kamen Valchanov

Echocardiography is an important part of cardiovascular imaging and presents the events in motion as they occur in real life. It utilises sonographic principles, and can be non-invasive, i.e. trans thoracic echocardiography (TTE), or semi-invasive, i.e. transoesophageal echocardiography (TOE).

The technology of ultrasound has evolved over the last century and is now so advanced that in many ways the images are so clear that they are almost as good as direct observations of the heart.

TTE has become an invaluable tool for elucidating derangements in cardiac morphology and physiology. The results can allow surgery to proceed and guide best intra-operative care for high-risk patients. Appropriate post-operative care can be planned in advance and complications anticipated.

The indications for pre-operative TTE are surgery specific, and patient specific.

Surgery specific indications for TTE are:

- All patients undergoing cardiac surgery. Some operations (e.g. mitral valve surgery, endocarditis surgery) also require TOE
- Operations where large blood loss or major intra-operative cardiovascular changes are expected (e.g. aortic surgery).

Patient-specific indications for pre-operative TTE are too many to discuss in detail. However, they can be grouped as follows:

- Patients with undiagnosed or symptomatic heart murmurs
- Patients with known heart murmurs but increasing symptoms
- All patients with congenital heart disease must have a recent TTE or TOE (unless they have had cardiac MRI)
- Advanced coronary artery disease listed for major elective surgery
- All patients with symptoms of heart failure (breathlessness, high jugular venous pressure, extensive pedal oedema)
- All patients with history of paradoxical embolism.

Some heart structures are better visualised by TOE because of their closer proximity to the oesophagus (where the probe is positioned). Mitral valve pathology, left atrial appendage and infective endocarditis vegetations are better investigated by TOE.

A Surgeon's Guide to Anaesthesia and Peri-operative Care, ed. Jane Sturgess, Justin Davies and Kamen Valchanov. Published by Cambridge University Press.

Importance of pre-operative echocardiography

The information from TTE and TOE can be used to guide peri-operative care.

Valvular pathology

Aortic valve stenosis, regurgitation and mixed aortic valvular disease are all very common in the ageing population. They need not be a reason for cancellation of elective surgery. The risk/benefit ratio of proceeding with surgery must be discussed with the patient, especially if surgery is minor, can be safely postponed, yet the valvular lesion is severe. In these circumstances it is worth seeking a cardiothoracic opinion.

If surgery is urgent, the results of the TTE can help the anaesthetist to choose the safest anaesthetic, and discuss risks openly with the patient:

- Spinal and epidural anaesthetics are less easy to control in patients with cardiac valvular abnormalities, and can result in complete cardiovascular collapse.
- Invasive blood pressure and central venous pressure monitoring are useful.
- Such patients may need vasopressor or inotropic support after major operations, and HDU/ICU can be arranged pre-operatively.

Mitral valve regurgitation is very common (Figure 26.1). All patients must be assessed by a cardiologist as some of the pathologies could benefit from early surgical correction. Asymptomatic patients could have uneventful peri-operative care but this must be assessed on an individual basis.

Mitral valve stenosis is now rare, and often of degenerative origin. If the patient is symptomatic, cardiac surgery should be recommended. Asymptomatic patients need to be maintained in sinus rhythm, and avoid changes in intravascular volume-loading conditions. It is essential to use invasive monitoring even for minor operations, as well as close post-operative observation.

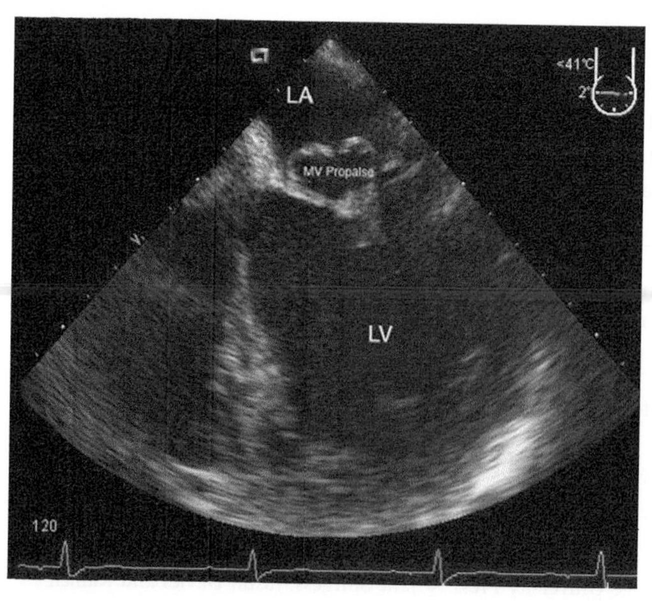

Figure 26.1 TOE. Four-chamber view of a heart with mitral valve prolapse. Both the anterior and posterior mitral leaflets are prolapsed in the shape of a heart. This pathology is likely to produce symptoms of breathlessness and is amenable to surgical correction. LA – left atrium, LV – left ventricle, MV Prolapse – mitral valve prolapse. (Source: Valchanov K, Wells F. You can love it so much. Case report. *Eur J Echo* 2008; **9**: 726.)

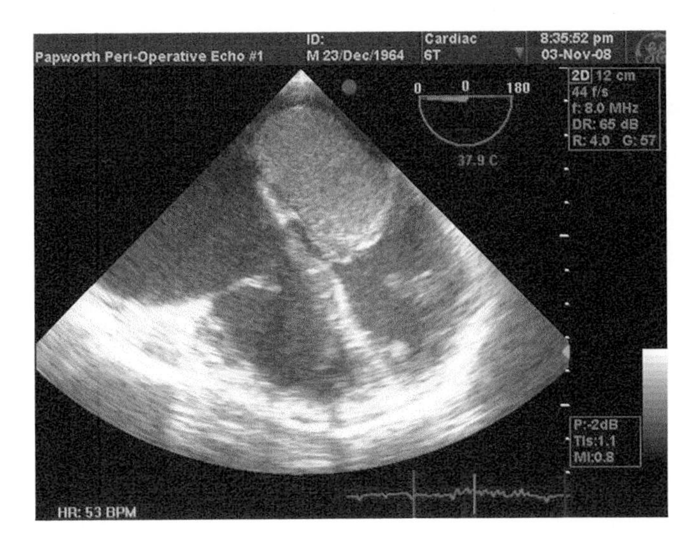

Figure 26.2 TOE. Four-chamber view showing a large left atrial myxoma. The patient presented with unexplained shortness of breath and was scheduled for elective thoracoscopic lung biopsy. Clinical examination led to suspicion of cardiac pathology and the echocardiography revealed the primary problem. The patient underwent myxoma removal rather than lung biopsy. (Source: Hallward G, Valchanov K. An unexpected pre-operative diagnosis. *Eur J Echo* 2010; **11**: 89–90.)

Tricuspid valve pathology is less of a problem, unless it is decompensated and leading to right heart failure.

Occasionally unexpected findings on a pre-operative echocardiography can change the plan for surgery (Figure 26.2).

Shunts

Intracardiac shunts: patent formaen ovale or ductus arteriosus, atrial or ventricular septal defects, or other congenital anomalies need to be assessed on an individual basis. They may require assessment by a cardiologist.

Myocardial function

Left ventricular systolic function:

- Poor left ventricular systolic function is a bad prognostic sign for the patient's life in general. It is not an outright reason for cancellation, as this may be the best condition the patient could achieve.
- Poor left ventricular function does not always equate to heart failure, which is a clinical diagnosis.
- Patients with poor systolic function need to be carefully assessed by a cardiologist, have a good intra-operative surgical and anaesthetic management plan, receive appropriate monitoring and adequate post-operative observations.

Left ventricular diastolic function:

- Impaired left ventricular diastolic function can be more challenging to manage than the systolic derangement.

- This is pathology of ventricular relaxation (which is an energy- consuming process), and can present with post-operative pulmonary oedema as a first sign.
- Diastolic dysfunction is very common in the elderly and hypertensive patients.

Echocardiography is one of the most useful pre-operative tools, and should be sought readily and well in advance of admission.

The results should be interpreted carefully in the context of patient symptoms, and the type and magnitude of proposed surgical intervention.

Section III At a glance

Chapter 27

Common drugs and doses

Jane Sturgess

Type	Drug	Action	Where	Doses	Presentation	Concentration
Vasopressor/ inotropes	Adrenaline	Vasopressor Inotrope Chronotrope	Sympathetic α and β	1:1,000 1:10,000 1:100,000 1:200,000 Max for infiltration 2 mcg/kg	1 ml 10 ml	1 mg/ml 0.1 mg/ml 0.01 mg/ml 0.005 mg/ml
	Dopamine	Inotrope	Sympathetic naturally occurring. α_1, β_1 and dopaminergic	2–10 mcg/kg/min		
	Dobutamine	Inotrope and chronotrope	Sympathetic β_1 and β_2	2.5–10 mcg/kg/min		
	Noradrenaline	Vasopressor	Sympathetic α	2–20 mcg/kg/min		
	Vasopressin	Vasopressor	Synthetic ADH	1–4 U/h		
Local anaesthetics	*l*-Bupivacaine	Long acting	Na channel nodes of Ranvier	2 mg/kg	0.25% 0.5% 0.75%	2.5 mg/ml 5 mg/ml 7.5 mg/ml
	Lidocaine	Intermediate acting	Na channel nodes of Ranvier	3 mg/kg or 7 mg/kg when mixed with adrenaline	1% 2%	10 mg/ml 20 mg/ml
	Prilocaine	Short acting	Na channel nodes of Ranvier	6 mg/kg/h (8 mg/kg/h with adrenaline)	0.5% 2%	5 mg/ml 20 mg/ml
	Ropivacaine	Long acting	Na channel nodes of Ranvier	3–4 mg/kg/h	0.2% 1.0%	2 mg/ml 10 mg/ml
Induction agents	Propofol	Induction and maintenance of anaesthesia Sedation	Multi action but $GABA_A$ agonism predominates Multi action	1–2 mg/kg 0.1–2 mcg/kg/min	1% 2%	10 mg/ml 20 mg/ml
	Etomidate			0.08 mg/kg		2 mg/ml

A Surgeon's Guide to Anaesthesia and Peri-operative Care, ed. Jane Sturgess, Justin Davies and Kamen Valchanov. Published by Cambridge University Press.

(cont.)

Type	Drug	Action	Where	Doses	Presentation	Concentration
		Induction of anaesthesia	Multi action but $GABA_A$ agonism predominates			
	Ketamine	Induction of anaesthesia	Non-competitive NMDA receptor antagonist centrally	1.5–2 mg/kg (i.v. infusions at 50 mcg/kg/min)	Can be used as an infusion	10 mg/ml OR 100 mg/ml
		Analgesia	NMDA receptors	0.1-0.5 mg/kg		
	Thiopentone	Induction of anaesthesia	Barbituate with $GABA_A$ agonism	2.5–5 mg/kg	Powder for reconstitution with saline	
Simple analgesics	Paracetamol	Analgesia, antipyretic, anti-inflammatory	COX-3 inhibitors	12 mg/kg	PO, IV, PR	Care in neonates and low-weight children
	Ibuprofen		COX inhibitors	5 mg/kg	PO	
	Diclofenac		COX inhibitors	1 mg/kg	PO, IV	
Opiate analgesics	Morphine	Strong analgesic	μ or OP1 receptors	0.1 mg/kg	IV, IM	Check dose range for PO
	Fentanyl	Strong analgesic	μ or OP1 receptors	1–2 mcg/kg	IV, sublingual, topical, PO	
	Oxycodone	Strong analgesic	μ or OP1 receptors	0.05–0.15 mg/kg 6 hourly	PO	
	Buprenorphine	Strong analgesic	Partial agonist/partial antagonist μ or OP1 receptors		Topical patch	
	Tramadol	Medium analgesic	μ or OP1 receptors, and $5HT_3$ agonist	1 mg/kg	IV, PO	
	Meptazinol	Strong analgesic, fast onset, short duration. Lower risk of dependence	Partial agonist/partial antagonist μ or OPI receptors	PO 200 mg 3–6 hourly IM. 75–100 mg 2–4 hourly IV 50–100 mg 2–4 hourly	Can be given PO, IM, IV	Not for children
	Codeine	Medium analgesic	Metabolised to morphine, some patients unable to metabolise codeine and will receive no analgesic effect. Some are 'super' metabolisers and gain excessive analgesia and sedation	1 mg/kg	PO, PR	
	Dihydro-codeine	Strong analgesic	As tramadol		PO	

(cont.)

Type	Drug	Action	Where	Doses	Presentation	Concentration
Anxiolytics and sedatives	Gabapentin	Analgesic, anxiolytic	Multiple sites of action, but increases available GABA	300–900 mg up to tds or 1.2 g 1 hour pre-op		
	Midazolam	Anxiolytic	Potentiates $GABA_A$	0.1–0.2 mg/kg	Can be given IV, PO, IM	
	Lorazepam	Anxiolytic, terminates seizures	Potentiates $GABA_A$	0.1 mg/kg	IV, PO, IM	
	Diazepam	Anxiolytic, terminates seizures	Potentiates $GABA_A$	0.2–0.3 mg/kg	Can be given rectally	
	Chlorpromazine	Sedation	α antagonist	0.1–-1.0 mg/kg at 1 mg/mn	PO, IV	
	Haloperidol	Sedation	Multiple action sites but post-synaptic dopamine $_{1\&2}$ antagonism predominate. Butyrophenone derivative	2–10 mg 8 hourly	PO, IM, IV	
Vagolytics	Atropine	Vagolytic, anti-sialogogue	Central and peripheral parasympathetic	20 mcg/kg	1 mg in mini jets 600 mcg/ml	
	Glycopyrrolate	Vagolytic, anti-sialogogue	Peripheral parasympathetic	4–10 mcg/kg	200–600 mcg	
Anti-emetics	Cyclizine	Sedative anti-emetic	H_1 antagonist	1 mg/kg	50 mg/ml	
	Dexametha-sone	Anti-inflammatory, anti-emetic	Central effects at the medulla	0.1-0.2 mg/kg	Multiple but in theatre 4 mg/ml	
	Metoclopramide	Prokinetic	Dopamine antagonist	0.1 mg/kg	10 mg/ml	
	Ondansetron	Anti-emetic	$5HT_3$ antagonist	0.1 mg/kg	4 mg/ml	
Other	Mannitol	Diuretic	Osmotic diuretic	0.25–1 g/kg	10% 20%	100 mg/ml 200 mg/ml
	Flumazenil	Reversal agent for benzodiazepines. Acts within a minute. Lasts for 15–140 minutes. Beware rebound seizures	Competitive antagonist at central benzodiazepine receptors	0.1 mg repeated to a total dose of 1 mg IV infusion 100–400 mcg/h	100 mcg/ml	
	Naloxone	Reversal agent for opioid-induced respiratory depression or opioid overdose. Acts within 2 minutes and lasts about 20 minutes	Competitive antagonist at μ, κ, δ, σ opioid receptors	0.1–0.2 mg up to 2 mg	0.02 mg/ml or 0.4 mg/ml	

Physiology and risk in special circumstances

Jane Sturgess

The following tables aim to give the reader an overview of the changes that occur to a patient's vital organ physiology in commonly adopted positions for surgery. Each table is followed by a summary of the important risks specific to the position adopted.

Pneumoperitoneum

System		Increased	Decreased	No change
Respiratory	Tidal volume		X	
	FRC		X	
	Oxygenation	X		
	$ETCO_2$	X		
Cardiovascular	Heart rate	X	(X initially)	
	Cardiac output		X	
	SVR	X		
	BP		X	
	Pre-load		X	
Renal/GI	GFR		X	
	Gastric emptying		X	
CNS	CBF		X	
	Venous drainage		X	
	ICP	X		

Specific risks of the pneumoperitoneum:

- Diaphragmatic splinting and raised airway pressures. A problem in patients with severe respiratory disease. There is a potential for pneumothorax. Minute ventilation needs to be increased to avoid the development of a respiratory acidosis
- Cardiac decompensation in patients with cardiac failure or those who are hypovolaemic
- Risks of initial hypertension and bradyarrhythmias
- Intra-abdominal compartment syndrome if sustained high-inflation pressures required. Can lead to acute kidney injury
- Reflux of abdominal contents

A Surgeon's Guide to Anaesthesia and Peri-operative Care, ed. Jane Sturgess, Justin Davies and Kamen Valchanov. Published by Cambridge University Press.

Prone

System		Increased	Decreased	No change
Respiratory	Tidal volume		X	
	FRC	X		
	Oxygenation	X		
	$ETCO_2$	X		
Cardiovascular	Heart rate	X		
	Cardiac output		X (some studies/some positions, e.g. prone jack knife)	X
	SVR	X		
	BP			X
	Pre-load		X	
Renal/GI	GFR		X	
	Gastric emptying		X	
CNS	CBF		X	
	Venous drainage		X	
	ICP	X		

Specific risks of prone position:

- Injury on turning
- Respiratory problems related to:
  - i. Poor diaphragmatic excursion if abdominal movement is not free
  - ii. Movement of the endotracheal tube on turning – either accidental extubation or endobronchial intubation
- Compression of the great vessels by poor positioning causing cardiovascular collapse
- Cerebrovascular accident in patients with occlusive cerebral artery disease if the head is turned to one side for prolonged periods, or if the neck is over-extended
- Hepatic congestion and potential liver failure if there is prolonged pressure on the right upper quadrant
- Difficulty accessing the airway intra-operatively
- Oropharyngeal swelling, if surgery is prolonged, placing the airway at risk following extubation
- Blindness – not necessarily related to pressure on the globe
- Nerve injuries, especially to the brachial plexus, median and ulnar nerve
- Shoulder injury

Sitting/beach chair

System		Increased	Decreased	No change
Respiratory	Tidal volume	X		
	FRC	X		
	Oxygenation	X		
	$ETCO_2$			X
Cardiovascular	Heart rate			X
	Cardiac output			X
	SVR			X
	BP		X	
	Pre-load		X	
Renal/GI	GFR			X
	Gastric emptying			X
CNS	CBF		X	
	Venous drainage	X		
	ICP	X		

Specific risks of sitting/beach chair position:

- Venous air embolism
- Cardiovascular collapse if no 'anti-gravity suit' utilised
- Pneumocephalus in neurosurgical procedures
- Cardiovascular accident in the elderly patient with carotid artery occlusive disease
- Difficulty accessing the airway intra-operatively
- Oropharyngeal swelling, placing the airway at risk following extubation

Lateral

System		Increased	Decreased	No change
Respiratory	Tidal volume			X
	FRC			X
	Oxygenation			X
	$ETCO_2$			X
Cardiovascular	Heart rate			X
	Cardiac output			X
	SVR			X
	BP			X
	Pre-load			X
Renal/GI	GFR			X
	Gastric emptying			X
CNS	CBF			X
	Venous drainage			X
	ICP			X

Specific risks in the lateral position:

- Ventilation–perfusion mismatch in the dependent and non-dependent lungs. Overall normal oxygenation
- Venous hypertension in the dependent arm
- Nerve injury to exposed peripheral nerves, e.g. ulnar, common peroneal
- Brachial plexus injury to the upper arm
- Electrical burns if metal arm supports are not adequately padded, and prevented from touching the patient's skin directly

Trendelenburg (head down)

System		Increased	Decreased	No change
Respiratory	Tidal volume		X	
	FRC		X	
	Oxygenation		X	
	$ETCO_2$	X		
Cardiovascular	Heart rate		X	
	Cardiac output	X		
	SVR		X	
	BP	X		
	Pre-load	X		
Renal/GI	GFR			X
	Gastric emptying		X	
CNS	CBF	X		
	Venous drainage		X	
	ICP	X		

Specific risks in the Trendelenburg position:

- Regurgitation of gastric contents
- Confusion from cerebral oedema secondary to venous congestion
- Potential fluid overload in patients with brittle cardiac function
- Theoretical risk of raised intra-ocular pressure, especially in those with glaucoma
- 'Slipping on the table' – supports and strapping are often required for steep Trendelenburg. These supports and strapping can cause pressure injuries themselves

Reverse Trendelenburg (head up)

System		Increased	Decreased	No change
Respiratory	Tidal volume			X
	FRC			X
	Oxygenation			X
	$ETCO_2$			X
Cardiovascular	Heart rate			X
	Cardiac output		X	
	SVR			X
	BP		X	
	Pre-load		X	
Renal/GI	GFR			X
	Gastric emptying			X
CNS	CBF			X
	Venous drainage	X		
	ICP		X	

Specific risk's of reverse Trendelenburg position:

- Venous air embolism
- Cardiovascular collapse, especially in combination with pneumoperitoneum
- Cerebrovascular accident in patients with occlusive carotid artery disease
- 'Slipping on the table' – supports and strapping are often required for steep reverse Trendelenburg. These supports and strapping can cause pressure injuries themselves

Lithotomy/legs up/Lloyd Davies

System		Increased	Decreased	No change
Respiratory	Tidal volume			X
	FRC			X
	Oxygenation			X
	$ETCO_2$			X
Cardiovascular	Heart rate			X
	Cardiac output	X		
	SVR			X
	BP	X		
	Pre-load	X		
Renal/GI	GFR			X
	Gastric emptying			X
CNS	CBF			X
	Venous drainage			X
	ICP			X

Specific risks of lithotomy/legs up/Lloyd Davies position:

- Volume overload in susceptible individuals, raise legs slowly and inform the anaesthetist
- Rebound hypotension as patient returned to supine position and pre-load temporarily decreases
- Compartment syndrome in calves because of direct pressure and hypoperfusion (especially in combination with pneumoperitoneum and Trendelenburg positions)
- Injury to femoral and common peroneal nerves
- Difficult for the anesthetist to access the airway and the circulation intra-operatively

Medicolegal aspects of consent

Kamen Valchanov

Medicine, surgery and anaesthesia offer services to patients, to which they need to agree, and it has to be in their best interests. Therefore, consent for surgery takes a critical place in the legal position of interventional treatments.

In medical terms consent is the provision of approval or agreement to a medical treatment. As such medical consent is a contract between caregivers and patients. In this chapter we will discuss the types of consent, the mechanisms of obtaining consent and the ethical issues surrounding it.

All medical interventions have intended benefits, success rates and complication rates. In addition the consequences of omitting a medical intervention have to be considered, as well as any potential alternative treatment options.

Consent is a process, and has several potential aspects to it:

Written consent

Written consent is a document, which explains that a competent medical practitioner offers an intervention to a patient, explains the intended benefits, with their success rates, as well as possible complications and alternatives. The document has to be signed and dated by both parties, preferably after sufficient time to allow the patient to assimilate the relevant information that will allow a fully informed decision to be made. This then begs the question: who is deemed a competent medical practitioner? In theory this could be a doctor who could potentially carry out the intervention, but ideally it should be the operator. It is important this documentation is carefully stored for medicolegal reasons.

Verbal consent

Verbal consent is given by using verbal communication. Interestingly, written consent for general anaesthesia is not mandatory in UK, and indeed implied in the surgical consent by stating the procedure will be carried out under general anaesthetic. There has been a movement to change this practice in the future.

Implied consent

Implied consent is a controversial term. It refers to consent given to a procedure, carrying a particular risk, which is presumed as known to the patient. This presumed knowledge of a

A Surgeon's Guide to Anaesthesia and Peri-operative Care, ed. Jane Sturgess, Justin Davies and Kamen Valchanov. Published by Cambridge University Press.

risk is not documented in the consent. A typical example is consent for minor surgical procedure carried out under general anaesthesia, which has an inherent risk of death.

Elaine Bromiley's case

In 2005 Elaine Bromiley died as a result of problems that developed during anaesthesia for elective sinus surgery. She developed a serious airway complication resulting in hypoxia, brain injury and death 13 days later. Since then, and in part because of the creation of the Clinical Human Factors Group by her husband, an airline pilot, errors have become culturally more accepted as something to be expected, managed and learnt from. Another issue is whether she would have consented for surgery knowing that there was a risk of death because of an anaesthetic complication.

Informed consent

Informed consent is important to define. It is important there is trust between the patient and medical practitioner, as the medical practitioner acts in the best interests of the patient and up to the current standards of medical practice. There are few elements to the informed consent:

1. Explain in simple terms, i.e. terms ensuring patient's comprehension of the procedure. Explain the necessary steps taken during the intervention.
2. Explain the intended benefit.
3. Explain the success rate.
4. Explain common and unavoidable risks and their treatment.
5. Explain rare but serious complications, e.g. paralysis after an epidural.
6. Explain any potential alternative treatments or interventions.
7. Invite the patient to ask questions.
8. Answer honestly and to the best of medical knowledge.

To what extent a medical practitioner needs to explain the details of a procedure and complications is less easy to define. A typical example is explaining to a patient prior to consenting for aortic valve replacement and coronary bypass grafting with a Logistic Euroscore of 5 that they have 5% or 1 in 20 chance of dying from this operation. Anaesthetists inform patients of post-dural puncture headache of 1 in 200 prior to epidural analgesia.

Answering patient's questions is the most difficult part of the consenting process. It relies on the consentor having adequate medical knowledge and a sufficient degree of expertise. Many patients would have read negative articles in newspapers and the internet prior to their procedure and would ask questions regarding the incidence of particular complications. It is important to answer questions honestly. If the consenter has performed a limited number of these operations they can honestly say so. Awareness under general anaesthesia is commonly quoted as 1 in 500, but one can declare they are not aware a patient of theirs has suffered from this complication. This does not mean any of their patients could not have suffered from a provoked recall.

Bolam test

The informed consent definitions have been tested in British law on several occasions. In this context the first point to discuss is the Bolam test: Bolam was a voluntary patient in a mental health institution. He agreed to electroconvulsive therapy. He was given an electroconvulsive shock without muscle relaxation or appropriate restraint, resulting in severe injuries, including acetabular fractures. He sued the Trust for negligence. The general medical opinion was that the electroconvulsive shock was acceptable practice, and hence there was no negligence. Henceforth the Bolam principle states that if a doctor reaches the standard of a responsible body of medical opinion, he/she is not negligent.

Conditions of consenting

Ideally informed consent for elective procedures should be unhurried, in advance of the proposed procedure, in a location suitable for private discussions, and in the presence of the next of kin. The process starts with information, preferably written as well as verbal, given to the patient about the risks, benefits and alternatives to the treatment, culminating in the signing of the consent form prior to the procedure itself. This process may go on over several weeks, with the patient able to ask any questions in the intervening time. This is not always practical, and in case of emergencies could not be complied with. A typical example is obtaining consent from a patient with a ruptured aortic aneurysm, where time is of the essence, and consent is usually discussed in brief terms in the emergency department.

Ethical issues of consenting

Capacity

It is important to observe the right of the patient to self-determination. In other words because we can carry out a procedure, and believe it would benefit the patient, this does not mean we should carry it out. A competent patient can refuse treatment, and hence in the absence of consent it must not be carried out. For a patient with capacity, the information that should be provided about a particular intervention as part of the consent process should include a discussion of the potential benefits, risks, alternatives and the consequences of omitting treatment. Information must be imparted in a way that takes account of a patient's level of knowledge and understanding of what is being proposed.

However, not all patients are deemed competent. 'Competent' means a patient who can understand the consequences of the proposed actions. Typically, children under the age of 16 cannot consent, and it is their parents and legal guardians who can sign the consent form for them. Certain psychiatric patients lacking mental capacity are unable to consent, as well as unconscious patients. In these circumstances the decisions for carrying out surgical procedures rely on the medical profession making the best decision for the patient. Where possible such procedures should be explained to the next of kin. In circumstances where the patient has left a power of attorney those nominated are legally competent to make informed decisions for the patient.

Gillick competence

In 1984 Mrs Victoria Gillick ran an active campaign against a new policy to allow doctors discretion in prescribing contraceptives to children under the age of 16 without parental consent. Mrs Gillick sought a declaration that prescribing contraception was illegal because the doctor would commit an offence of encouraging sex with a minor, and that it would be treatment without consent as consent rested in the parent.

This case prompted the judgement: As a matter of law the parental right to determine whether or not their minor child below the age of 16 will have medical treatment terminates if and when the child achieves sufficient understanding and intelligence to understand fully what is proposed.

Jehovah's Witness

Jehovah's Witness patients present common difficulty in informed consent. Their beliefs mean that they generally refuse to receive transfusion of blood and blood products. The members of the religion are heterogeneous in their attitudes towards transfusional medicine. Some are willing to accept particular blood products, and some refuse any blood having left their body, including through a cardiopulmonary bypass machine. It is the duty of the consenting practitioner to understand and document the exact beliefs of the patient, and follow their instructions in order to follow legal consent.

Unconscious patients

With the advances of organ support in Critical Care Medicine it is possible to support patients for a long time and extend the boundaries of medicine. Patients in renal failure and cardiac failure who used to die in the past are now supported to recovery or transplantation. However, not all conditions are recoverable in the current standards of medicine. Hence, it is the duty of the medical team to make decisions in the patient's best interests, including undergoing emergency procedures. In such cases, where the patient is not competent, or unable to sign, written informed consent cannot be obtained. The medical profession has a duty to carry out procedures to save their lives. In these cases a discussion with the family explaining the situation and intended plan for management is a part of good communication, but cannot yield valid consent, unless the patient has an advanced directive. Family assent, rather than consent, is obtained. The decision should also be discussed with and counter-signed by a fellow medical professional in these challenging circumstances.

Further reading

General Medical Council guidance for doctors. *Consent: Patients and Doctors Making Decisions Together*. London: GMC Publications, 2008.

Royal College of Surgeons. Advancing Surgical Standards: Consent for Blood Transfusion. London: RCS, 2010.

Wheeler, R. Consent in surgery. *Ann R Coll Surg Engl* 2006; **88**: 261–4.

Section III At a glance

Nerve injury

Jane Sturgess

Nerve injury is one of the leading causes for settled cases of litigation. Medical Protection Services data have shown that of all the cases that are recorded, 75% proceed to a claim for medical negligence. The incidence of nerve damage has been described as between 1:1,000 or as frequent as 1:350 cases.

The nerves most often affected are ulnar (30–43%), brachial plexus (25%), lumbosacral roots (16%) and common peroneal (11%). It has historically been considered that stretch and pressure effects on nerves are the predominant cause for nerve injury. Many retrospective studies looking at closed claims analysis have called this in to question, yet it remains the most often blamed cause for injury. Analysis of cases in studies has shown that many factors play a contributing role in the development of nerve injury. Some patients (the elderly, frail, diabetic, hypertensive, anaemic patient) can be identified as at greater risk, and extra care and attention can be placed on reducing the additive problems of pressure and stretch.

It is also interesting to note that cases of peripheral nerve injury may have a delayed presentation and are not often apparent in the recovery room. Most present within the first 24 hours, and over 90% present within seven days post-operatively. About 60% of patients with a nerve injury will recover within a year, but a quarter will suffer persistent pain.

Nerve injury can be caused by excessive stretch of nerves or plexi; pressure injury because of poor positioning; direct injury by needles or sharp surgical instruments; chemical injury because of local anaesthetics or antiseptic solutions.

Prevention

Protection from injury is the responsibility of both the surgeon and the anaesthetist. Even though many cases of nerve injury occur without pressure or stretch, there is no excuse for failing to pay attention to pressure areas while positioning the patient. Choosing a position which will allow good surgical exposure but does not subject the patient to unreasonable risk of injury is important. Careful padding of pressure areas and regularly checking, or movement of the area, during long cases is essential. When operating near important nerve structures careful dissection and location of nerve structures can prevent most of the injuries.

Nerve injury can be central or peripheral. Central nerve injury is a result of damage to the spinal cord, and peripheral nerve injury results from damage to peripheral nerves.

A Surgeon's Guide to Anaesthesia and Peri-operative Care, ed. Jane Sturgess, Justin Davies and Kamen Valchanov. Published by Cambridge University Press.

Central nerve injury

Table 30.1 Summary of the causes of central nerve injury

Anaesthetic	1. Needle damage – typical areas are lumbar and thoracic spine because of spinal and epidural injections, as well as cervical spine because of brachial plexus blocks 2. Skin preparation contamination – when no other reason for the nerve injury following neuraxial blocks can be found, it is assumed that the reason for the injury is the skin cleansing antiseptic used prior to the procedure 3. Incorrect drug – injecting incorrect medication intrathecally (e.g. vincristine) can lead to permanent neurological deficit and painful demise. As these events continue over the years new non-Luer-Lock systems for intrathecal injections have been introduced 4. Catheter related – small intrathecal and epidural catheters can directly injure spinal cord or cauda equina 5. Infection (arachnoiditis/encephalitis/compression) – sterile or bacterial infections because of epidural and intrathecal manipulations can produce both systemic effects and local spinal cord compression with devastating and sometimes permanent deficit 6. Haematoma (compression by space occupying lesion) – haematoma in the spinal canal occurs because of excessive manipulations and poor coagulation. If this emergency is not treated within hours the neurological deficit can be permanent
Surgical	1. Cord hypoperfusion – typically resulting from aortic cross-clamping reducing spinal arterial supply. Monitoring of these effects intra-operatively and using partial bypass techniques can reduce its incidence 2. Manipulation of unstable spinal injury could sever the spinal cord or produce neuropraxia 3. Haematoma – this needs early recognition and evacuation

Peripheral nerve injury

Table 30.2 Summary of the causes of peripheral nerve injury

Anaesthetic	Needle damage from regional anaesthetic techniques Skin preparation contamination during regional techniques Incorrect drug Intraneural injection (most troublesome if intra-fascicular injection) Toxicity of local anaesthetics in high concentration caused by inappropriate dose/equipment failure or pooling of anaesthetic Pressure from airway devices on nerves supplying the airway
Surgical	Accidental (or deliberate) ligation causing direct neural injury Compression with surgical instruments Secondary damage from LASERs/thermal insults from diathermy/ultrasonic ablation Tourniquet pressure effects Compression from haematoma Radiotherapy injury

Surgical-specific	Acoustic nerve injury can be unavoidable with some surgical approaches Accidental laryngeal nerve injury during neck surgery can produce vocal cord palsy (e.g. thyroid surgery) Phrenic nerve injury during intrathoracic procedures has serious consequences for complicated patients like lung transplant recipients Vagal nerve injury is often accidental as planned surgical vagotomies are rarely performed
Positioning	Pressure Stretch Superficial nature of the nerve
Patient factors	Extremes of BMI Increasing age Pre-existing peripheral neuropathy Diabetes Males > females Peripheral vascular disease
Peri-operative factors	Hypovolaemia/dehydration Prolonged hypotension (or occasionally limited) Hypoxia Induced hypothermia Electrolyte disturbance Prolonged procedure

Specific types of peri-operative nerve injury

Traumatic nerve injury

In cases of major and complicated trauma, major peripheral nerves can be affected but not diagnosed until after life- or limb-saving surgery is completed. In such cases careful documentation of all steps taken by surgical and anaesthetic teams is important to avoid further litigation.

Visual loss

Visual loss because of nerve injury has a special place in this section because of its devastating consequences. Optic injury and blindness can occur after prone positioning and was originally thought to be because of pressure on the globe. Visual loss is presumed to be caused by retinal artery occlusion, but there are increasing numbers of cases where this is not the mechanism. The most commonly accepted current theory for this alternative cause of blindness is a 'compartment like syndrome' affecting the blood supply and drainage of the globe, leading to ischaemic optic neuropathy. Neither has a good prognosis.

Pain and nerve injury

Little is known of the long-term consequences of peripheral nerve block complications. In the 1980s and 1990s there was a vogue for central neuraxial blocks where the enthusiasts popularised these techniques as safer and producing benefits in terms of reducing mortality, post-operative complications and reducing hospital stay. It was later clear that while in some cases central neuraxial blocks are beneficial, they are not necessarily safer than general anaesthetics and many of the stipulated benefits have been questioned and dismissed. Similarly, because of much improved quality of ultrasound, peripheral nerve blocks are gaining popularity. Undoubtedly, these provide excellent post-operative pain control. However, the long-term effects of these techniques need evaluating in time. In many cases peripheral nerve blocks produce prolonged motor block and analgesia. However, in some, chronic pain in the distribution of the blocked nerve can be detected. Data on long-term nerve damage would have to be evaluated in the next decade before a conclusion on risk/ benefit can be drawn.

Neuropathic pain

Neuropathic pain can result from division of a nerve or compression during retraction by means of pathological nerve healing. It has to be borne in mind that injuring a nerve can not only produce loss of function but also pathological healing that leads to neuropathic pain. As such the latter can worsen patient's quality of life dramatically, and may lead to litigation. A typical example is the neuropathic pain post-thoracotomy. Conventional thoracotomy involves costotomy and therefore division of an intercostal nerve. Healing of the injured intercostal nerves is frequently pathological, and chronic pain incidence post-operatively is quoted as high as 25% or more. In a case of bullectomy or lobectomy the patient can be technically cured but their quality of life may subsequently worsen because of the devastating effects of neuropathic pain. Thoracoscopic approaches avoid the costotomy phase and could help reduce these problems.

Summary

Peri-operative nerve injury is more common than perceived. In many of the cases it improves and can completely heal. In cases when it remains permanent it dramatically impairs quality of life, and therefore is a subject of litigation. Preventing nerve injury is often possible and good team work between surgeons, anaesthetists and theatre personnel, as well as attention to detail is necessary. Prompt detection is likely to offer the best chance of recovery.

Further reading

Bogod D, Szypula K. Injury during anaesthesia. *Anaesthetic and Peri-operative Complications*. Cambridge: Cambridge University Press, 2011; pp. 119–29.

Sawyer RJ, Richmond MN, Hickey JD, Jarratt JA. Peripheral nerve injuries associated with anaesthesia. *Anaesthesia* 2000; **55**: 980–91.

Warner MA, Warner ME, Martin JT. Ulnar neuropathy. Incidence, outcome and risk factors in sedated or anesthetized patients. *Anaesthesiology* 1994; **81**(6): 1332–40.

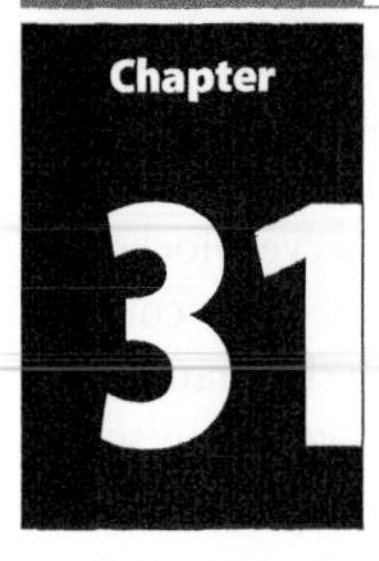

Pre-operative investigations

Joseph E. Arrowsmith

Introduction

Among the many roles that the anaesthetist has, risk assessment and risk modification are perhaps the most important. In order to manage peri-operative risk, the anaesthetist must have an understanding of the impact of co-existing medical conditions and concomitant drug therapy on normal physiology, and an appreciation of their likely interactions with both anaesthesia and surgery. When conducted effectively, pre-operative assessment decreases the risk of cancellations on the day of surgery and has the potential to reduce peri-operative morbidity and mortality.

Taking a detailed medical history and performing a competent physical examination remain the most efficient and effective ways of predicting and detecting significant co-morbid conditions. Pre-operative investigations should therefore be considered an adjunct to, rather than a substitute for, basic medical vigilance. Many pre-operative clinical investigations are justifiable on the grounds that they aid diagnosis (e.g. CT scan), assist in surgical planning (e.g. coronary angiography), permit more accurate risk stratification (e.g. exercise testing), guide risk-modification strategies or provide a 'baseline' before major surgery. A significant number of tests, however, are ordered 'routinely' without any clinical indication or justification.

The laws of probability dictate that ordering multiple tests will eventually yield abnormal results. For continuous variables, such as sodium, potassium and haemoglobin concentration, the so-called 'normal' or reference range quoted by clinical laboratories is typically the mean ±1.96 standard deviations. By definition, therefore, 5% of normal individuals will have a test result that lies outside the reference range (i.e. 2.5% above and 2.5% below). Given the probability that a test result will lie within the normal range is 0.95, the likelihood of obtaining twenty normal test results is only 36% (i.e. 0.95^{20}). The more tests that are ordered, the more likely it is that an abnormal result will be reported – even in completely healthy individuals.

The important questions are:

- What is the significance of the finding of an abnormal test result in an otherwise healthy and asymptomatic patient?
- In a patient with symptomatically stable chronic disease, how likely is a test result to be significantly different for previous results?
- How might a test result lead to an alteration in patient management?
- Will an alteration in patient management improve the clinical outcome?

A Surgeon's Guide to Anaesthesia and Peri-operative Care, ed. Jane Sturgess, Justin Davies and Kamen Valchanov. Published by Cambridge University Press.

Guidelines

The Association of Anaesthetists of Great Britain and Ireland (AAGBI) published updated guidance on pre-operative assessment and patient preparation in 2010. In the section on investigation, it is stated that *'Routine pre-operative investigations are expensive, labour intensive and of questionable value, especially as they contribute to morbidity or cause additional delays because of spurious results.'* Citing guidelines published by the National Institute for Health and Clinical Excellence, the authors go on to recommend that some tests should be undertaken routinely in a number of specific patient groups before most types of surgery – even procedures typically performed on a day-care basis (Tables 31.1 and 31.2).

Despite the publication of clinical guidelines, healthcare professionals and patients harbour fundamental misunderstandings about the utility of routine pre-operative testing. Believing that they are erring on the side of caution, clinicians seemingly order tests in the

Table 31.1 Pre-operative tests recommended by the National Institute for Health and Clinical Excellence

Test	Indication(s)
Electrocardiograph (ECG)	Patients >80 years old Patients >60 years old undergoing grade 3 or 4 surgery Patients with *any* cardiovascular disease Patients with *severe* renal disease (creatinine >150 μmol l^{-1})
Full blood count	Patients >60 years old undergoing grade 2, 3 or 4 surgery All adults undergoing grade 3 or 4 surgery Patients with *severe* renal disease (creatinine >150 μmol l^{-1}) *Anaemia should be investigated and treated before planned surgery*
Urea, electrolytes and creatinine	Patients >60 years old undergoing grade 3 or 4 surgery All adults undergoing grade 4 surgery Patients with *any* renal disease Patients with *severe* cardiovascular disease (CCS class III or IV angina pectoris with marked limitation of ordinary activity, myocardial infarction within the last month, decompensated cardiac failure, severe symptomatic valvular disease)
Pregnancy test	All women who may be pregnant
Sickle cell test	Members of families with homozygous disease or heterozygous trait Patients with African, Afro-Caribbean, Asian, Middle-Eastern or east-Mediterranean ancestry
Chest radiograph	Patient scheduled for post-operative admission to critical care unit
Exercise ECG **Cardiopulmonary exercise testing (CPX)** **Myocardial perfusion studies**	According to severity of cardio-respiratory disease, functional capacity and grade of planned surgery

Source: National Collaborating Centre for Acute Care. *Pre-operative Tests. The Use of Routine Pre-operative Tests for Elective Surgery. Evidence, Methods And Guidance.* London: NICE, 2003. Available at http://guidance.nice.org.uk/CG3/Guidance/pdf/English. See Table 31.2 for examples of surgical complexity grade. CCS, Canadian Cardiovascular Society.

Table 31.2 Surgical complexity

Grade	Examples
1	Diagnostic endoscopy, diagnostic laparoscopy, breast biopsy, cataract surgery
2	Inguinal hernia repair, varicose vein surgery, adenotonsillectomy, knee arthroscopy
3	Total abdominal hysterectomy, transurethral resection of prostate, lumbar discectomy, thyroidectomy
4	Total knee or hip replacement, arterial reconstruction/bypass, colonic resection, radical neck dissection

belief that they are an effective opportunistic screen for disease that cannot be detected or predicted on the basis of history and examination. Moreover, it is widely believed (correctly or incorrectly) that ordering a comprehensive battery of tests will 'cover all the bases' and somehow 'appease' even the most exacting anaesthetist – providing sufficient time to rectify any unexpected problems before surgery. As recently stated in an editorial, *'One could be forgiven for thinking that routine testing has acquired its own therapeutic value and, at least in part, replaced the need for taking a clinical history and performing a competent physical examination.'*

Routine testing

Ordering tests routinely, without sound clinical indication, is a potentially risky strategy – especially on the day of surgery itself when the results may not available to the operating team at the scheduled start of surgery. Strictly speaking, an anaesthetist would be perfectly justified in delaying or even cancelling a procedure because the result of a pre-operative test was unavailable. To do otherwise, at least in theory, exposes the entire medical team to medicolegal risk. More often than not, however, an unexpectedly abnormal test result has little or no impact on the conduct of anaesthesia and surgery, or indeed the clinical outcome. The obvious question is: why subject a patient to the assault (and associated expense) of an unnecessary test and then disregard the result?

Regardless of the indication, the finding of an abnormal test result carries with it the obligation to evaluate its clinical significance and decide upon the need for further investigation. This burden of clinical responsibility may not be immediately obvious to well-intending non-medical personnel that have ordered tests that are not clinically indicated. It should come as no surprise to learn that, in up to 60% of cases, the discovery of an abnormal test result before elective surgery leads to no further investigation. In many instances, this might actually be in a patient's best interests because acting on a clinically insignificant result may lead to needless postponement of surgery and expose the patient to the unnecessary risk of further investigations, treatment or procedures (Table 31.3).

The truth is that, when used to screen for disease, the positive predictive value of individual tests is low. In a study of 9,584 American Society of Anesthesiologists (ASA) class I or 2 patients undergoing low-risk, day-case surgery, routine pre-operative testing revealed anaemia (haemoglobin concentration $<90\ \text{gl}^{-1}$) in 75 (0.8%) patients. The finding of anaemia resulted in no alteration in peri-operative management. Four other patients with

Table 31.3 Routine pre-operative testing

Test	Findings
Chest X-ray	Abnormal in 7.4% (2.5–37.0%) patients Change in management in 0.5% (0–2.1%) patients Abnormality rates increase with patient age Usefulness as predictor of post-operative complications – uncertain
Electrocardiograph	Abnormal in 12.4% (4.6–31.7%) patients Change in management in 0.6% (0.2.2%) patients Abnormality rates increase *exponentially* with patient age Usefulness as predictor of post-operative complications – little or no value
Haemoglobin	Abnormal in 1.1% (0.7–4.8%) patients Change in management in 0.2% (0.1–2.7%) patients Usefulness as predictor of peri-operative complications – none
Platelet count	Abnormal in 0.9% (0–8.0%) patients Change in management – rare, if ever
White cell count	Abnormal in 0.3% (0.1–0.9%) patients Change in management – rare, if ever
Haemostasis	***Bleeding time*** abnormal in 1.9% (0–3.8%) patients ***Prothrombin time*** abnormal in 0.2% (0–4.8%) patients ***Partial thromboplastin time*** abnormal in 1.9% (0–15.6%) patients Change in management – rare Usefulness as predictor of peri-operative bleeding – none
Biochemistry	Serum ***sodium*** concentration abnormal in 0.5% patients Serum ***potassium*** concentration abnormal in 0.8% (02.-1.4%) patients Change in management in 0.2% (0–0.4%) patients Serum ***urea*** concentration abnormal in 1.3% patients Serum ***creatinine*** concentration abnormal in 0.7% patients Change in management – rare Blood ***glucose*** concentration abnormal in 1.9% (1.1–5.2%) patients Change in management in 0.1% (0–0.2%) patients
Urine testing	***White blood cells*** present in 7.3% (4.3–10.6%) patients Change in management in 2.4% (0.1–2.8%) patients ***Red blood cells*** present in 4.0% (1.7–4.9%) patients Change in management – rare ***Glucose*** present in 3.3% (2.2–5.7%) patients Change in management – rare ***Glucose*** present in 13% patients Change in management – rare

Source: Munro J, Booth A, Nicholl J, *et al.* Routine pre-operative testing – estimates of frequency of abnormal findings and likelihood of subsequent change in clinical management extracted from 82 studies. *Health Technol Assess* 1997; 1(12): i-iv; 1–62.

haemoglobin concentration >90 gl^{-1} received red cell transfusions on the basis of symptoms (e.g. dyspnoea) or physical signs (e.g. third heart sound) alone.

The superiority of history and examination over routine pre-operative testing was demonstrated in a prospective study of over 17,000 day-care surgical patients. Clinical risk factors such as obesity, asthma, gastro-oesphageal reflux, hypertension, and smoking were much better predictors of adverse post-operative events than abnormal pre-operative test results.

In a study of 513 elderly patients undergoing non-cardiac surgery, 386 (75%) had at least one abnormality on their pre-operative electrocardiograph (ECG). Multivariate analysis revealed that predictors of post-operative cardiac complications included physical status and a history of congestive cardiac failure. The finding of an abnormal ECG was not associated with an increased risk of post-operative cardiac complications.

A systematic review of three studies in which a total of 21,531 patients undergoing cataract surgery were randomised to either routine testing or to selective or no testing revealed that testing reduced the risk of neither intra-operative nor post-operative adverse events.

More recently, the authors of a systematic review of the effectiveness of non-cardiac investigation in patients undergoing non-cardiac surgery concluded that there was no evidence to support routine pre-operative testing in healthy adults undergoing non-cardiac surgery. Of interest, it was concluded that the evidence for testing on the basis of medical history and physical examination was 'scarce'.

Targeted investigation

The roles of targeted investigation in patients with known or suspected co-morbid disease are: documentation of the presence, severity and progression of disease; detection of active or unstable conditions that require further evaluation; determination of the need for additional testing or therapeutic intervention and quantification of peri-operative risk. This is well illustrated by patients with cardiac disease scheduled to undergo non-cardiac surgery. In this situation the risks of proceeding to surgery without delay have to be balanced against the risks of delay and the inherent risks of the tests themselves. Published in 2009, the European Society of Cardiology (ESC) *Guidelines for Pre-operative Cardiac Risk Assessment and Peri-operative Risk Management in Non-Cardiac Surgery* recommend that the Lee Revised Cardiac Risk Index (RCRI) be used for peri-operative risk stratification and to guide pre-operative testing. Unfortunately cardiac risk indices, particularly those that include only pre-operative factors, have their limitations. A recent study failed to confirm that all of the Lee RCRI risk factors were independent predictors of outcome, and identified additional pre-operative and *intra-operative* predictors of outcome (Table 31.4). More recently still, a more simplified risk index has been shown to have superior predictive power. Large overlaps between the 95% confidence intervals of the risk classes dictate that they are better suited for comparing risk in different populations rather than predicting risk to an individual (Table 31.5). Details of a systematic, step-wise approach to pre-operative cardiac risk assessment and investigation can be found elsewhere.

While this guideline-based approach appears to serve low- and high-risk patients reasonably well, the role of pre-operative testing in intermediate-risk patients is less clear. In the second Dutch Echocardiographic Cardiac Risk Evaluation Applying Stress Echocardiography (DECREASE II) study, 770 intermediate-risk patients scheduled to undergo vascular surgery were randomised to no additional testing or to have surgery delayed to permit further testing. Patients in the latter group had either dobutamine stress echocardiography or stress perfusion scintigraphy, and (if indicated) coronary angiography. There

Table 31.4 Independent predictors of cardiovascular complications

Lee, 1999 (RCRI)	Kheterpal, 2009	Davis, 2013
High-risk surgery History of ischaemic heart disease History of congestive heart failure History of cerebrovascular disease Pre-operative treatment with insulin Pre-operative serum creatinine concentration >177 µmol/l (2.0 mg/dl)	Emergency surgery Previous cardiac intervention Active congestive heart failure Cerebrovascular disease Age >68 years BMI >30 kg/ m^2 Hypertension Duration of surgery ≥3.8 hours PRBC transfusion ≥1 unit	High-risk type of surgery History of ischaemic heart disease Congestive heart failure Cerebrovascular disease GFR <30 ml/min

RCRI, Revised Cardiac Risk Index; BMI, body mass index; PRBC, packed red blood cells; GFR, glomerular filtration rate. From: Lee TH, Marcantonio ER, Mangione CM, *et al. Circulation* 1999; 100(10): 1043–9, Kheterpal S, Tremper KK, Englesbe MJ, *et al. Anesthesiology* 2009; 110(1): 58–66 and Davis, *et al. Can J Anaesth* 2013; 60(9): 855–863.

Table 31.5 Risk classes and incidence of cardiac complications

		Adverse cardiovascular events				
		Lee, 1999 (RCRI)		Kheterpal, 2009		
Risk class	Risk factors	n	% (95% CI)	n	%	HR (95% CI)
I	0	2/488	0.4 (0.05–1.5)	5/2,222	0.2	-
II	1	5/567	0.0 (0.3–2.1)	13/2,531	0.5	2.3 (0.8–6.4)
III	2	17/258	6.6 (3.9–10.3)	25/1,885	1.3	6.0 (2.3–15.6)
IV	≥3	12/109	11.0 (5.8–18.4)	40/1,102	3.6	16.7 (6.6–42.4)

RCRI, Revised Cardiac Risk Index; CI, confidence interval; HR, hazard ratio. Source: Priebe (2012) after Lee *et al.* (1999) and Kheterpal *et al.* (2009).

was no statistically significant difference in the primary end-points (myocardial infarction or cardiac death at 30 days and two years after surgery). Additional testing caused an average delay to surgery of 19 days. Frustratingly, the suspension of the senior DECREASE investigator in 2011 for misconduct has cast doubt over the validity of the findings.

The question of whether pre-operative cardiac testing alters medical or surgical management was investigated in 235 consecutive patients aged >60 years with hip fractures undergoing surgery at a level 1 trauma centre. A total of 35 (15%) patients underwent pre-operative cardiac testing – 16 (6.9%) for a newly diagnosed cardiac problem and 19 (8.1) for known, stable cardiovascular disease. Although cardiovascular complications were more common in tested patients (15% *vs.* 0.5%), pre-operative cardiac testing did not change surgical management and no patient underwent coronary revascularisation as a result of the testing. In only half (52%) of patients were changes in medical treatment for known cardiac disease recommended. Cardiac testing resulted in significant delay (3.3 vs. 1.9 days) and increased cost (>$1,200/ >£780/ >€900 per patient tested).

In a retrospective study conducted in Canada, the impact of non-invasive pre-operative cardiac stress testing on length of hospital stay and mortality was investigated in a cohort of 271,082 patients, aged 40 years or over, undergoing elective intermediate and high-risk non-cardiac surgery. Compared to 23,060 propensity-matched untested patients, the 23,991 (8.9%) patients who underwent stress testing had greater one-year survival and shorter length of hospital stay. Sub-group analysis revealed that testing was of benefit in patients undergoing intra-abdominal or intrathoracic surgery, but of questionable value in orthopaedic and vascular patients. Testing in low-risk patients was associated with harm. Interestingly, stress testing was more likely to be undertaken in males; in patients with several co-morbid conditions; at moderate- to high-volume, non-teaching medical centres; and in patients undergoing vascular, hepatic, pancreatic, pulmonary, renal and oesophageal surgery.

Conclusions

Obtaining a comprehensive medical history and performing a competent physical examination remains the most efficient and accurate way to detect significant disease. Pre-operative testing should be considered *after* the history and examination, using established clinical guidelines and common sense.

In patients with known co-morbidity, many of whom will be under routine medical follow-up, the results of recent investigations should be sought before ordering unnecessarily repetitive tests.

Pre-operative tests that do not aid diagnosis, assist in surgical planning, aid risk stratification and risk-modification strategies or provide a useful 'baseline' before major surgery are a waste of time, effort and money.

Pre-operative tests should not be ordered if the results will not be available at the time of surgery.

Pre-operative tests have no inherent therapeutic value.

Further reading

Chung F, Mezei G, Tong D. Pre-existing medical conditions as predictors of adverse events in day-case surgery. *Br J Anaesth* 1999; **83(2)**: 262–70.

Johansson T, Fritsch G, Flamm M, *et al.* Effectiveness of non-cardiac pre-operative testing in non-cardiac elective surgery: a systematic review. *Br J Anaesth* 2013; **110(6)**: 926–39.

Klein AA, Arrowsmith JE. Should routine pre-operative testing be abandoned? *Anaesthesia* 2010; **65(10)**: 974–6.

Priebe HJ. Cardiovascular disease and non-cardiac surgery. In Mackay JH, Arrowsmith JE, eds., *Core Topics in Cardiac Anesthesia, 2nd edn.* Cambridge: Cambridge University Press, 2012; pp. 469–78.

Ricci WM, Della Rocca GJ, Combs C, Borrelli J. The medical and economic impact of pre-operative cardiac testing in elderly patients with hip fractures. *Injury* 2007; **38 (Suppl. 3)**: S49–52.

Smetana GW, Macpherson DS. The case against routine pre-operative laboratory testing. *Med Clin North Am* 2003; **87(1)**: 7–40.

Task Force for Pre-operative Cardiac Risk Assessment and Peri-operative Cardiac Management in Non-cardiac Surgery; European Society of Cardiology (ESC),

Poldermans D, Bax JJ, Boersma E, *et al.* Guidelines for pre-operative cardiac risk assessment and peri-operative cardiac management in non-cardiac surgery. *Eur Heart J* 2009; **30(22)**: 2769–812.

Valchanov KP, Steel A. Pre-operative investigation of the surgical patient. *Surgery (Oxford)* 2008; **26(9)**: 363–8.

Wijeysundera DN, Beattie WS, Austin PC, Hux JE, Laupacis A. Non-invasive cardiac stress testing before elective major non-cardiac surgery: population-based cohort study. *BMJ* 2010; **340**: b5526.

Working Party of the Association of Anaesthetists of Great Britain and Ireland. *AAGBI Safety Guideline. Pre-operative Assessment and Patient Preparation: The Role of the Anaesthetist 2.* London: AAGBI, 2010. Available at http://www.aagbi.org/sites/default/files/preop2010.pdf.

Enhanced recovery

Jane Sturgess

The enhanced recovery project has been embraced by almost all surgical specialties. The programme purports to offer benefits to all end users. What is apparent is that it involves, and requires engagement of every person involved in the patient pathway. The success of the programme does not exclude the patient nor their care-givers.

Proposed benefits of employing an enhanced recovery programme

General practice

- Closer working relationships between the acute and primary care sectors – with recognition of good care from local commissioning groups
- Family physician able to start the process of preparation for surgery, and get ready to receive the patient back with good information post-operatively

Patient

- More involved in their care
- Earlier return to home and/or work
- Purported to have less exposure to hospital-acquired infection, and lower complication rates post-operatively

Staff

- Education and training
- Implementation of technology to support care
- Sense of achievement and recognition about providing excellent care with reduced lengths of stay, and improved patient experience

Quality

- Allegedly improved clinical outcomes, faster detection of complications and standard care across the UK
- It is certainly something that can be measured by both hospital mangers and inspecting bodies

A Surgeon's Guide to Anaesthesia and Peri-operative Care, ed. Jane Sturgess, Justin Davies and Kamen Valchanov. Published by Cambridge University Press.

Table 32.1 Summary of the key elements of a successful enhanced recovery programme

Pre-operative	**General practice** Control of co-morbidities, e.g. diabetes, hypertension Correction of anaemia **Pre-assessment** Consent/information about the procedure and likely patient pathway Optimise medical conditions Prescribe carbohydrate load Pre-habilitation Start discharge plans	*Peri-operative*	**Surgical factors** Laparoscopic/ minimally invasive surgery where possible Minimal drains and drips **Anaesthetic factors** Multimodal analgesia – opiate-sparing Goal-directed fluid therapy Normothermia/ normoglycaemia Anti-emesis	*Post-operative*	Minimal drains Early mobilisation Early eating and drinking Regular oral analgesia and avoid strong opiates Use of typical care pathway Therapy support – dietician, stoma nurse, physiotherapist 24-hour telephone follow-up (if appropriate) Early targeted mobilisation

Hospital management

- Helps to keep procedures within national tariff and patient bed days to a minimum
- Improves hospital reputation when comparing length of stay in statistical analysis (e.g. Dr Foster)
- May come with additional payment for adhering to certain guidelines (e.g. CQUIN for using oesophageal Doppler)
- Each surgical specialty has made contributions to their own enhanced recovery programmes. Across the UK colorectal, gynaecological and orthopaedic programmes are well established

Further reading

Department of Health. Delivering Enhanced Recovery. Helping patients to get better sooner after surgery. Enhanced recovery partnership programme. London: Department of Health, 2010.

Section III At a glance

Post-operative cognitive dysfunction

Ram Adapa

Introduction

Advances in peri-operative care over the past several decades have resulted in a significant reduction in patient mortality and morbidity. This has contributed to an increasing focus on sometimes subtle changes in cognition that are associated with surgery, especially in the elderly. These changes can be transient or permanent, or can also modify the course of long-standing cognitive decline. Although more common, or more pronounced in the elderly, such cognitive impairment is not uncommon in all age groups. When persistent, cognitive decline after surgery can lead to an increased risk of disability and mortality, which can result in loss of employment or independence, and reduction in quality of life. An increasingly aged population also means that such cognitive impairments can have a significant societal impact too.

Types of cognitive disturbances following surgery

Post-operative cognitive impairment can be either because of exacerbation of a previously existing condition, or new-onset. It is clinically important to distinguish between the various types of new-onset impairment, as the time course of each condition is different. Delirium is probably the most common cause of such deterioration, occurring either in the immediate post-operative period (emergence delirium) or a few days later. This is distinct from the condition called post-operative cognitive dysfunction (POCD), defined on the basis of a cognitive test battery performed before and at several times after anaesthesia and surgery. Early POCD, i.e. impairment of cognition around seven days post-operatively, must be distinguished from late POCD, which is diagnosed at least three months post-operatively. The occurrence of POCD after anaesthesia may also represent the cognitive decline in the elderly (MCI, mild cognitive impairment) that precedes the dementia of Alzheimer's disease. The main differences between the two conditions are summarised in Table 33.1.

Delirium

Delirium is characterised as an acute and transient disturbance of mental functions that may be accompanied by changes in awareness. The incidence of post-operative delirium

A Surgeon's Guide to Anaesthesia and Peri-operative Care, ed. Jane Sturgess, Justin Davies and Kamen Valchanov. Published by Cambridge University Press.

Table 33.1 Types of cognitive disturbances following surgery

	Post-operative delirium (PD)	Post-operative cognitive dysfunction (POCD)
Onset	Immediate (emergence delirium), or acute (1–3 days after surgery)	Subtle onset, often first identified by relatives, onset variable, from between 2 weeks to 2 months after surgery
Duration	A few days to weeks	Up to 3 months, could become permanent in a small subset of patients
Symptoms	Fluctuating level of consciousness associated with inattention, change in cognition	Impairment of memory, concentration and information processing
Diagnosis	Confusion Assessment Method (CAM); DSM-IV remains gold standard	Failure on more than 2 tests affecting different cognitive domains on a neuropsychological test battery
Prognosis	Usually reversible, but may contribute to POCD	Usually reversible, but a prolonged course, some evidence of permanence

(PD) following general surgery is reported from 5 to 15%, ranging up to 65% for patients with hip fractures.

Clinical features and diagnosis

Patients with delirium can be restless, irritable, combative and agitated (hyperactive delirium), or lethargic with decreased alertness/motor activity and unawareness (hypoactive delirium), or present with mixed features. The gold standard for diagnosing delirium remain the DSM-IV criteria; however, this is time consuming for routine clinical practice, and rapid assessment tools such as the Confusion Assessment Method (CAM) and Delirium Detection Scale (DDS) are more commonly employed.

Risk factors

Although the mechanism underlying delirium is incompletely understood, there are several well-recognised risk factors that predispose to delirium in the post-operative period. These include patient factors such as dementia and reduced cognitive reserve related to advancing age, severe co-morbidities (including renal impairment, pulmonary disease, atherosclerotic disease, diabetes, atrial fibrillation), pre-existing sensory impairment, malnutrition, dehydration, alcohol abuse and smoking. The presence of the apolipoprotein E4 genotype is also associated with a greater risk of developing post-operative delirium. Several peri-operative factors also contribute to the development of delirium. These include prolonged surgical time, the need for blood transfusion, major or emergency surgery, infection, the presence of a urinary catheter, and the use of drugs such as benzodiazepines, anticholinergics, antiarrhythmics, and possibly opioids. Other correctable factors that may predispose to PD include post-operative pain, hypoxaemia and electrolyte abnormalities. The peri-operative period is commonly associated with sleep/wake disturbances that can also precipitate/worsen delirium in some patients.

Post-operative cognitive dysfunction (POCD)

In contrast to delirium, POCD is characterised by subtler and longer-lasting changes in cognition unaccompanied by alteration in awareness level. The reported incidence of POCD varies substantially, depending on the patient population, time of measurement and the neuropsychological tests used. The International Study of POCD (ISPOCD), a large multicentre trial including more than 1,200 patients, identified a 10% incidence of POCD in the elderly, three months after surgery. Post-operative cognitive dysfunction is highly prevalent up to three months post-operatively, especially in elderly patients.

Clinical features and diagnosis

Post-operative cognitive dysfunction is considered a mild form of cognitive dysfunction, and is a diagnosis of exclusion. It is defined on the basis of a cognitive test battery performed before and at several times after anaesthesia and surgery. The most common cognitive functions affected include memory (especially visual and verbal recall), attention, and language and visuospatial processing.

Causal/contributory factors

It is important to recognise that post-operative impairment in cognitive function can be multifactorial in origin. The greater the number of risk factors a patient has, the more likely he/she is to develop POCD. The strongest predictors for developing POCD include a reduction in cognitive reserve of the patient (because of increased age, or other underlying cognitive disorders), lower level of education and a history of previous cerebrovascular accident. Post-operative delirium is also associated with an increased chance of developing POCD. Similar to delirium, prolonged anaesthesia, respiratory or infectious complications, and the need for second operation add to the risk of developing POCD. It is also possible that cognitive decline could be related to the illness itself rather than being causally related to surgery and anaesthesia.

Mechanisms of cognitive dysfunction following surgery

The pathophysiology of POCD remains incompletely understood, although recent evidence points to a disease continuum involving MCI, POCD and Alzheimer's dementia. Animal and laboratory evidence points to several potential mechanisms for the development of POCD and delirium. Volatile anaesthetic agents have been demonstrated to cause neurotoxicity in in vitro and murine models. Another proposed mechanism is neuroinflammation with increased secretion of systemic inflammatory mediators and enhanced production of Alzheimer-related biomarkers (ß amyloid and tau protein phosphorylation). Increase in anticholinergic activity, intra-operative micro-emboli in the cerebral circulation and decrease in cerebral oxygenation have also been shown in some small studies to be associated with the development of POCD. Magnetic resonance imaging in affected patients often shows an extensive range of brain regions affected including prefrontal, frontal, parietal, temporal, occipital, hippocampal, insular, cingulate, thalamic and cerebellar regions.

Management of post-operative cognitive impairment

There is no definitive treatment for cognitive dysfunction following surgery and treatment is largely supportive. However, it is imperative to exclude organic causes since these are often reversible. Clinical investigation should initially focus on identification of metabolic causes of delirium (e.g., electrolyte disturbances, evaluation for infection). The medication list should also be reviewed and drugs that are likely to cause/exacerbate delirium or confusion should be stopped whenever possible.

The mainstay of pharmacological management of post-operative delirium remains haloperidol, an antipsychotic agent that can be administered orally, intramuscularly and intravenously. An initial dose of 1 to 2 mg of haloperidol is recommended with doses of 0.25 to 0.5 mg every four hours for maintenance dosing in elderly patients. Haloperidol can cause extrapyramidal side effects and prolongation of the QTc interval in the ECG. Risperidone is an atypical antipsychotic that has also been shown to reduce the incidence and severity of post-operative delirium, and both drugs have been demonstrated to reduce length of hospital stay in small studies.

Prevention

A multimodal strategy should be employed in patients identified to be at risk of developing cognitive impairment. This should be aimed at both optimising preventative measures in addition to pharmacologic management. A pre-operative assessment of surgical patients at risk for POCD should include information about the condition and its mostly transient nature, pre-operative psychological assessment to establish baseline cognitive function, and pre-operative correction of metabolic function. Environmental and supportive interventions shown to be of benefit include an orientation protocol to provide the patient with repeated orientation to their surroundings and careteam members, ensuring uninterrupted night time sleep, early mobilisation in the post-operative period and vision/hearing protocol to allow easy access to glasses and hearing aids. Care should be taken to avoid dehydration, and urinary catheters, nasogastric tubes, or intravenous catheters should be removed when not required to reduce the risk of delirium. The use of short-acting and rapidly metabolised drugs during anaesthesia and keeping the surgery as short and as minimally invasive as possible in patients at risk may also reduce the risk of POCD. Studies on several neuroprotective drugs (piracetam, remacemide and ketamine) have shown no consistent benefits for the prevention and treatment of POCD.

Prognosis

Post-operative delirium and POCD are considered reversible conditions, although the time course of POCD tends to be longer. Most patients who suffer from POCD up to three months post-operatively eventually recover. Recent studies have suggested a link between post-operative delirium and POCD and long-term cognitive dysfunction. Post-operative cognitive impairment results in functional decline and longer hospital stay. Delirium also increases the risk of complications such as falls, pulled lines/tubes and aspiration pneumonia. Patients who develop delirium during their hospitalisation have a higher six-month mortality and patients with POCD at three months have significantly increased mortality. It is currently unclear whether POCD itself causes an increase in mortality, or if this is a consequence of pre-existing co-morbidities.

Further reading

Alcover L, Badenes R, Montero MJ, *et al.* Post-operative delirium and cognitive dysfunction. *Trends in Anaesthesia and Critical Care* 2013; **3**: 199–204.

Grape S, Ravussin P, Rossi A, *et al.* Post-operative cognitive dysfunction. *Trends in Anaesthesia and Critical Care* 2012; **2**: 98–103.

Lloyd GW, Ma D, Vizcaychipi MPl. Cognitive decline after anaesthesia and critical care. *Continuing Education in Anaesthesia, Critical Care & Pain* 2012; **12(3)**: 105–9.

Newman S, Stygall J, Hirani S, *et al.* Post-operative cognitive dysfunction after noncardiac surgery. *Anesthesiology* 2007; **106**: 572–90.

Abbreviations

AAA: abdominal aortic aneurysm
AAGBI: Association of Anaesthetists of Great Britain and Ireland
ACC: American College of Cardiologists
ACE inhibitor: angiotensin converting enzyme inhibitor
ACLS: advanced cardiac life support
ACT: activated clotting time
ACTH: adrenocorticotropic hormone
ACoTS: acute coagulopathy of trauma - shock
ADH: antidiuretic hormone
ADP: adenosine diphosphate
AHA: American Heart Association
AKI: acute kidney injury
ALS: advanced life support
ALT: alanine aminotransferease
AMP: adenosine monophosphate
AMPA: α-amino-3-hydroxy-5-methyl-4-isoxazolepropionic acid
AMPLE: allergies, medications, past medical history, last oral intake and last menstruation, events leading up to the injury
APLS: advanced paediatric life support
APTT: activated partial thromboplastin time
ARDS: acute respiratory distress syndrome
ASA: American Society of Anesthesiologists
AST: aspartate transaminase
ATMIST: age, time of incident, mechanism of injury, vital signs, treatment, expected time of arrival
ATP: adenosine triphosphate
AVM: arterio-venous malformation
AVPU: alert, verbalising, painful stimulus, unresponsive
AVR: aortic valve replacement
BAEP: brainstem auditory evoked potentials
BAETS: British Association of Endocrine and Thyroid Surgeons
BLS: basic life support
BMI: body mass index
BMS: bare metal stents
BMV: bag mask ventilation
CABG: coronary artery bypass graft
CAM: Confusion Assessment Method
CBF: cerebral blood flow
CCS: Canadian Cardiovascular Society
CF: cystic fibrosis
CHD: congenital heart disease
$CMRO_2$: cerebral metabolic rate for oxygen
CNB: central neuraxial block
CNS: central nervous system
COX: cyclo-oxygenase
COPD: chronic obstructive pulmonary disease
CPAP: continuous positive airway pressure
CPB: cardiopulmonary bypass
CPP: cerebral perfusion pressure
CPX/CPET: cardiopulmonary exercise testing
CQUIN: commissioning for quality and innovation
CRASH-2: clinical randomisation of an antifibrinolytic in significant haemorrhage
CRH: corticotrophin-releasing hormone
CSE: combined spinal and epidural injection
CSF: cerebrospinal fluid
CT: computed tomography
CUSA: cavitron ultrasonic aspirator
CXR: chest X-ray
DDAVP: 1-desamino-8-D-arginine vasopressin
DES: drug-eluting stents
DDS: Delirium Detection Scale
DI: diabetes insipidus
DIEP: deep inferior epigastric perforator flap
DLT: double-lumen tube
DSE: dobutamine stress echocardiography
DSM Criteria: Diagnostic and Statistical Manual of Mental Disorders
ECG: electrocardiogram
ECHO: echocardiogram
ECMO: extracorporeal membrane oxygenation
ED: emergence delirium
EMLA: eutectic mixture of local anaesthetics
EP: electrophysiology
ERP: enhanced recovery program
ETT: endotracheal tube
EVAR: endovascular aortic reconstruction
FAST: focused assessment with sonography for trauma
FBC: full blood count
FEV_1: forced expiratory volume
FFP: fresh frozen plasma
FHH: familial hypocalciuric hypercalcaemia
FLACC: face, legs, activity, cry, consolability scales
FOB: fibre-optic bronchoscope
FRC: functional residual capacity
FVC: forced vital capacity

GALA Trial: general anaesthetic local anaesthetic trial
GCS: Glasgow Coma Scale
GFR: glomerular filtration rate
GORD: gastro-oesophageal reflux disease
GTN: glyceryltrinitrate
HAS: human albumin solution
HDU: high-dependency unit
HES: hydroxyethyl starch
HLA: human leucocyte antigens
HMG: HMG-CoA-3 hydroxy-3-methylglutaryl-coenzyme A
HOCM: hypertrophic obstructive cardiomyopathy
HoLEP: holmium laser enucleation of the prostate
HPV: hypoxic pulmonary vasoconstriction
5HT3: 5-hydroxytryptamine
IABP: invasive arterial blood pressure
ICH: intracranial haematoma
ICP: intracranial pressure
ICU/ITU: intensive therapy unit
IGAP: inferior gluteal artery perforator flap
IHD: ischaemic heart disease
INR: international normalise ratio
IPF: idiopathic pulmonary fibrosis
IPPV: intermittent positive pressure ventilation
IVC: inferior vena cava
IVRA: intravenous regional anaesthesia
JVP: jugular venous pressure
LA: left atrium
LABS: longitudinal assessment of bariatric surgery
LD: latissimus dorsi
LDF: latissimus dorsi flap
LEA: lumbar epidural analgesia
LIA: local infiltration anaesthesia
LMA: laryngeal mask airway
LMWH: low molecular weight heparin
LODS: Logistic Organ Dysfunction Score
MAOI: monoamine oxidase inhibitors
MAP: mean arterial pressure
MCA: middle cerebral artery
MDT: multi-disciplinary team
MELD: model for end-stage liver disease
MEN: multiple endocrine neoplasia
MEP: motor evoked potentials
METs: metabolic equivalents
MEWS: Modified Early Warning Score
MI: myocardial infarction
MIBI: methoxy-isobutyl-isonitrile scan for myocardial perfusion
MLB: microlaryngoscopy bronchoscopy
MODS: Multiple Organ Dysfunction Score
MRI: magnetic resonance imaging
MRSA: methicillin resistant *Staphylococcus aureus*
MTC: medullary thyroid carcinoma
MVD: microvascular decompressions
NCA: nurse-controlled analgesia
NEMS: Nine Equivalents of Nursing Manpower Use Score
NEWS: National Early Warning Score
NG: nasogastric
NHSLA: National Health Service Litigation Authority
NICE: National Institute for Health and Clinical Excellence
NIPS: neonatal infant pain scale
NIV: non-invasive ventilation
NMDA: N-methyl-D-aspartate
NO: nitric oxide
NSAIDs: non-steroidal anti-inflammatory drugs
NYHA: New York Heart Association
ODP: operating department practitioner
OLV: one-lung ventilation
OS-MRS: The Obesity Surgery Mortality Risk Score
PA: pulmonary artery
PAH: pulmonary arterial hypertension
PAWP: pulmonary arterial wedge pressure
PCA: patient-controlled analgesia
PC: pressure control (method of ventilatory support)
PCC: prothrombin complex concentrates
PEEP: positive end expiratory pressure
PD: post-operative delirium
PH: pulmonary hypertension
PHA: primary hyperaldosteronism
PHPT: primary hyperparathyroidism
PICC: peripherally inserted central catheters
PNB: peripheral nerve block
PO: *per os* (by mouth)
POCD: post-operative cognitive dysfunction
PONV: post-operative nausea and vomiting
POSSUM: Physiological and Operative Severity Score for the enUmeration of Mortality and morbidity
PS: pressure support (method of ventilatory support)
PRAE: peri-operative adverse respiratory events
PRBC: packed red blood cells
PRN: *pro re nata* (as required)
PT: prothrombin time
PTC: percutaneous transhepatic cholangiography
PTH: parathormone
PTFE: polytetrafluoroethylene (a material used to make synthetic bypass grafts)

PUJ: pelvi-ureteric junction
PVR: pulmonary vascular resistance
RBC: red blood cell
REM: rapid eye movement sleep
RER: respiratory exchange ratio
RLN: recurrent laryngeal nerve
RS: respiratory system
RSI: rapid sequence induction
RV: right ventricle
SAH: subarachnoid haemorrhage
SCS: spinal cord stimulation
SGAP: superior gluteal artery perforator flap
SIADH: syndrome of inappropriate antidiuretic hormone production
SIGN: Scottish Intercollegiate Guidelines Network
SIMV: synchronised intermittent mandatory ventilation
SIRS: systemic inflammatory response syndrome
SSEP: somatosensory evoked potentials
SVR: systemic vascular resistance
TAP block: transversus abdominis plane block
TAVI: transcatheter aortic valve implantation
TBI: traumatic brain injury
TBSA: total body surface area
TCD: transcranial Doppler
TEA: thoracic epidural analgesia
TEMS: transanal endoscopic microsurgery
TENS: transcutaneous electrical nerve stimulation
TEVAR: thoracic endovascular aneurysm repair
TFT: thyroid function test
TIA: transient ischaemic attack
TIPS(S): transjugular intrahepatic portosystemic shunt
TIVA: total intravenous anaesthesia
TISS: Therapeutic Intervention Scoring System
TME: total mesorectal excision
TNF: tumour necrosis factor
TOE: transoesophageal echocardiography
TPN: total parenteral nutrition
TRAM: transverse rectus abdominus myocutaneous flap
TSH: thyroid stimulating hormone
TTE: transthoracic echocardiography
TURBT: transurethral resection of bladder tumour
TURP: transurethral resection of the prostate
UKELD: UK model for end-stage liver disease
URTI: upper respiratory tract infection
VACTERL: vertebral anomalies, anal atresia, cardiac defects, transoesophageal fistula (or atresia), renal anomalies, limb defects
VAD: ventricular assist device
VATS: video assisted thoracoscopy
VC: either volume control (method of ventilation) or vital capacity (lung volume)
VF: ventricular fibrillation
VMA: vanillyl mandelic acid
V/Q: ventilation perfusion ratio
VT: ventricular tachycardia
VTE: venous thromboembolism

Index

abdominal wall defects, 177
acid–base balance, 7, 24
regulation, 1
acidosis, 7
acromegaly, 204
acute respiratory distress syndrome (ARDS), 18–19
adenomas, cortical, 133–4
adrenalectomy
cortical tumors, 133–4
phaeochromocytoma, 134–6
adrenaline, 41
solution terminology, 188
with lignocaine, 164
adrenocorticotrophic hormone (ACTH), 41
airway obstruction, 161–2, 211
albumin 4.5% solution, 11
alkalosis, 7
allodynia, 38
AMPLE history, 210
anaemia, 92
urological surgery patients, 237
analgesia. *See also specific drugs*
cardiothoracic surgery patients, 80
colorectal surgery patients, 97
neurosurgery patients, 200
obese patients, 256–7
pain/analgesic ladder, 46
pre-emptive use, 46
strategies, 39
analgesic response, 40
aneurysm
aortic, 144
endovascular aortic reconstruction (EVAR), 142–3
hybrid procedures, 144
open repair, 141–3
ruptured, 142–3
intracranial, 201–3
angina, refractory, 89–90
angiotensin converting enzyme (ACE) inhibitors, 140
angiotensin II, 27, 41
ankle blocks, 56
ankle surgery, 231–3
ankylosing spondylitis, 227
anticoagulants, 280
antidiuretic hormone (ADH), 41
anti-emesis, 96. *See also* nausea; vomiting
fundoplication patients, 104–5
posterior fossa surgery patients, 203
antiplatelet therapy, 139–40, 280
antithrombotic drugs, 280
anxiety, pain adverse effects, 43
anxiolysis, 59
aortic cross-clamping, 141
aortic stenosis, 93
aortic surgery, 85
aortic valve disease, 282
APACHE (Acute Physiology and Chronic Health Evaluation) score, 266
apnoea
infants, 175
sleep, 161, 248–9
argon beam coagulation, 74
arrhythmias, 93
pre-operative management, 109
arterial blood gas analysis, 6–8
arteriovenous malformation (AVM), 206–7
ASA (American Society of Anesthesiology Physical Status Classification System), 259–60
ascites, 118
aspirin, 139–40
atherosclerosis, 138, *See also* vascular surgery
ATMIST handover, 209
atrial fibrillation, 93
autonomic dysreflexia, 206
axillary brachial plexus block, 55
balanced resuscitation, 209, *See also* haemostatic resuscitation
trauma patients, 1
bariatric surgery, 246
anaesthesia principles, 252–3
deep versus standard neuromuscular blockade, 255–6
drug dosing, 253
multi-disciplinary teams, 251
patient positioning, 253–4
pneumoperitoneum, 254–5
muscle relaxants and, 255
post-operative care, 256–7
analgesia, 256–7
mobilisation, 257
monitoring, 256
pre-operative assessment, 251–2
basal metabolic rate, 4
base excess/deficit, 8
beach chair position, risks of, 290
benzodiazepines, 60
reversal agent, 60
safety in pregnancy, 61
trauma patients, 219
beta blockers, 100, 140
Bier's block, 57
bladder perforation, 245
blood flow, 68–9. *See also* cerebral blood flow (CBF)
blood gas analysis, 6–8, 71
blood gas transport, 71
blood pressure
control, 21–2
pathological influences, 23
invasive measurement, 69–70
mean arterial pressure (MAP), 79
neurosurgery, 200–1
vasodilator effects, 79
blood transfusion, .11, 96 *See also* haemostatic resuscitation
massive transfusion protocol, 213–14

body mass index (BMI), 247. *See also* obesity
boiling point, 66
Bolam test, 296
brain. *See* central nervous system physiology
brain relaxation, 198–9
aneurysm surgery, 202–3
breast augmentation surgery, 191
breast reconstruction, 192–6
free flap surgery, 193–6
latissimus dorsi pedicled flap, 192–3
bupivacaine, 171
burns patients, 221–2
fluid replacement, 275

calcitonin measurement, 127
capacitors, 72–3
capacity for consent, 296
Gillick competence, 297
carbohydrate metabolism, 4–6
carbon monoxide poisoning, 221–2
cardiac output, 10, 78–9
control of, 19–21
cardiac tamponade, 213
cardiopulmonary exercise testing (CPET), 94–5
cardiothoracic surgery, 77
anaesthetic change during surgery, 81–2
aortic surgery, 85
cardiac risk assessment, 306–8
cardiorespiratory pharmacology, 79–80
cardiorespiratory physiology, 78–9
coagulation management, 82–3
complications, 307
heart and lung transplantation, 84
heart failure management, 84
invasive monitoring, 81
lung isolation, 81
minimally invasive surgery, 85
post-operative care, 83–4
pulmonary hypertension (PH), 84–5
requirements of the anaesthetist, 77–8
team working, 78
without cardiopulmonary bypass (CPB), 82
cardiovascular physiology, 19–22
autoregulation, 19
blood pressure control, 21–2
cardiac output, 10
control of, 19–21
cardiac pressure cycle, 19
cardiothoracic surgery and, 78–9
pain adverse effects, 42
carotid endarterectomy, 144–5
caudal anaesthesia, 240
CCS (Canadian Cardiovascular Society grading of angina pectoris), 260
central nervous system physiology, 29–34
autoregulation, 32–4
head injury effects, 33
mean arterial blood pressure, 32
space occupying lesions, 30
central neuraxial blockade (CNB), 52–4
complications, 51–4
spinal versus epidural blockade, 53
cerebral blood flow (CBF), 32
head injury patients, 220
$PaCO_2$ relationship, 33
PaO_2 relationship, 34
cerebral perfusion pressure (CPP) maintenance, 200
cerebrovascular disease, 94
Child-Pugh scoring system, 117–18
children. *See* paediatric patients
cholecystectomy, 121–2. *See also* obese patient case study
clopidogrel, 139–40
coagulation
assessment, 218
management, cardiothoracic surgery, 82–3
coagulation defects
liver disease patients, 118
trauma patients, 209
cocaine, 164
cognitive impairment, post-operative, 312–13
management, 315
mechanisms, 314–15
prevention, 315
prognosis, 316
types of, 312
delirium, 312–14
post-operative cognitive dysfunction (POCD), 314
colloid solutions, 10–11, 274
colorectal surgery, 91
anaesthetic considerations, 98–9
analgesia, 96–7
patient position, 98–9
pelvic bleeding, 99
transanal endoscopic microscopy (TEMS), 99
operative management, 95–6
post-operative management, 99–100
pre-operative assessment, 91–5
coronary disease, 92–3
fluid balance, 92
haemoglobin, 92
nutrition and electrolytes, 92
pneumoperitoneum, 91
respiratory disease, 93–4
thromboembolic disease, 92
compartment syndrome, 98, 232, 234
conductive heat loss, 64
confusion, post-operative, 31
congenital anomalies, 176–7
congenital heart disease (CHD), 177–8
Conn's syndrome, 133–4
consciousness assessment, 216
consent issues, 294
conditions of consenting, 296
ethical issues, 296–7
capacity, 296
Jehovah's Witness patients, 297
implied consent, 294–5
informed consent, 295–6
paediatric patients, 168–9
unconscious patients, 297
verbal consent, 294
written consent, 294
continuous positive airway pressure (CPAP), 270–1

convective heat loss, 64
coronary artery stents, 225–6
coronary disease
See also cardiothoracic surgery
post-operative risk management, 100
pre-operative assessment, 92–3
corticotrophin-releasing hormone (CRH), 41
cortisol, 41
cosmetic surgery, 185, See also plastic surgery
critical pressure, 66
critical temperature, 66
cryoprecipitate, 277
crystalloid solutions, 10–11, 273
Cushing Reflex, 30
Cushing syndrome, 133–4, 204
cystectomy, radical, 243

damage control resuscitation, 208–9, 213
Davenport diagram, 7
deep vein thrombosis (DVT). See also thromboembolism
obese patients, 249–50
paediatric patients, 173
defibrillators, 72
definitive airway, 211
delirium, 312–14
diagnosis, 313
emergence (ED), 176
prognosis, 316
risk factors, 313–14
dementia, 94
desflurane, 220
Detsky's Modified Cardiac Risk classification, 261
dexamethasone suppression test, 133
dextrose 5% solution, 11
dextrose saline solution, 11
diaphragmatic hernia, congenital, 177
diazepam, 47
difficult airway, 212–13
dorsal horn, 38

ear surgery, 166–7
ear, nose and throat (ENT) surgery. See ear surgery; head and neck surgery
echocardiography, 281–2
importance of, 282–5
myocardial function, 283–4
shunts, 283
valvular pathology, 282–3
elbow surgery, 233–4
elderly patients
pain management, 47
sedation, 61
electricity, 72–5
capacitors, 72–3
charge, 72
current, 72
direct and alternating current applications, 73–4
electrical resistance, 72
impedance, 73
electrocautery, 279
electrosurgery, 74, 279
emergence delirium (ED), 176
emergency airway, 162
encephalins, 38, 40
encephalopathy, 118–19
endocrine surgery, 125–6
neuroendocrine surgery, 204–5
endorphins, 38, 40
endovascular aortic reconstruction (EVAR)
abdominal, 142
ruptured aneurysm, 142–3
thoracic (TEVAR), 143–4
energy metabolism, 4
enhanced recovery, 91, 100, 310
benefits, 310–11
hip surgery, 231
key elements, 311
Entonox®, 60
epidural analgesia
See also central neuraxial blockade (CNB)
complications, 51–2
oesophagectomy patients, 110
paediatric patients, 171
epinephrine solution terminology, 188. See also adrenaline
etomidate, 218–19
EuroSCORE (European System for Cardiac Operative Risk Evaluation), 266
evaporative heat loss, 65
extracorporeal membrane oxygenation (ECMO), 87–9
extubation, 167
neurosurgery patients, 207

facelift, 188–9
factor VII, 215
recombinant factor VIIa, 277
familial hypocalciuric hypercalcaemia (FHH), 131
fatty liver, 249
femoral nerve blocks, 56
fever, 3
fibrin sealants, 279
fibrinogen replacement, 215
fight or flight response, 40
flow metabolism coupling, 32
flow volume loops, 15
fluid balance, 10
daily requirements, 274
pre-operative assessment, 92
urological surgery patients, 237
fluid replacement, 10
balanced resuscitation, 209
burns patients, 221, 275
choice of fluid, 274–5
colloid solutions, 10–11, 274
crystalloid solutions, 10–11, 273
massive blood loss, 11–12
paediatric patients, 172–3, 276
special circumstances, 275
fluids, 65
flow, 67–70
laminar flow, 67
turbulence, 67–9
flumazenil, 60
foot surgery, 231–3
foreign body removal, 165
Frank–Starling law, 19
fresh frozen plasma (FFP), 215, 277
Functional Status Assessment/ Duke Activity Status Index, 262
fundoplication. See laparoscopic oesophageal fundoplication case study

gabapentin, 87
gases, 65. See also fluids
properties of, 65–7
partial pressure, 66–7

gastrointestinal surgery
See colorectal surgery, upper gastrointestinal surgery
gastro-oesophageal reflux disease (GORD), 103. *See also* laparoscopic oesophageal fundoplication case study
gastroparesis, 42
gastroschisis, 177
gelatin matrix/thrombin sealants, 279
gelatin solutions, 11
general anaesthesia, 59. *See also specific types of surgery*
Gillick competence, 297
Glasgow Coma Score (GCS), 263
Glasgow Outcome Scale, 264
glaucoma, 94
glucagon, 41
glutamate, 38
glycine toxicity, 241–2
goitre, 127
Goldmann Risk Classification, 260
Graves' ophthalmopathy, 127
growth hormone, 41

haemophilia, 227
haemopneumothorax, 213
haemorrhage
control, 214. *See also* hypotensive resuscitation
massive blood loss, 11–12
neurosurgery patients, 200–1
subarachnoid (SAH), 201–2
haemostasis, neurosurgery patients, 200–1
haemostatic agents, 279
haemostatic resuscitation, 209, 213
trauma patients, 214–16
haemothorax, 213
haloperidol, 315
hand surgery, 233–4
harmonic scalpel, 74, 280
Hartmann's solution, 10
head and neck surgery, 161. *See also* thyroid surgery
anaesthesia maintenance, 164
hypotensive anaesthesia, 164
local anaesthesia and vasoconstrictors, 164
muscle relaxation, 164
ear surgery, 166–7
emergency airway, 162
extubation, 167
foreign body removal, 165
intubation, 163–4
positioning, 163–4
throat pack, 163
laser surgery, 165
major reconstructive surgery, 166
microlaryngobronchoscopy (MLB), 165
neck dissection, 166
post-operative care, 167
pre-operative assessment, 161–2
airway obstruction, 161–2
day case surgery, 162
head and neck malignancy, 161
secreting tumors, 162
tracheostomy, 166
ventilation, 164–5
head injury, 33, 220–1. *See also* neurosurgery
heart failure
management, 84
obese patients, 249
heart transplantation, 154–7
donor considerations, 154
operative considerations, 155–6
anaesthetic management, 156
surgical approach, 156
post-operative considerations, 157
pre-operative considerations, 154–5
assessment, 161–2
preparation, 155
heart-lung transplantation, 84, 160
heat, 63–5, *See also* thermo-regulation
as energy, 64–5
intra-operative heat loss, 64–5
conduction, 64
convection, 64
evaporation, 65
radiation, 64
measurement, 63–4
heparin, 82, 279
bariatric surgery and, 249–50
hepatectomy, 152
hepatobiliary surgery, 116
cholecystectomy, 121–2
hepatic resection, 120–1
porto-systemic shunts, 123–4
post-operative management, 124
pre-operative factors, 116–17
pre-existing liver disease, 117
transjugular intrahepatic portal shunt (TIPS), 123
Whipples resection, 122–3
hepato-pulmonary syndrome, 120
hepato-renal syndrome, 120
hernia repair, 94
hip surgery, 229–31
holmium laser enucleation of the prostate (HoLEP), 242
homeostasis, 1–4
neurosurgery patients, 200
osmosis, 3
thermoregulation, 3–4
Hunt and Hess scale, 264
hydrocoele, 179
hypercalcaemia, 131–2
hyperdynamic circulation, 119–20
hyperglycaemia, 201
hyperkalaemia, 215
hypernatraemia, 204
free water deficit estimation, 275
hyperparathyroidism
primary, 131
peri-operative care, 132–3
post-operative care, 133
pre-operative assessment, 131–2
secondary, 131
tertiary, 131
hyperthyroidism, 126
hypocalcaemia, 130–1, 215
hyponatraemia, 200, 204
hypospadias, 178
hypotension. *See* hypotensive anaesthesia, permissive hypotension
hypotensive anaesthesia

hypotensive anaesthesia (cont.)
contra-indications, 184
drugs used for hypotension induction, 184
head and neck surgery, 164
plastic surgery, 183
hypothermia, 3–4, 63, 183
neuroprotection, 201
surgical exposure relationship, 217
trauma patients, 216–17
hypothyroidism, 126
hypovolaemic shock, 28

implied consent, 294–5
infection control, orthopaedic surgery, 229
informed consent, 295–6, *See also* consent issues
infra-clavicular nerve block, 55
inguinal hernia, 179
insulin, 5
intercostal nerve blocks, 56–7, 86
interleukin 1, 41
intermittent positive pressure ventilation (IPPV), 271
interscalene nerve block, 54
intestinal atresia, 177
intracranial pressure (ICP), 30
management, 198–201
aneurysm surgery, 202–3
fluids, 275
head injury patients, 220
reduction, 30–1, 33
space occupying lesion effects, 30
intravenous regional anaesthesia (IVRA), 57
intubation, 163–4
burns patients, 221
ease of intubation assessment, 212
neurosurgery patients, 198
positioning, 163–4
trauma patients, 211–13
intussusception, 179
ischaemic heart disease, 93
isoflurane, 220

jaundice, obstructive, 119
jaw thrust, 211
Jehovah's Witness patients, 297

ketamine, 60, 218
kidney, 23. *See also* renal physiology
anatomy, 25
hormonal function, 25
loop of Henle, 24–6
nephron, 23, 25
outflow obstruction, 29
stones, 29
kidney position, problems with, 244
kidney transplantation, 147–50
closure, 150
donor considerations, 147–8
deceased donor kidneys, 148
live donor kidneys, 147–8
patient preparation, 148–9
post-operative management, 124
pre-operative assessment, 148
reperfusion, 149
surgical approach, 149
paediatric patients, 47
knee surgery, 231–3

laminar flow, 67
laparoscopic oesophageal fundoplication case study, 102–5
anaesthesia induction and maintenance, 103–4
case history, 103
pneumoperitoneum, anaesthetic considerations, 104
post-operative nausea and vomiting, 104–5
pre-operative assessment, 103
laparoscopic surgery risks, 240–1
laryngeal mask airway (LMA), 129, 142, 145
laser coagulation, 279
laser surgery, 165
lateral position, risks of, 290–1
latissimus dorsi pedicled flap, 192–3
Lee Modified Cardiac Risk Index, 262, 306
left ventricular function, 283–4
failure, 93
lethal triad, 208–9
LigaSure, 74
liposuction, 189–91
liquids, 65. *See also* fluids
lithotomy position, risks of, 292–3

liver disease, .95, 116–17
See also hepatobiliary surgery
Child–Pugh scoring system, 118
morbidity, 118–20
anaesthesia and, 119
ascites, 118
coagulation defects, 118
encephalopathy, 118–19
hepato-pulmonary syndrome, 120
hepato-renal syndrome, 120
hyperdynamic circulation, 119–20
obstructive jaundice, 119
liver transplantation, 151–4
donor considerations, 152
operative considerations, 152–3
anhepatic phase, 152–3
hepatectomy, 152
reperfusion, 153
patient preparation, 152
post-operative management, 154
pre-operative assessment, 152
Lloyd Davies position, risks of, 292–3
local anaesthetics, 48–9
complications, 49–52
central neuraxial blockade (CNB), 51–2
lipid rescue, 50
nerve damage, 50–2
peripheral nerve blockade (PNB), 50–1
systemic toxicity, 49–50, 186–7
toxic levels, 186
paediatric patients, 171
pharmacology, 48–9
plastic surgery, 185–6
safe doses, 49, 186
terminology, 187
urological surgery, 239–40
LODS (Logistic Organ Dysfunction Score), 267
loop of Henle, 24–6
lower limb surgery, 231–3
lumbar plexus blockade, 55
lung functions, 14–15
flow volume loops, 15
lung volumes, 16
spirometry, 15

lung transplantation, 157–60. *See also* heart-lung transplantation
donor considerations, 157
operative considerations, 159–60
post-operative considerations, 160
pre-operative considerations, 157–9

magnesium, 47
Mallampati classification, 212
mannitol, 199, 202
massive blood loss, 11–12
mastectomy, breast reconstruction. *See* breast reconstruction
mastopexy, 191–2
maxillofacial surgery. *See* head and neck surgery
mean arterial pressure (MAP), 79
neurosurgery, 200–1
mechanical ventilation, 269
invasive, 270–2
non-invasive, 270
medullary thyroid carcinoma (MTC), 127
MELD (Model for End-stage Liver Disease), 117, 118
MEN2 syndrome, 129
metabolic pathways, 4–6
metabolic syndrome, 248
MEWS (Modified Early Warning Score), 267
microlaryngobronchoscopy (MLB), 165
midazolam, 60, 219
mitral valve regurgitation, 282
mitral valve stenosis, 282
MODS (Multiple Organ Dysfunction Score), 267
monoamine oxidase inhibitors (MAOIs), 227
multiple organ failure, 250
muscle relaxants
cardiothoracic surgery, 80
obese patients, 255
deep versus standard neuromuscular blockade, 255–6
trauma patients, 219–20
muscle spasm, 43
management, 47
myocardial function, 283–4
myocardial infarction, 140
myocardial ischaemia, 140

naloxone, 60
nasogastric tube (NG tube), 163
nausea
pain adverse effects, 43
post-operative
fundoplication patients, 103–5
plastic surgery patients, 183–4
risk factors, 184
neck dissection, 166
NEMS (Nine Equivalents of Nursing Manpower Use Score), 268
nephrectomy, 243–4
nerve injury, 298
central, 299
pain and, 301
neuropathic pain, 301
peripheral, 299
prevention, 298–9
traumatic, 300
visual loss, 300
neural tube defects, 178
neuroendocrine system, 41–2
pain adverse effects, 43
neurogenic shock, 206
neuropathic pain, 301
neuroprotection, 201–2
aneurysm surgery, 203
spinal cord, 205
neurosurgery, 197
anaesthesia induction, 198
anaesthesia maintenance, 198–200
aneurysm surgery, 201–3
AVM surgery, 206–7
awake craniotomies, 205
brain relaxation, 198–9
cerebral perfusion pressure (CPP) maintenance, 200
extubation, 207
intracranial pressure (ICP) management, 198–9
intubation, 198
mean arterial pressure (MAP) management, 200–1
pituitary/neuroendocrine surgery, 204–5
posterior fossa surgery, 203–4
post-operative care, 207
pre-operative assessment, 197–8
spinal surgery, 205–6
NEWS (National Early Warning Score), 268
nimodipine, 201
N-methyl-D-aspartate (NMDA) receptors, 38
nociception. *See* pain
non-steroidal anti-inflammatory drugs (NSAIDs), 87, 227
noradrenaline, 41
NYHA (New York Heart Association Classification of heart failure symptoms), 260

obese patients
anaesthesia principles, 252–3
case study, 105–7
causes of peri-operative mortality and morbidity, 249–51
anastomotic breakdown, 250–1
cardiac, 249
multiple organ failure, 250
thromboembolic, 249–50
deep versus standard neuromuscular blockade, 255–6
drug dosing, 253
patient positioning, 253–4
pneumoperitoneum, 254–5
post-operative care, 256–7
pre-operative assessment, 251–2
Obesity Surgery Mortality Risk Score (OS-MRS), 251–2
obesity, 246. *See also* obese patients
co-morbidities, 248–9
fatty liver, 249
metabolic syndrome, 248
sleep apnoea, 248–9
fat distribution significance, 247–8
health risks, 246–7
oesophageal atresia, 176–7
oesophagectomy, 107–14

oesophagectomy (cont.)
  anaesthesia induction and maintenance, 109, 119
    one lung anaesthesia, 111–13
  case history, 108
  peri-operative pain management, 109–10
  post-operative management, 113–14
  pre-operative assessment, 108–9
omphalocoele, 177
oncotic pressure, 3
one-lung anaesthesia, 111–13
  physiology, 111–12
  ventilatory strategies, 112–13
opioids
  cardiothoracic surgery, 80
  post-thoracotomy analgesia, 86–7
  reversal agent, 60
  sedation, 60
  spinal injections, 86
  trauma patients, 219
  urological surgery patients, 238
organ transplantation, 147. *See also specific organs*
  post-transplant surgery, 227
orthopaedic surgery, 223
  complicating co-morbidities, 224–8
    anticoagulation and anti-platelet therapy, 225–6
    cardiac disease, 224–5
    pacemakers, 226
    respiratory disease, 226
  early mobilisation and rehabilitation, 227–8
  hip surgery, 229–31
  intra-operative management, 229
  lower limb surgery, 231–3
  paediatric patients, 179
  pain control, 227
  post-operative care, 234
  pre-operative assessment, 223–9
  upper limb surgery, 233–4
  venous thromboembolism risk management, 228, 230
osmosis, 3
oxidised regenerated cellulose, 279
pacemakers, 226
paediatric patients
  anaesthetic considerations, 174–6
    cardiovascular and respiratory reserve, 175
    emergence delirium (ED), 176
    maximum doses, 171
    need for general anaesthesia, 168
    neurotoxicity, 175
    post-operative apnoea, 175
    recent upper respiratory tract infection, 175
    regional anaesthesia, 171
    syndromes, 176
  common surgical procedures, 179–80
    hydrocoele, 179
    inguinal hernia, 179
    intussusception, 179
    pyloric stenosis, 179
    testicular torsion, 180
  consent issues, 168–9
  definitions, 180
  examination, 174
  fluid management, 172–3, 276
  history taking, 173–4
  kidney transplantation, 47
  nutritional requirements, 173
  pain management, 47, 171–2
  peri-operative considerations, 169–71
    thermoregulation, 170–1
  post-operative care, 171–3
  pre-operative care, 168–9
  sedation, 61
  surgical issues, 176–9
    congenital heart disease (CHD), 177–8
    correctable congenital anomalies, 176–7
    neural tube defects, 178
    orthopaedic surgery, 179
    urological anomalies, 178
    vascular access, 176
  weight estimation, 180
pain, 35–6
  acute, 36–7
  adverse effects of, 42–3
    cardiovascular effects, 42
    gastrointestinal effects, 42–3
    immune suppression, 43
    musculoskeletal effects, 43
    neuroendocrine/metabolic effects, 43
    psychological and cognitive effects, 43
    respiratory effects, 42
    urinary effects, 42
  analgesic response, 40
  anatomy and physiology, 37–40
  assessment, 44–5
    aggravating factors, 44
    associated symptoms, 45
    impact, 45
    intensity, 44–5
    nature of pain, 45
    neutralising factors, 45
    place and pattern of pain, 44–5
  chronic, 36–7, 43
  definition, 36–7
  fast pain, 37
  gate theory, 38
  management
    analgesic strategies, 39
    deficiencies, 37
    elderly patients, 47
    muscle spasm, 47
    orthopaedic surgery, 227
    paediatric patients, 47, 171–2
    pain/analgesic ladder, 46
    role of anaesthetist and surgeon, 36
    services, 47
  nerve injury and, 301
    neuropathic pain, 301
  post-operative
    modifying factors, 43–4
    oesophagectomy patients, 109–10
    thyroid surgery patients, 131
  pre-emptive therapy, 46
  receptors, 40
  slow pain, 37
pancreas transplantation, 150–1
paracetamol, 87
paraganglioma, 134
parathyroid hormone (PTH) levels, 132
parathyroid surgery, 131–3
paravertebral blocks and infusions, 86

parenteral nutrition, paediatric patients, 173
Parsonnet additive risk stratification model, 265
partial pressure, 66–7
blood gases, 71
peripheral nerve blockade (PNB). *See also specific nerve blocks*
intravenous regional anaesthesia (IVRA), 57
lower limb blocks, 55–6
nerve damage, 50–1
nerve location, 52
truncal blocks, 56–7
upper limb blocks, 102
peripheral vascular disease, 145–6
permissive hypotension, 213, *See also* hypotensive anaesthesia
trauma patients, 214
pH, 7
regulation, 1
phaeochromocytoma, 134–6
pituitary surgery, 204–5
plastic surgery, 181
bleeding control, 183
breast surgery, 191–6
breast augmentation, 191
onco-plastic surgery, 192–6
reduction mammoplasty and mastopexy, 191–2
intra-operative patient access, 182
liposuction, 189–91
local anaesthesia, 185–6
multiple team involvement, 182
post-operative nausea and vomiting management, 183–4
prolonged surgery, 182–3
rhinoplasty, 188
rhytidectomy (facelift), 188–9
pleural effusion, 94
pneumoperitoneum, 65, 91
anaesthetic considerations, 104
obese patients, 254–5
muscle relaxants and, 255
physiological effects, 240–1
risks of, 288–9
pneumothorax, 191, 213
portal hypertension, 116
porto-systemic shunts, 123–4
positive end expiratory pressure (PEEP), 271
positive pressure ventilation, 271
POSSUM (Physiological and Operative Severity Score for the enUmeration of Mortality and morbidity), 263
posterior fossa surgery, 203–4
post-operative cognitive dysfunction (POCD), 312–14
diagnosis, 314
mechanisms, 314–15
prevention, 315
prognosis, 316
risk factors, 314
post-operative nausea and vomiting (PONV). *See* nausea; vomiting
pregabalin, 87
pregnant patients, sedation, 61
premedication, 96
pre-operative investigations, 302–3. *See also specific types of surgery*
guidelines, 303–4
routine testing, 304–6
targeted investigation, 306–8
pressure, 65
partial pressure, 66–7
pressure control ventilation (PC), 271
pressure support (PS), 271
primary hyperaldosteronism (PHA), 133
prone position, risks of, 289–90
prophylactic antibiotics, 229
propofol, 60, 201, 219
cardiothoracic surgery, 79, 81
fundoplication surgery, 103
overload syndrome, 79
plastic surgery, 184
prostatectomy, radical, 244–5
protamine, 82, 278
prothrombin complex concentrate, 277
pulmonary embolus, 94
pulmonary hypertension (PH), 84–5
pyloric stenosis, 179
radiative heat loss, 64
recombinant factor VIIa, 277
recurrent laryngeal nerve (RLN) palsy, 131
reduction mammoplasty, 191–2
reflex escape response, 40
remifentanil, 219
renal disease, 95
renal failure, 237
anaesthetic drugs and, 238–9
causes, 27–9
pharmacodynamic changes, 238
pharmacokinetic changes, 237
types of, 29
acute kidney injury (AKI), 29
chronic renal failure, 29
renal physiology, 23–9
acid–base balance, 24
autoregulation, 26
counter-current multiplier, 24–6
renin, 27, 41
renin–angiotensin system, 27
respiratory disease
oesophagectomy patients, 114
pre-operative assessment, 93–4
respiratory failure, 18, 114
causes, 17
respiratory physiology, 13–15
cardiothoracic surgery and, 78–9
lung functions, 14–15
pain adverse effects, 42
ventilation control, 13–14
RET gene mutation, 129
reverse Trendelenberg position, risks of, 292
rhinoplasty, 188
rhytidectomy, 188–9
Ringer's lactate solution, 10
risk scoring, 137–8
risperidone, 315
robotic surgery risks, 240–1
rocuronium, 219
ROTEM® test, 218

saline, 10
SAPS (Simplified Acute Physiology Score), 267
sciatic blocks, 56

sedation
  complications, 62
  definition, 59
  drugs used, 59–60
  elderly patients, 61
  levels of, 59
  monitoring, 61
  paediatric patients, 61
  pregnant patients, 61
  requirements for, 61–2
  safety guidelines, 60
seizures, 198, 205
sepsis, 8–9
septic shock, 8–10, 28
shock, 27
  cardiogenic, 28
  hypovolaemic, 28
  septic, 8–10, 28
shoulder surgery, 233–4
sickle cell disease, 227
sitting/beach chair position, risks of, 290
sleep apnoea, 161, 248–9
SOFA (Sequential Organ Failure Score), 267
solubility, 70–2
spinal anaesthesia, urological surgery, 239–40
spinal analgesia. *See* central neuraxial blockade (CNB)
spinal arthritis, 95
spinal injury, 221
spinal shock, 206
spinal surgery, 205–6
spirometry, 15
starch solutions, 11
statins, 140
sternotomy, analgesia, 80
subarachnoid haemorrhage (SAH), 201–2
substance P, 38
supraclavicular nerve block, 54–5
surgical complexity, 304
surgical exposure, hypothermia and, 217
surgical risk score, 138
suxamethonium, 219
sympathetic nervous system, 41
synchronised intermittent mandatory ventilation (SIMV), 271
systemic inflammatory response syndrome (SIRS), 8–10
tapentadol, 87
targeted investigation, 306–8
temperature, 63–5. *See also* thermoregulation
tension pneumothorax, 213
testicular torsion, 180
thermistors, 63
thermocouples, 63
thermopiles, 64
thermoregulation, 3–4. *See also* heat; temperature
  intra-operative management, 96
  paediatric patients, 170–1
thoracic anaesthesia, 86
thoracotomy
  analgesia, 80, 86–7
  post-operative pain, 301
throat pack, 163
thrombin sealants, 279
thromboembolism
  obese patients, 249–50
  orthopaedic surgery and, 225–6, 228
    hip surgery, 230
  pre-operative assessment, 92
  pulmonary embolus, 94
  urological surgery patients, 239
thyroid function tests (TFTs), 126–7
thyroid surgery, 126–31, 165–6
  anaesthetic technique, 129–30
  post-operative care, 130
  post-operative complications, 130–1
    haemorrhage, 130
    hypocalcaemia, 131
    pain, 131
    recurrent laryngeal nerve (RLN) palsy, 131
    tracheomalacia, 131
  pre-operative assessment, 126–9, 131–2
    anaesthetic assessment, 129
TISS (Therapeutic Intervention Scoring System), 268
total parenteral nutrition, paediatric patients, 173
tourniquet, 231–2
tracheomalacia, 131
tracheostomy, 163, 166
tramadol, 87
tranexamic acid, 278
  trauma patients, 215
transanal endoscopic microscopy (TEMS), 99
transcranial Doppler (TCD), 145
transjugular intrahepatic portal shunt (TIPS), 123
transoesophageal echocardiography (TOE), 83, 281
transthoracic echocardiography (TTE), 281
transurethral resection of bladder tumour (TURBT), 243
transurethral resection of the prostate (TURP), 241–2
transversus abdominus plane (TAP) blocks, 57
trauma patients, 208–9
  airway management, 210–13
  anaesthetic drugs, 218–20
  burns, 221–2
  circulation management, 213–16
  consciousness assessment, 216
  head injury, 220–1
  hypothermia, 216–17
  initial assessment, 209–10
  monitoring, 217–18
  spinal injury, 221
traumatic brain injury (TBI). *See* head injury
Trendelenburg position, risks of, 291–2
trisomy 21, 175
turbulence, 67–9
TURP syndrome, 241–2. *See also* transurethral resection of the prostate (TURP)

ultrasound activated scalpel, 280
upper gastrointestinal surgery, 102
  laparoscopic oesophageal fundoplication case study, 102–5
  obese patient case study, 105–7
  oesophagectomy case study, 107–14
upper limb surgery, 233–4

upper respiratory tract infection (URTI), paediatric patients, 175
urological surgery, 236
anaesthetic drugs used, 238–9
bladder perforation, 245
intra-operative management, 239–40
anaesthesia, 239–40
deep vein thrombosis prophylaxis, 239
hypothermia prevention, 239
laparoscopic/robotic surgery risks, 240–1
post-operative care, 245
pre-operative management, 236–8
anaemia, 237
fluid balance, 237
pre-assessment, 236
radical cystectomy, 243
radical/partial nephrectomy, 243–4
radical prostatectomy, 244–5
transurethral resection of bladder tumour (TURBT), 243
transurethral resection of the prostate (TURP), 241–2
vascular access
paediatric patients, 176
trauma patients, 210
vascular patients, 138
pharmacotherapy, 139–40
vascular surgery, 137
anaesthesia general principles, 140–1
carotid endarterectomy, 144–5
endovascular aortic reconstruction (EVAR), 142–3
thoracic (TEVAR), 143–4
hybrid procedures, 144
open aortic aneurysm repair, 141–3
peripheral vascular disease, 145–6
pre-operative assessment, 138–9
risk scoring, 137–8
ruptured aortic aneurysm, 142–3
vasopressin, 41
venous gas embolism, 241
venous thromboembolism (VTE). *See* thromboembolism
ventilation. *See also* mechanical ventilation
control, 13–14
head and neck surgery, 164–5
verbal consent, 294
video assisted thoracoscopic surgery (VATS), 86
visual loss, 300
vitamin K, 277
deficiency, 119
vocal cord palsy, 127
volume control ventilation (VC), 271
vomiting
pain adverse effects, 43
post-operative
fundoplication patients, 103–5
plastic surgery patients, 183–4
posterior fossa surgery patients, 203
prevention, 96
risk factors, 184

warfarin, 225
weight estimation, paediatric patients, 180
WFNS SAH grading scale, 264
Whipples resection, 122–3
written consent, 294

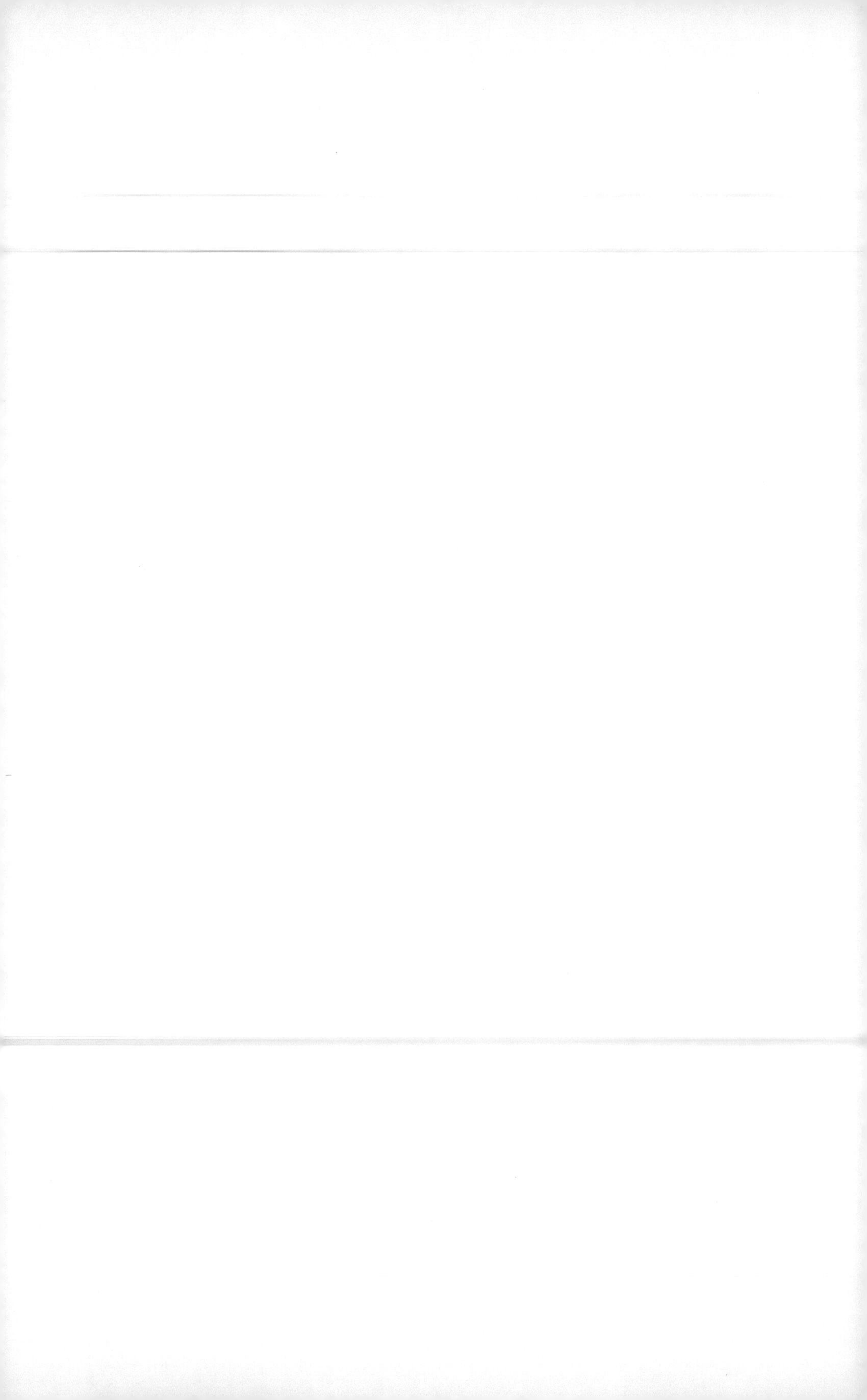

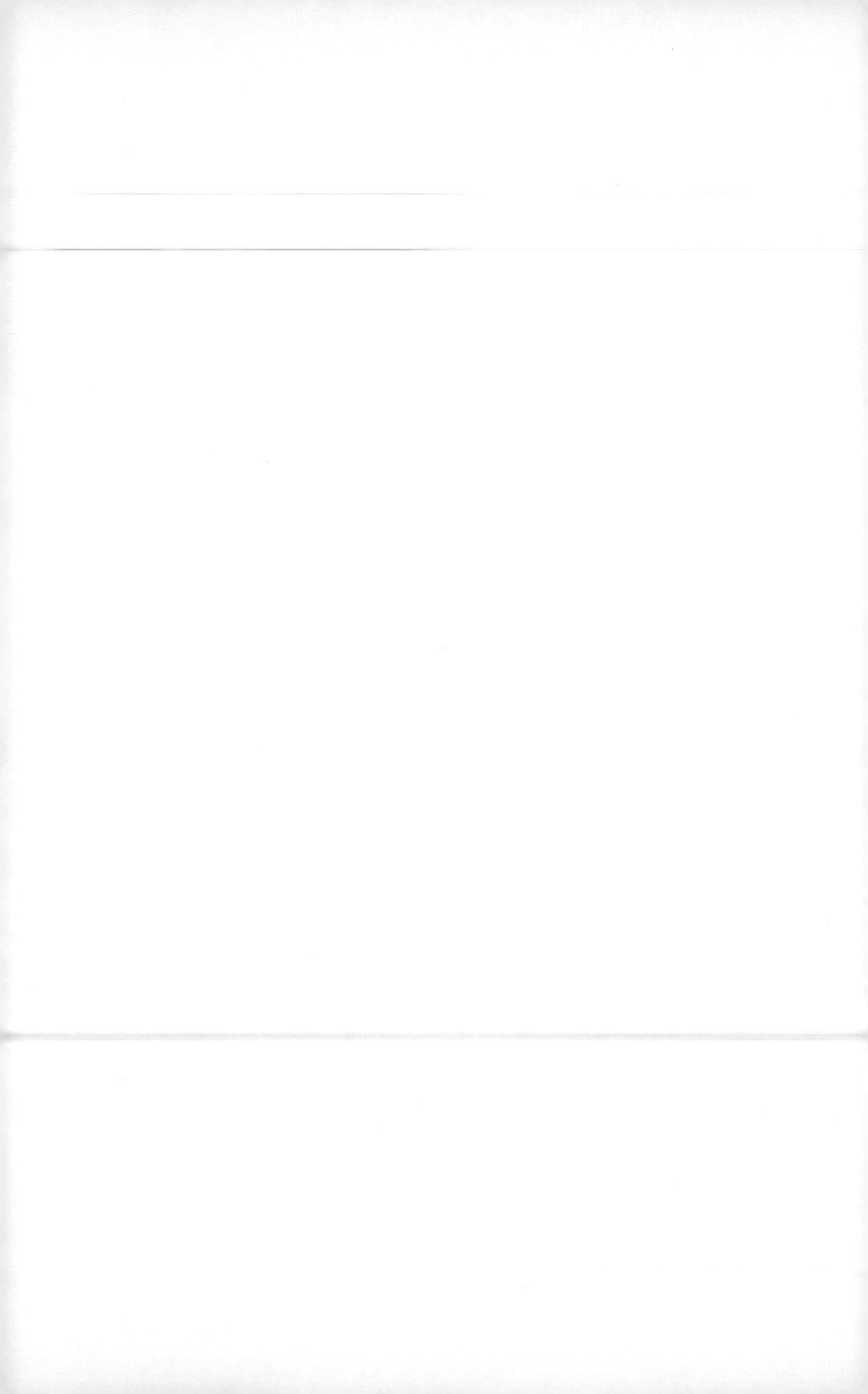